Concepts and methods in infectious disease surveillance

Concepts and methods in infectious disease surveillance

EDITED BY

Nkuchia M. M'ikanatha

Surveillance Epidemiologist
Pennsylvania Department of Health
Harrisburg, PA, USA

John K. Iskander

CAPT, United States Public Health Service
Senior Medical Consultant
Office of the Associate Director for Science
Centers for Disease Control and Prevention
Atlanta, GA, USA

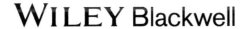

Registered office: John Wiley & Sons, Ltd, The Atrium, Southern Gate, Chichester, West Sussex, PO19 8SQ, UK

Editorial offices: 9600 Garsington Road, Oxford, OX4 2DQ, UK

The Atrium, Southern Gate, Chichester, West Sussex, PO19 8SQ, UK

111 River Street, Hoboken, NJ 07030-5774, USA

For details of our global editorial offices, for customer services and for information about how to apply for permission to reuse the copyright material in this book please see our website at www.wiley.com/wiley-blackwell

Library of Congress Cataloging-in-Publication Data

Concepts and methods in infectious disease surveillance / edited by Nkuchia M. M'ikanatha, John K. Iskander.
      p. ; cm.
   Includes bibliographical references and index.
   ISBN 978-0-470-65939-7 (paper)
   I. M'ikanatha, Nkuchia M., editor.   II. Iskander, John K., editor.
   [DNLM: 1. Communicable Disease Control.   2. Disease Notification.   3. Disease Outbreaks–prevention & control.
4. Public Health Surveillance–methods. WA 110]
   RC111
   616.9–dc23
                                          2014017664

A catalogue record for this book is available from the British Library.

Wiley also publishes its books in a variety of electronic formats. Some content that appears in print may not be available in electronic books.

Cover image: Left-hand image: adapted from Snow, John. *On the Mode of Communication of Cholera*, 2nd edition. London: John Churchill, New Burlington Street, England, 1855. Reproduced with permission of Ralph R. Frerichs, University of California, Los Angeles School of Public Health Department of Epidemiology. Right-hand image: developed by Louisa Chapman with the Situational Awareness Unit of the Centers for Disease Control and Prevention Emergency Operations.
Cover design by Andy Meaden

Set in 8.5/12 pt MeridienLTStd by Toppan Best-set Premedia Limited

1   2015

Contents

List of contributors

Lennox K. Archibald
Hospital Epidemiologist
Malcom Randall Veterans Administration Medical Center
North Florida/South Georgia Veterans Health System
Gainesville, FL, USA

Lori R. Armstrong
Epidemiologist
Division of Tuberculosis Elimination
Centers for Disease Control and Prevention
Atlanta, GA, USA

David S. Barnes
Associate Professor
Department of History and Sociology of Science
University of Pennsylvania
Philadelphia, PA, USA

Casey Barton Behravesh
Commander, U.S. Public Health Service
Deputy Branch Chief
Outbreak Response and Prevention Branch
Division of Foodborne, Waterborne, and Environmental
Diseases
National Center for Emerging and Zoonotic Infectious
Diseases
Centers for Disease Control and Prevention
Atlanta, GA, USA

Kyle T. Bernstein
Director
Applied Research, Community Health Epidemiology, and
Surveillance
Population Health Division
San Francisco Department of Public Health
San Francisco, CA, USA

David L. Blazes
Director, Military Tropical Medicine
US Navy Specialty Leader for Infectious Diseases
Uniformed Services University of the Health Sciences,
Bethesda, MD, USA

Eric Brenner
Medical Epidemiologist
South Carolina Department of Health and Environmental
Control
Columbia, SC, USA

Louisa E. Chapman
Captain, U.S. Public Health Service
Medical Epidemiologist
Public Health Surveillance Program Office
Office of Surveillance, Epidemiology, and Laboratory Services
Centers for Disease Control and Prevention
Atlanta, GA, USA

Elizabeth Chuang
Assistant Professor
Department of Family and Social Medicine
Palliative Care Services
Montefiore Medical Center
Bronx, NY, USA

Daniel R. Church
Epidemiologist/Viral Hepatitis Coordinator
Bureau of Infectious Disease
Hinton State Laboratory Institute
Massachusetts Department of Public Health
Jamaica Plain, MA, USA

Bruno Christian Ciancio
Head, Epidemiological Methods Section
Surveillance and Response Support Unit
European Centre for Disease Prevention and Control
Stockholm, Sweden

Alfred DeMaria, Jr.
State Epidemiologist, Medical Director
Bureau of Infectious Disease
Hinton State Laboratory Institute
Massachusetts Department of Public Health
Jamaica Plain, MA, USA

Rebecca J. Eisen
Research Biologist
Division of Vectorborne Diseases
Centers for Disease Control and Prevention
Fort Collins, CO, USA

Lars Eisen
Associate Professor
Department of Microbiology, Immunology and Pathology
Colorado State University
Fort Collins, CO, USA

James J. Gibson
Director of Disease Control and State Epidemiologist (Retired)
South Carolina Department of Health and Environmental Control
Columbia, SC, USA

Carolyn Greene
Deputy Commissioner
Division of Epidemiology
New York City Department of Health and Mental Hygiene
Queens, NY, USA

Gillian A. Haney
Director
Integrated Surveillance and Informatics Services
Bureau of Infectious Disease
Hinton State Laboratory Institute
Massachusetts Department of Public Health
Jamaica Plain, MA, USA

Lee H. Harrison
Infectious Diseases Epidemiology Research Unit
Division of Infectious Diseases
University of Pittsburgh Graduate School of Public Health and School of Medicine
Pittsburgh, PA, USA

Richard S. Hopkins
Department of Epidemiology
Colleges of Public Health and Health Professions and of Medicine
University of Florida
Gainesville, FL, USA

Gail Horlick
Senior Legal Analyst
Office of Scientific Integrity
Centers for Disease Control and Prevention
Atlanta, GA, USA

John K. Iskander
CAPT, United States Public Health Service
Senior Medical Consultant
Office of the Associate Director for Science
Centers for Disease Control and Prevention
Atlanta, GA, USA

Ruth A. Jajosky
Epidemiologist
Division of Health Informatics and Surveillance
Center for Surveillance, Epidemiology and Laboratory Services
Office of Public Health Scientific Services
Centers for Disease Control and Prevention
Atlanta, GA, USA

Bridget J. Kelly
Health Communication Research Scientist
RTI International
Washington, DC, USA

Monina Klevens
Medical Epidemiologist
Epidemiology and Surveillance Branch
Division of Viral Hepatitis
Centers for Disease Control and Prevention
Atlanta, GA, USA

Piotr Kramarz
Deputy Chief Scientist
European Centre for Disease Prevention and Control
Stockholm, Sweden

Gayle Fischer Langley
Medical Epidemiologist
Respiratory Diseases Branch
National Center for Immunization and Respiratory Diseases
Centers for Disease Control and Prevention
Atlanta, GA, USA

Sheri Lewis
Global Disease Surveillance PM
Johns Hopkins University Applied Physics Laboratory
Columbia, MD, USA

Theresa J. McCann
Associate Dean of Basic and Allied Health Sciences
Director, Simulation Center Education and Research
Epidemiologist and Professor, Department of Behavioral Sciences
School of Medicine, St. George's University
Grenada

Nkuchia M. M'ikanatha
Surveillance Epidemiologist
Pennsylvania Department of Health
Harrisburg, PA, USA

Roque Miramontes
Epidemiologist, Surveillance Team Lead
Division of Tuberculosis Elimination
Centers for Disease Control and Prevention
Atlanta, GA, USA

Eve D. Mokotoff
Managing Director
HIV Counts
Ann Arbor, MI, USA

Jennifer B. Nuzzo
Senior Associate
UPMC Center for Health Security
Baltimore, MD, USA

Jean O'Connor
Director
Health Promotion and Disease Prevention
Georgia Department of Public Health and Rollins School of
Public Health
Atlanta, GA, USA

Daniel C. Payne
Epidemiologist
Division of Viral Diseases
National Center for Immunization and Respiratory Diseases
Centers for Disease Control and Prevention
Atlanta, GA, USA

Linda Capewell Pimentel
Acting Chief
Animal Care and Use Program Office
Office of Scientific Integrity, Office of the Associate Director
for Science
Centers for Disease Control and Prevention
Atlanta, GA, USA

Elaine Scallan
Assistant Professor
Department of Epidemiology
Colorado School of Public Health
University of Colorado Denver
Aurora, CO, USA

Brian G. Southwell
Program Director
Science in the Public Sphere Program
RTI International
Research Triangle Park, NC, USA

Ethel V. Taylor
Veterinary Epidemiologist
Health Studies Branch
National Center for Environmental Health
Centers for Disease Control and Prevention
Atlanta, GA, USA

Elizabeth A. Torrone
Epidemiologist
Division of STD Prevention
Centers for Disease Control and Prevention
Atlanta, GA, USA

James N. Tyson
Chief, Situation Awareness Unit
Division of Emergency Operations
Office of Public Health Preparedness and Response
Centers for Disease Control and Prevention
Atlanta, GA, USA

Jennifer Ward
Epidemiologist
Communicable and Environmental Diseases and Emergency
Preparedness
Tennessee Department of Health
Nashville, TN, USA

Foreword

If you don't know where you are going, any road will get you there.

Lewis Carroll

When I was young, my family used to take the occasional long-distance road trip. During the 1960s, these trips required months of planning and preparation. Requests were sent to tourism divisions in the states we would pass through, in the hope that maps and brochures would be sent so that we could plot our route and identify things to do and see along the way. Booklets were also requested from major motel chains to reserve places to stay based on our anticipated route and daily driving distances. Sometimes a package of information came quickly in the mail; but, just as often, nothing arrived or the material came too late. Afterward, the well-worn maps and booklets were tossed in a drawer for future use, even though the information was often out of date. Once on the road, if car trouble, bad weather, or road closures disrupted our itinerary, we'd spread out the maps to plot an alternative route, seek out pay phones to cancel lodging reservations, and take a chance on finding a place to stay overnight on the new route. International trips were more involved, and pretravel information was much more difficult to obtain.

Our road trip experiences could be a metaphor for the state of infectious disease surveillance during that era. Back then, implementing and sustaining surveillance took significant time, effort, and patience. Sources of surveillance data were not easy to locate and available information was difficult to access. Physicians and laboratories, the primary sources of infectious disease data, often complied poorly with disease reporting requirements. These providers were often unaware of what diseases to report and how to report them, or they were disinclined to fill out tedious reports. If submitted at all, forms or cards were filled in by hand or typed; and when they reached the correct officials at the health department days later, forms were often incomplete, difficult to read, damaged, or incorrect. Reports were stored in file cabinets or on shelves where they were susceptible to damage, decay, or misplacement. Summary statistics were calculated by hand with the aid of an adding machine and periodically disseminated in hard copy. All of these factors made disease surveillance inefficient, insensitive, inflexible, and highly variable in place and time. International surveillance efforts were even less dependable, when they existed at all.

It is remarkable to realize how much both the way we arrange travel and the way we conduct infectious disease surveillance have evolved in only a few decades. Hard-copy maps are now quaint anachronisms. Instead, we rely on the Internet or global positioning systems (GPS) to plot our trips. We punch in our intended destination and in seconds have preferred and alternative routes accompanied by stunningly detailed satellite and ground images. Travel arrangement websites and applications provide exquisite details on the destination, transport and lodging options, room and restaurant availability, and prices in even the remotest corner of the world.

Similarly, paper disease report forms previously used for surveillance have been supplanted by encrypted Web-based or smart-phone data entry that includes range and consistency checks to reduce errors. Electronically entered data are easily transmitted by designated disease reporters to the correct recipient. Reporting requirements, forms, and formats are easily accessed online by any provider or laboratory. Electronic health records and electronic laboratory reports allow automated, highly accurate data extraction coupled with direct computer-to-computer transfer from source providers to public health authorities. Once received, these data are assessed using computerized algorithms that manipulate and perform complex analyses and produce outputs on a near–real-time basis. Aberration software detects atypical disease patterns and unusual case reports; and, through automatic alerts, it flags such deviations so they can be immediately investigated. Databases are housed in server farms and cloud-based storage systems for easy retrieval, transfer, and analysis. Surveillance analyses can be shared with providers and the public via the Web and through social media.

With such a rapidly evolving landscape, it is critically important that students of public health and epidemiology have a sound understanding of the concepts and principles that underpin modern surveillance of infectious diseases. Students should be acquainted with the major surveillance systems used to collect and report infectious disease data domestically and internationally, and they should understand the strengths and limitations of these systems. Every practitioner or organization working in the field of infectious diseases uses surveillance data. That is true whether they provide direct patient care, conduct fundamental or applied research, or implement programs to prevent, control, or eradicate disease. Surveillance information is used to assure science-based decision making, to allocate resources for maximum impact, and to determine whether we have achieved desired outcomes. Only through high-quality surveillance can we measure the burden of and trends in infectious diseases, which today continue to be major contributors to global morbidity, mortality, disability, and social upheaval.

Concepts and Methods in Infectious Disease Surveillance lays out infectious disease surveillance for the student in several ways. First, it familiarizes the reader with basic surveillance concepts; the legal basis for surveillance in the United States and abroad; and the purposes, structures, and intended uses of surveillance at the local, state, national, and international level. This information is important for those who seek to understand our current surveillance systems, their strengths, and their limitations.

Once these broad-based principles are addressed, the text introduces the approaches to surveillance for various categories of infectious diseases. The student will quickly discover that surveillance goals and methods differ radically by infectious disease. Surveillance approaches to healthcare-associated infections or antimicrobial resistance are completely different from those used for vectorborne infections, rabies, or influenza. For many (but not all) infectious diseases, it is important to count individual cases of the disease of interest (e.g.,

HIV, measles, salmonellosis, tuberculosis). However, the methods used to find these cases will vary; and, often, additional types of information are collected to complete the picture. As examples, for vaccine preventable diseases, systems are in place to collect data on vaccine coverage and vaccine-related adverse events; and, for HIV, systems collect data on testing trends, treatment, disease outcomes, coinfections, and risk behaviors.

The student must also understand noncategorical, or nondisease specific, approaches to collection and analysis of surveillance data. Increasingly, these methods have been established as core surveillance practices, especially for emergency preparedness. One example is syndromic surveillance, where the generic patterns of respiratory illness, rash illness, or gastrointestinal disease seen in healthcare settings are monitored. Another example is the monitoring of prescription dispensing or over-the-counter purchases of antidiarrheal medications or cough suppressants in pharmacy settings. Yet another example is the use of social media or websites to observe trends in mentions of, or searches for, infectious disease–related terms like influenza, tick bites, or antibiotics.

It is also necessary for public health practitioners to have a grasp of disciplines like laboratory analytic methods and information technology concepts that play important roles in infectious disease surveillance. In particular, subtyping (or fingerprinting) methodologies in widespread use in public health laboratories, from simple bacterial serotyping to whole genome sequencing of microbes, have revolutionized our ability to identify links among human, animal, and environmental pathogens and to detect and control outbreaks. Geospatial analysis is another emerging technology that has allowed previously unrecognizable or underappreciated patterns of illness to be revealed. The final sections of this book introduce the student to methods of communicating the findings derived from analyses of surveillance data. This is every bit as important as data collection and data analysis. If the findings of surveillance systems are not disseminated to those who can use them, the public health benefits of surveillance cannot be realized.

This text demonstrates the infectious disease landscape and roadmap of today; but we are in an era of dynamic change marked by personal medicine and genomics, the human microbiome, metadata, supercomputation, and other trends that will profoundly impact our approach to disease surveillance. In another generation, how we now travel and conduct surveillance may appear as antiquated to public health practitioners as hard-copy road maps and mail-in disease reports of the past generation appear to us today. This illustrates that all of us will be learning new disease surveillance concepts and methods throughout our professional careers.

Stephen M. Ostroff, MD
Acting Chief Scientist at the U.S. Food and
Drug Administration

Preface

A functional surveillance system is essential in providing information for action on priority communicable diseases; it is a crucial instrument for public health decision-making in all countries.

World Health Organization, 2000

During the past century, all regions of the world have made significant, but uneven, progress in prevention and control of infectious diseases. Microbial agents inflict widespread suffering on humans and the diseases they cause can disrupt trade and restrict travel resulting in unfavorable economic impacts. The emergence of severe acute respiratory syndrome (SARS) in 2003 and the 2009 pandemic H1N1 influenza virus outbreak are stark reminders that human pathogens are a serious threat to public health. The rapid spread of both SARS and pandemic H1N1 influenza demonstrated the need for effective systems to track, detect, and respond to disease outbreaks at various levels.

At the beginning of this century, many countries, including the United States, scaled up investments in infrastructure to monitor infectious diseases. Those investments have benefited enormously from the widespread use of electronic information systems in clinical laboratories, which enabled creation of new modalities for timely submission of reportable test results to public health authorities. Incentives that are aimed at accelerating adoption of useful electronic health records are expected to increase reporting of designated diseases to public health jurisdictions. Implementation of such systems, however, is complex and requires close collaboration among information technologists and public health professionals with necessary backgrounds in surveillance and epidemiology.

Advances in molecular subtyping methods, including pulsed-field gel electrophoresis and multilocus sequence typing, have increased the specificity and power of laboratory-based surveillance to detect outbreaks. Use of geographic information systems can better clarify pathogen transmission dynamics than methods used in the past, and statistical algorithms can be applied to Internet-based data to monitor evolving public health crises. In addition, social media and mobile technologies have expanded both data sources and means for dissemination of surveillance findings. Novel methods for conducting surveillance, however, raise unresolved legal concerns.

A desire for a readily accessible, concise resource that detailed current methods and challenges in disease surveillance inspired the collaborations that resulted in this volume. Written by colleagues with hands-on experience in conducting surveillance and teaching applied public health, the book has three sections. Section I provides an overview of legal considerations for surveillance and a description of multilevel systems that are the cornerstones for infectious disease surveillance in the United States. Section II presents chapters on major program-area or disease-specific surveillance systems including those that monitor bacterial infections, foodborne diseases, healthcare-associated infections, and HIV/AIDS.

Section III is devoted to methods for conducting surveillance and approaches for data analysis. There are chapters focused on methods used in global surveillance and global disease detection, practical considerations for electronic laboratory reporting, and approaches for analysis and interpretation of surveillance data. Section IV includes a chapter on approaches for communication and use of social media and a concluding chapter on lessons learned from the New York City Department of Health and Mental Hygiene's 50-year experience in surveillance and applied epidemiology training.

The book covers major topics at an introductory-to-intermediate level and was designed to serve as a resource or class text for instructors. It can be used in graduate level courses in public health, human and veterinary medicine, as well as in undergraduate programs in public health–oriented disciplines. We hope that the book will be a useful primer for frontline public health practitioners, hospital epidemiologists, infection-control practitioners, laboratorians in public health settings, infectious disease researchers, and medical informatics specialists interested in a concise overview of infectious disease surveillance. We are delighted by the growing interest in use of surveillance to inform public health practice, in addition to its use as a tool for early detection of epidemics. Our hope is that this volume will contribute to this endeavor.

Nkuchia M. M'ikanatha
John K. Iskander

Acknowledgments

We are grateful to many individuals and institutions that embraced the vision for this book. It is a privilege for us to participate in surveillance and the broad field of applied epidemiology at state (NMM) and federal (JKI) levels in the United States. We are grateful for all the direct and indirect support we received from our own institutions and from the institutions represented by contributors to this volume.

Wiley-Blackwell, our publisher, invited us to develop this textbook and supported us throughout the process; we are grateful for the opportunity. In particular, we thank Maria Khan, our Commissioning Editor; Deirdre Barry, and Claire Brewer for their efforts and guidance during various stages of the book.

Contributors to this volume invested enormous time and energy during the writing process—we thank each of them for their collaborative spirit and friendship. A number of individuals provided significant help in either reviewing initial drafts for the overall book or specific chapters. In particular, we thank Chris Carr,

Harry Sultz, Jaclyn Fox, Natalie Mueller, and Jacqueline Wyatt for their invaluable feedback. We are grateful to Sameh Boktor for wide-ranging editorial assistance, including the amazing job he did in finalizing many of the illustrations in this book.

Our separate journeys to public health careers and to this specific work began with the love and guidance each of us received at an early age from our parents: Mama Ciomwereria and Kaithia M'ikanatha, and Michel and Betty Iskander. We are eternally grateful for their invaluable gifts. NMM would also like to thank D. A. Henderson for sharing with him insights gained in the application of surveillance in the successful eradication of smallpox. NMM also expresses gratitude to Brian L. Strom for encouragement and opportunities to participate in academic aspects of public health. During our work on this book, we received love and nourishment from our families: the M'ikanatha family: Kathleen and Isaac; and the Iskander family: Susan Duderstadt, Eleanor, and Jonas.

Acronyms and abbreviations

AAP	American Academy of Pediatrics
AAVLD	American Association of Veterinary Laboratory Diagnosticians
ABCs	Active Bacterial Cores
ACA	Affordable Care Act
ACIP	Advisory Committee on Immunization Practices
ACOG	American College of Obstetricians and Gynecologists
ADAP	AIDS Drug Assistance Program
AFB	Acid-fast bacillus
AGE	Acute gastroenteritis
AIDS	Acquired immunodeficiency syndrome
ALT	Alanine transaminase
AMA	American Medical Association
APACHE II	Acute Physiology and Chronic Health Evaluation
APEC EIN	Asia Pacific Economic Council's Emerging Infections Network
APHA	American Public Health Association
ARCHES	Applied Research, Community Health Epidemiology, and Surveillance
ARI	Acute respiratory infection
ART	Antiretroviral treatments
ASA	American Society of Anesthesiologists
ASC	Area surveillance coordinators
ASM	American Society of Microbiology
AST	Aspartate transaminase
AVMA	American Veterinary Medical Association
BPHT	Bureau of Public Health Training
BSE	Bovine spongiform encephalopathy
CCs	Collaborating centres
CDA	Clinical Document Architecture
CDC	Centers for Disease Control and Prevention
CHD	County health department
CHIP	Comprehensive Hospital Infections Project
CIR	Citywide Immunization Registry
CQI	Continuous quality improvement
CSTE	Council of State and Territorial Epidemiologists
DADE	Division of Acute Disease Epidemiology
DALYs	Disability-adjusted life years
DHEC	Department of Health and Environmental Control
DIS	Disease intervention specialist
DoD	U.S. Department of Defense
DOH	Department of health

DOHMH	Department of Health and Mental Hygiene (New York City)
DoI	Data of interest
DOT	Directly observed therapy
DRC	Democratic Republic of Congo
DSMB	Data safety monitoring board
EAIDSNet	East African Integrated Disease Surveillance Network
EARS	Early Aberration Reporting System
ECDC	European Centre for Disease Prevention and Control
ED	Emergency department
eHARS	Enhanced HIV/AIDS Reporting System
EHR	Electronic health record
EID	Emerging infectious disease
EIP	Emerging Infections Program
EIS	Epidemic Intelligence Service
EISN	European Influenza Surveillance Network
ELC	Epidemiology and Laboratory Capacity for Infectious Diseases
ELR	Electronic laboratory reporting
EMR	Electronic medical record
EMRO	Regional Office for Eastern Mediterranean
EPI	Expanded Program on Immunization
EPT	Emerging Pandemics Threat
ERL	Essential Regulatory Laboratory
ESSENCE	Electronic Surveillance System for the Early Notification of Community-based Epidemics
EU	European Union
EURO	The Regional Office for Europe
FAO	Food and Agriculture Organization
FDA	Food and Drug Administration
FELTP	Field Epidemiology Laboratory Training Program
FETP	Field Epidemiology Training Program
FLDOH	Florida Department of Health
FU-1	Follow-up 1 form of the RVCT
FU-2	Follow-up 2 form of the RVCT
GABG	Coronary artery bypass graft
GAS	Group A *Streptococcus*
GBS	Group B *Streptococcus*
GDD	Global Disease Detection Program
GDDER	Global Disease Detection Program and Emergency Response
GEIS	Global Emerging Infections Surveillance and Response System
GGT	Gamma glutamyl transpeptidase

GIS	Geographic information system
GISP	Gonococcal Isolate Surveillance Project
GISRS	Global Influenza Surveillance and Response System
GLEWS	Global Early Warning and Response System
GoARN	Global Outbreak Alert and Response Network
GPHIN	Global Public Health Intelligence Network (Public Health Agency of Canada)
GPS	Global Positioning System
GRASP	Geospatial Research, Analysis and Service Program
HAA	Hepatitis-associated antigen
HAART	Highly active antiretroviral therapy
HAI	Healthcare-associated infections
HAV	Hepatitis A virus
HBsAg	Hepatitis B surface antigen
HCV	Hepatitis C virus
HDV	Hepatitis D virus
HEV	Hepatitis E virus
HI	Hemagglutination inhibition
HIPAA	Health Insurance Portability and Accountability Act
HIV	Human immunodeficiency virus
HL7	Health Level 7 International
HPV	Human papillomavirus
HRTP	Health Research Training Program
IAP	Intrapartum antibiotic prophylaxis
ICD	International Classification of Diseases
ICU	Intensive care units
IDSA	Infectious Diseases Society of America
IDU	Intravenous drug users
IGRA	Interferon-gamma release assay
IHR	International Health Regulations
IHSP	Influenza Hospitalization Surveillance Project
ILI	Influenza-like illness
IPD	Invasive pneumococcal disease
IS	Intussusception
ISO	International Organization for Standardization
IT	Information technology
IVR	Interactive voice response
JCAHO	Joint Commission on Accreditation of Healthcare Organizations
LIMS	Laboratory information management systems
LOINC	Logical Observation Identifiers Names and Codes
LQAS	Lot quality assessment sampling
LTBI	Latent TB infection
MBDS	Mekong Basin Disease Surveillance
MDR-TB	Multidrug-resistant tuberculosis
MECIDS	Middle East Consortium on Infectious Disease Surveillance
mHealth	Mobile health
MLST	Multilocus sequence typing
MLVA	Multiple-locus variable number tandem repeat analysis

MMP	Medical Monitoring Project
MMR	Measles, mumps, rubella
MMWR	Morbidity and Mortality Weekly Report
MRSA	Methicillin-resistant *Staphylococcus aureus*
MSM	Men who have sex with men
MSPH	Mailman School of Public Health (Columbia)
MSPP	Ministry of Public Health and Population (Ministère de la Santé Publique et de la Population) (Haiti)
MSSP	Monitoring Sexually Transmitted Infections Survey Program
MTB	*Mycobacterium tuberculosis*
NAAT	Nucleic acid amplification test
NAHRS	National Animal Health Reporting System
NARMS	National Antimicrobial Resistance Monitoring System
NARSA	Network on Antimicrobial Resistance in *Staphylococcus aureus*
NASA	National Aeronautics and Space Administration
NBIC	National Biosurveillance Integration Center
NBS	NEDSS-based system
NEDSS	National Electronic Disease Surveillance System
NETSS	National Electronic Telecommunications System for Surveillance
NHANES	National Health and Nutrition Examination Survey
NHBS	National HIV Behavioral Surveillance
NHS	National Health Service
NHSN	National Healthcare Safety Network
NICs	National Influenza Centers
NNC	Nationally Notifiable Conditions
NNDSS	National Notifiable Diseases Surveillance System
NNIS	National Nosocomial Infections Surveillance
NPSTF	National Preventive Services Task Force
NSC	National Security Council
NTA	National Tuberculosis Association
NTM	National Tuberculosis Indicators Project
NTM	Nontuberculosis mycobacteria
NYC	New York City
NYDOH	New York State Department of Health
OCR	Optical character recognition
ODS	Operational data store
OI	Opportunistic illness
OIE	World Organization for Animal Health (Office International des Epizooties)
ORV	Oral rabies vaccine
PAHO	Pan American Health Organization
PCIP	Primary Care Information Project
PCR	Polymerase chain reaction
PCV	*Porcine circovirus*
PCV13	13-valent pneumococcal conjugate vaccine
PCV7	7-valent pneumococcal conjugate vaccine

PEP	Postexposure prophylaxis		SISS	Severity of Illness Scoring Systems
PFGE	Pulsed-field gel electrophoresis		SMS	Short message service
PHCR	Public health case reporting		SNOMED CT	Systematized Nomenclature of Medicine— Clinical Terms
PHEIC	Public Health Emergency of International Concern		SNOMED	Systematized Nomenclature of Medicine
PHI	Protected health information		SPHL	State public health laboratories
PHLIP	Public Health Laboratory Interoperabilty Project		SSI	Surgical site infection
			SSuN	STD Surveillance Network
PHPS	Public Health Prevention Service		STARHS	Serologic Testing Algorithm for Recent HIV Seroconversion
PHSA	Public Health Service Act			
PIP	Pandemic Influenza Preparedness		STD	Sexually transmitted disease
PPD	Purified protein derivative		SUA	Sokoine University of Agriculture
PPV	Positive predictive value		TB	Tuberculosis
PrEP	Pre-exposure prophylaxis		TIMS	Tuberculosis Information Management System
PV	Polio virus		TSS	Toxic shock syndrome
RCMT	Reportable Condition Mapping Table		TST	Tuberculin skin test
RCT	Randomized clinical trials		UN	United Nations
RDB	Reporting database		USAHA	U.S. Animal Health Association
RIDR	Routine Interstate Duplicate Review		USAID	U.S. Agency for International Development
RT-PCR	Reverse transcriptase polymerase chain reaction		USAMRU–K	U.S. Army Medical Research Unit–Kenya
			USDA	United States Department of Agriculture
RVCT	Report of verified case of tuberculosis		USGS	United States Geological Survey
SACIDS	Southern African Centre for Disease Surveillance		USPHS	U.S. Public Health Service
			VAP	Ventilator-associated pneumonia
SARI	Severe acute respiratory infections		VCPV	Vaccine-derived polio virus
SARS	Severe acute respiratory syndrome		VPD	Vaccine preventable disease
SEARO	Regional Office for South-East Asia		VRE	Vancomycin-resistant enterococcus
SENIC	Study on the Efficacy of Nosocomial Infection Control		WAHID	World Animal Health Information Database
			WHO	World Health Organization
sFTP	Secure file transfer protocol		WNV	West Nile virus
SHEA	Society for Healthcare Epidemiology of America		WPRO	Western Pacific Regional Office
			XDR-TB	Extensively drug-resistant TB

SECTION I

Introduction to infectious disease surveillance

CHAPTER 1

Surveillance as a foundation for infectious disease prevention and control

Nkuchia M. M'ikanatha[1] and John K. Iskander[2]

[1] Pennsylvania Department of Health, Harrisburg, PA, USA
[2] Centers for Disease Control and Prevention, Atlanta, GA, USA

Background and rationale

Throughout human history, infectious diseases have caused human suffering, disrupted trade, restricted travel, and limited human settlement. Today the emergence of new pathogens and reemergence of new strains of old pathogens in different parts of the world illustrates the continuing threat of infectious diseases to the public's health. A combination of globalization of the food supply and travel within countries and across international borders makes it easy for an outbreak in one location to spread rapidly within and beyond national borders. Endemic infectious diseases, including sexually transmitted diseases (STDs) like gonorrhea, foodborne illnesses like campylobacteriosis, and blood-borne pathogens such as hepatitis B and C remain problems in North America, Europe, and other regions of the world. Table 1.1 lists the ten most commonly reported communicable diseases in the United States, which include multiple types of STDs, infections transmitted by food and water, vaccine-preventable diseases, and a vectorborne disease transmitted by ticks. (The United States population was estimated at 314 million in 2013.) The cumulative morbidity from these 10 diseases, in a single wealthy country, is nearly 2 million cases a year or approximately 32 cases of a communicable disease per 10,000 persons. Given that underreporting occurs in many surveillance systems, the real human toll in terms of cases and attendant suffering and healthcare costs is undoubtedly higher.

Surveillance can provide timely information crucial to public health interventions in an evolving situation. For example, during the 2009–2010 H1N1 influenza pandemic, surveillance data were used to prioritize vaccination to specific high-risk groups such as pregnant women because the supply of vaccine was limited [1]. Surveillance data also form the bases for disease-specific treatment guidelines; in the United States, for example, public health authorities now recommend use of injectable third-generation cephalosporins for treatment of gonococcal infections because of increasing resistance to oral cephalosporins [2]. Information from carefully designed and implemented surveillance systems can also inform the allocation of resources to public health programs and reassure the public in face of public health crises resulting from natural disasters such as the Sichuan earthquake in China in 2008 [3]. Epidemiologic data generated through disease surveillance serve as the bases for research and development of drugs, vaccines, and other therapeutic and prophylactic interventions.

Although central to disease prevention programs, public health surveillance infrastructure is inadequate or weak in many parts of the world. The need to strengthen capacity to conduct public health surveillance for infectious diseases is a priority for practitioners

Table 1.1 Ten diseases with the highest numbers of reported cases.

Name	Total
Chlamydia trachomatis infection	1,412,791
Gonorrhea	321,849
Salmonellosis	51,887
Syphilis, total (all stages)	46,042
HIV diagnoses	35,266
Lyme disease, total	33,097
Coccidioidomycosis	22,634
Pertussis	18,719
Streptococcus pneumoniae, invasive disease (all ages)	17,138
Giardiasis	16,747

Source: Adams DA, Gallagher KM, Jajosky RA, et al. Division of Notifiable Diseases and Healthcare Information, Office of Surveillance, Epidemiology, and Laboratory Services, CDC. Summary of notifiable diseases—United States, 2011. *MMWR Morb Mortal Wkly Rep* 2013; 5;60:1–117.

and policy makers in North America and Europe. The establishment of the European Centre for Disease Prevention and Control (ECDC) and the renewed focus on surveillance at the United States Centers for Disease Control and Prevention (CDC) [4,5] demonstrate the growing interest in this field. Furthermore, the current International Health Regulations explicitly call for establishment of functioning surveillance units in the public health systems in all countries. Contrary to the misconception that infectious diseases have been conquered by advances in medicine and technology, established and newly emerging pathogens will likely continue to be threats to public health for the foreseeable future.

Definitions

Public health disease surveillance
Public health surveillance is the ongoing systematic collection, analysis, and interpretation of health data essential to the planning, implementation, and evaluation of public health practice, closely integrated with the timely dissemination of these data to those who need to know.

Intended audiences for surveillance data may include public health practitioners, physicians, and other healthcare providers; policymakers; traditional media; and the general public. Depending on the primary target audience, the format and manner in which surveillance data are communicated may vary substantially. Contemporary communications channels for sharing surveillance information include various types of social media. The final and most-important link in the surveillance chain is the application of these data to disease prevention and control. A surveillance system includes a functional capacity for data collection, analysis, and dissemination linked to public health programs [6].

Newer types of surveillance
Biosurveillance has been defined as "the science and practice of managing health-related data and information so that effective action can be taken to mitigate adverse health effects from urgent threats" [7]. The Centers for Disease Control and Prevention defines syndromic surveillance as surveillance that uses health-related data that precede diagnosis and signal a sufficient probability of a case or an outbreak to warrant further public health response [8].

Historical development of infectious disease surveillance

The methods used for infectious disease surveillance depend on the type of disease. Part of the rationale for this is that there are fundamental differences in etiology, mode of transmission, and control measures between different types of infections. For example, surveillance for malaria (a vectorborne disease) is different from surveillance for influenza (a respiratory illness). Interventions may also vary greatly, from vector control and environmental interventions for malaria to vaccines, antivirals, and respiratory protections for influenza.

Despite the fact that much of surveillance is practiced on a disease-specific basis, it is worth remembering that surveillance is a general tool used across all types of infectious and, noninfectious conditions, and, as such, all surveillance methods share certain core elements. We advocate the view that surveillance should not be regarded as a public health "specialty," but rather that all public health practitioners should understand the general principles underlying surveillance.

Data derived from public health surveillance activities can provide important input into local, regional, national, and domestic policy making related to control of infectious diseases. Readers should bear in mind that other policy tools must be considered as well. For example, the values of populations affected by communicable diseases or their control measures should be taken into account when new or revised measures are contemplated. Legal, regulatory, and other policy-related considerations may be key factors in decision making. While we agree strongly with the premise that individuals representing public health data and science should have "a seat at the table" when disease control policies are discussed, we recognize that those sitting at other seats should have their views heard as well.

Conclusion

This book is designed to address concepts and methods used to conduct infectious disease surveillance at an introductory level in an easily accessible format. We hope that the book will also be a primer for frontline public health professionals interested in a concise overview of infectious disease surveillance. It is divided into four main parts covering surveillance organization and underlying principles, important categorical surveillance systems, methods applied across multiple types of infectious disease surveillance systems, and finally cross-cutting aspects of surveillance which go "beyond the data." "Stand-alone" or "categorical" programs for conditions such as HIV and foodborne diseases is still of importance, and this book gives expert practitioners in these areas a voice in explaining the day-to-day conduct, nuances, and broader implications of their work. An important example highlighted in this book is surveillance for healthcare-associated infections, a field in which public values—such as the need for transparency—are shaping which data elements are collected, selection of data sources, and how those data are used. Case studies and study questions that are provided as parts of chapters are intended to stimulate discussion and debate among students and practitioners. The questions can also be used by individuals or groups as part of self-directed study in order to strengthen understanding of the topics covered in the chapter.

Contributors to this volume include individuals practicing in academic and public health settings, many of whom are active participants in global health activities. The authors provide numerous examples of the achievements and obstacles encountered in the everyday course of creating and maintaining surveillance systems. Although the book draws on experiences from North America, discussions on how the lessons learned could be applied to strengthen surveillance in other parts of the world, including areas with limited resources, are provided. The book covers practical considerations in the use of new technologies to conduct surveillance, including mobile phones, molecular subtyping methods, and geographic information system (GIS) tools.

In areas such as biosurveillance and international surveillance, intelligence gathering and synthesis from nontraditional sources have become as important as analysis of established data. Infectious disease surveillance data increasingly will have implications not only for public health response, but also for policy development in other areas including healthcare delivery, security, and commerce. Practitioners of infectious disease surveillance are increasingly expected to play a key role in designing data systems, and in using data that emerges from diverse types of health information management systems (e.g., immunization registries and large linked databases). They will ultimately also need to be able to understand their data and its implications at a deep level and to communicate that to diverse audiences through traditional media, social media, the internet, and other communication modalities not yet conceived.

Ultimately, the quality and societal value of infectious disease surveillance depends on the diligence and expertise of those involved in its practice. Public health practitioners must be comfortable working in a technology-rich environment, but should also be aware of the limitations of relying too heavily on a technological approach to surveillance. The skillset of the contemporary infectious disease epidemiologist must include the ability to analyze and interpret complex data, communicate it clearly to diverse audiences, and understand the implications of surveillance for public health and broader health policy concerns.

References

1. Centers for Disease Control and Prevention. H1N1 vaccination recommendations. 2009. Available at http://www.cdc

.gov/h1n1flu/vaccination/acip.htm (accessed November 30, 2009).

2. Centers for Disease Control and Prevention. Update to CDC's sexually transmitted diseases treatment guidelines, 2010: Oral cephalosporins no longer a recommended treatment for gonococcal infections. *MMWR Morb Mortal Wkly Rep* 2012;**61**: 590–594.

3. Yang C, Yang J, Luo X, Gong P. Use of mobile phones in an emergency reporting system for infectious disease surveillance after the Sichuan earthquake in China. *Bull World Health Organ* 2009;**87**(8):619–623.

4. European Centre for Disease Prevention and Control (ECDC). The European Surveillance System (TESSy). Avail-able at http://www.ecdc.europa.eu/en/activities/surveillance/TESSy/Pages/TESSy.aspx (accessed April 2, 2014).

5. Buehler JW. Centers for Disease Control and Prevention. CDC's vision for public health surveillance in the 21st century. *MMWR Surveill Summ* 2012; **61** Suppl:1–2.

6. Thacker SB, Berkelman RL. Public health surveillance in the United States. *Epidemiol Rev* 1988;**10**:164–190.

7. Building BioSense 2.0: The Redesign. Available at http://www.cdc.gov/biosense/background.html (accessed April 2, 2014).

8. Eysenbach G. Infodemiology: Tracking flu-related searches on the web for syndromic surveillance. *AMIA Annu Symp Proc* 2006;**2006**:244–248.

CHAPTER 2

The legal basis for public health surveillance

Gail Horlick[1] and Jean O'Connor[2]

[1] Centers for Disease Control and Prevention, Atlanta, GA, USA
[2] Georgia Department of Public Health and Rollins School of Public Health, Atlanta, GA, USA

Introduction

Surveillance for diseases and conditions is one of the main means by which public health practitioners assess the health of the population. Public health surveillance is the "ongoing systematic collection, analysis, and interpretation of outcome-specific data for use in the planning, implementation, and evaluation of public health practice" [1]. Surveillance data are used for a variety of purposes including detecting emerging diseases and conditions; drawing conclusions about the causes of cases of diseases or illnesses; determining when to implement control measures; assessing the effectiveness of public health interventions and programs; and understanding the underlying causes of morbidity and mortality [2–4].

There are many approaches to and types of public health surveillance including passive, active, sentinel, special systems (e.g., syndromic surveillance), and statistical (e.g., sampling the population to infer the burden of a certain disease across a larger population) [5]. In each type of surveillance, data are collected or analyzed by different means. For example, passive surveillance involves direct reporting to a state or local health department of cases of diseases, most often infectious diseases such as HIV. However, generally speaking, public health surveillance involves the collection of information about *individual* cases of diseases or illnesses. These data are frequently collected along with identifying demographic information, such as name, age, sex, and county of residence. Because health authorities collect and use individually identifiable data, ethics and trust play a very important role in the relationship between health authorities and the public.

The unwarranted disclosure of personally identifiable healthcare information may adversely affect an individual's ability to obtain or maintain insurance, employment, or housing [6]. There may be financial harm as well, such as the inability to obtain a loan based on a diagnosis of cancer or another illness or condition. A person may also experience mental distress, social stigmatization, and discrimination [7]. In situations involving intimate partner violence, the disclosure of an address can be harmful to a person and their family. Individuals concerned about their immigration status may also avoid health care if they fear disclosure of their address. If a person avoids care or treatment because of these concerns, their health may deteriorate; in some cases, a person with a communicable disease may become a threat to the public's health.

De-identified health information neither identifies nor provides a reasonable basis to identify an individual [8]. The disclosure of de-identified information also may be harmful. Although de-identified data does not include names, de-identification of information does not usually remove information about race, ethnicity, gender, or religion [9]. Thus, all members of a group (e.g., ethnic) with an increased risk for developing a particularly stigmatizing condition (e.g., mental illness), could potentially suffer based on association with the group, even if an individual's health records are not identified [9].

Concepts and Methods in Infectious Disease Surveillance, First Edition. Edited by Nkuchia M. M'ikanatha and John K. Iskander.
Published 2014 by John Wiley & Sons, Ltd.

Table 2.1 Role of law in public health surveillance.

Privacy	An individual's claim to limit access by others to some aspect of her personal life
Health informational privacy	An individual's claim to control the circumstances in which personal health information is collected, used, stored, and transmitted
Confidentiality	A form of health information privacy that focuses on maintaining trust between two individuals engaged in an intimate relationship, characteristically a physician–patient relationship
Security	The technological, organizational, and administrative safety practices designed to protect a data system against unwarranted disclosure, modification, or destruction and to safeguard the system itself

Source: Gostin, LO. *Public Health Law: Power, Duty, Restraint.* California/Milbank Books on Health and the Public (2000). Reproduced with permission of University of California Press.

In the United States, law plays a very important role in public health surveillance and in protecting the privacy, confidentiality, and security of health information (Table 2.1). All surveillance, regardless of the type, is conducted based on a mandate from a legislative body. The legal mandate is either a general one granting health officials the broad authority to carry out the activities necessary to control disease or is specific to a certain disease. In some cases, the law also limits the information that can be collected by health authorities or limits disclosure of that information. The laws and the diseases and conditions covered by the laws vary significantly across jurisdictions in the United States [10]. Federal law also plays an important role in protecting individuals' privacy and the confidentiality of public health data.

This chapter elaborates on this legal basis for public health surveillance; examines the balance between individual rights and the common good; and explores the relationships among law, surveillance, and technology using examples from the past decade.

The roles of state and federal laws in infectious disease surveillance

To understand the role of law in disease surveillance, particularly infectious disease surveillance, it is helpful to have a basic understanding of the legal framework that defines public health practice in the United States. The U.S. Constitution divides power between the federal government and the states [11]. It limits the authority of the federal government to specific enumerated powers (e.g., the regulation of interstate commerce), some of which are closely connected to public health and disease surveillance, but it reserves to the states the primary authority to regulate the public's health.

These state powers are primarily in areas known as police powers, which include the power to take steps to protect and promote the public's health. States exercise police powers through the adoption of statutes, which are written laws that specifically and generally authorize public health and other government officials to take steps to carry out the core functions of public health, including assessing the health of the population through disease surveillance. These and other public health–related statutes are carried out by state agencies—usually the public health agency—through programs, licensure, and regulations that implement laws.

States also adopt laws that control the ways in which disease surveillance can be conducted. All states have some sort of broad statutory language that requires some reporting of diseases of public health significance. The specific diseases and conditions that must be reported are not uniform throughout the United States [10,12]. For example, some state statutes and regulations allow public health officials to collect only certain types of information regarding individual cases of diseases, such as HIV or tuberculosis; or they limit the use of the information collected [13]. Some states do not have complete reporting laws. A Centers for Disease Control and Prevention (CDC) study published in 2002 showed that many states have deficiencies in immediate reporting requirements for category A agents (e.g., anthrax, botulism, plague, smallpox, and tularemia) [14]. A 2011 survey of states found that at least three nationally notifiable infectious conditions were not explicitly reportable across all states [12].

Federal laws also play an important role in conduct of surveillance. Although the federal government does not possess police powers, exercise of very broad specific powers of the federal government can impact how states carry out infectious disease surveillance and use the resulting data. The sections that follow describe examples of federal laws that protect the confidentiality of health information.

Privacy Act of 1974

The Privacy Act of 1974, as amended in 2009, governs the collection, use, and dissemination of personally identifiable information about living individuals that is maintained by a federal agency in a system of records [15]. A system of records is a group of records under the control of the agency from which information is retrieved by the name of the individual or by some identifier that uniquely identifies the individual such as a Social Security number [16]. The Privacy Act requires that agencies notify the public about their systems of records by publishing a notice in the Federal Register whenever a system of records is developed or revised [17]. The notice must include the name and the location of the system of records, the categories of individuals on whom records are maintained, the routine uses of records contained in the system, and individuals' rights with regard to their records (e.g., the right to seek access to and request amendments to their records). The Privacy Act prohibits the disclosure of information from a system of records without the written consent of the individual, unless the disclosure is pursuant to one of 12 statutory exceptions. For example, the Privacy Act permits the disclosure of identifiable information pursuant to a court order or pursuant to a showing of compelling circumstances affecting the health or safety of an individual [18].

HIPAA Privacy Rule

The U.S. Department of Health and Human Services issued the HIPAA Privacy Rule [19] to implement the Health Insurance Portability and Accountability Act of 1996 (HIPAA) [20]. The Privacy Rule became fully effective in 2004; and it established, for the first time, a set of national standards for the protection of individually identifiable health information called protected health information (PHI). The Privacy Rule regulates the use and disclosure of PHI in any form (e.g., paper, electronic) by entities subject to the rule. These so-called "covered entities" include health plans, healthcare clearinghouses, and providers (and their business associates) who conduct certain healthcare transactions electronically [21].

The Privacy Rule generally prohibits the use or disclosure of PHI without the written authorization of the individual. There are several exceptions to this requirement including an exception for public health. The Privacy Rule expressly permits covered entities to dis-close PHI, without the authorization of the individual, to a public health authority that is authorized to collect or receive it for specified public health purposes, including prevention or control of disease, public health surveillance, public health investigations, and public health interventions [22]. The definition of a public health authority includes an entity working under a grant of authority from or a contract with public health [23]. In addition, the Privacy Rule permits covered entities to use and disclose PHI without individual authorization as required by law [24]. Thus, the Privacy Rule permits covered entities to report communicable diseases and other conditions to the state or local health department if a state law or regulation requires the reporting of the disease or condition.

The Privacy Rule also permits covered entities to use or disclose PHI to avert or lessen a serious threat to the health or safety of a person or the public [25]. In this case, the covered entity may disclose the information to a person or persons reasonably able to prevent or lessen the threat, including public health officials. The Privacy Rule requires that a covered entity make reasonable efforts to use, disclose, and request only the minimum amount of PHI necessary to accomplish the intended purpose [26].

Public Health Service Act

The Public Health Service Act (PHSA) provides additional protection for highly sensitive, research, epidemiological, and statistical data collected by the U.S. Department of Health and Human Services [27]. Some information is so sensitive (e.g., illegal conduct, intimate partner violence, hospital-associated infection rates) that individuals or institutions might be reluctant to participate in a study or to provide accurate information without an assurance that the data will be protected. An Assurance of Confidentiality, issued under Section 308(d) of the PHSA [28], and a Certificate of Confidentiality, issued under Section 301(d) of the PHSA [29], protect sensitive data from compulsory disclosure (e.g., subpoena); that protection lasts forever.

A Certificate of Confidentiality protects the identity of individuals who are the subjects of research studies. An Assurance of Confidentiality protects the identity of individuals and institutions, and the sensitive research and epidemiological and statistical data that they provide. For example, an Assurance of Confidentiality might be used to protect sensitive surveillance data such as information on pregnancy-related mortality. The statute states that no identifiable information may be used for any purpose other than the purpose for which it was supplied unless the individual or the institution has consented to the use for the other purpose [28]. It also states that statistical or epidemiological information may not be published or released if the establishment or institution supplying the information is identifiable, unless the individual or establishment has consented to the release.

Family Educational Rights and Privacy Act

The Family Educational Rights and Privacy Act (FERPA) was enacted in 1974 to protect the privacy of student education records [30]. This law applies to all schools that receive funds under an applicable U.S. Department of Education program. Healthcare information is part of the education record. FERPA generally prohibits the disclosure of any personally identifiable information contained in an education record without the written consent of the parent, the guardian, or the student (if he or she is over 18 years old). There are limited exceptions to this requirement. An exception permits schools to disclose individually identifiable information from the education record to protect the health or safety of the student or other persons [31]. In an emergency, school officials may disclose this information to any person whom they reasonably believe needs the information to protect the health or safety of the student or others. Guidance issued by the U.S. Department of Education indicates that this exception is limited to a specific situation that presents an imminent danger such as an outbreak of vaccine-preventable disease [32]. FERPA also gives parents certain rights with respect to their child's education record, including the right to inspect and request corrections to the record.

Freedom of Information Act

The Freedom of Information Act (FOIA), enacted in 1966, establishes the public's right to access to U.S. government records [33]. Upon written request, federal agencies are required to disclose those records, unless they can be lawfully withheld from disclosure under one of nine specific exemptions. One exemption permits an agency to withhold personnel and medical files that, if released, would constitute a clearly unwarranted invasion of personal privacy [34]. Another exemption prohibits the disclosure of information that is specifi-

cally exempted from disclosure by statute [35]. For example, information protected by a Certificate or an Assurance of Confidentiality issued under the PHSA would be exempt from disclosure.

State laws

State laws related to the use, disclosure, security, and privacy of surveillance data by public health authorities vary dramatically from state to state. Thus, an understanding of specific state laws related to surveillance is essential for state and local public health practitioners [13].

The limits of the law

There is currently no comprehensive federal law that protects all personally identifiable healthcare information in all settings. The Privacy Act and FOIA govern records maintained by federal agencies, and they may not protect information from compulsory disclosure. The HIPAA Privacy Rule regulates the use and disclosure of personally identifiable information by covered entities and their business associates. Other federal and state laws protect specific types of healthcare information (e.g., HIV, genetic) or information in specified settings (e.g., drug and alcohol treatment facilities). Federal and state privacy laws do not generally address the secondary use and disclosure of information by recipients of the information; however, the recipient of the data may be regulated by other privacy laws. It is also notable that federal privacy laws protect individually identifiable information; they do not protect de-identified information.

Technology advances much more rapidly than the law. Information technology now allows for the rapid collection and linking of data sources in ways that have dramatically advanced the science of infectious disease surveillance and ways that increase public health's ability to identify and control threats and improve health. Moreover, technology also makes it possible to engage in activities that raise important legal and ethical questions, particularly when data is released to the public. The ability to link data that is considered de-identified with the data in different computerized databases (e.g., voter registration records, hospital discharge records) could result in the unintended re-identification of an individual or an institution and a violation of their privacy [9].

Examples from recent infectious disease outbreaks

In the past decade, several major public health events have illustrated the importance of communicable disease surveillance and highlighted the role of law during our response to those events. Law played a key role in the global outbreak of severe acute respiratory syndrome (SARS) in 2003, when a previously unknown coronavirus was causing an atypical pneumonia and infected over 8000 people in more than 37 countries. The city of Toronto, where SARS was first present in North America, successfully contained the outbreak through public health control measures such as quarantine, isolation, and closure of public facilities. The law in Toronto served a very important purpose as it allowed health officials to compel or coerce compliance with these measures. It is notable that, in most cases, the public voluntarily complied with the control measures and health officials only had to use their legal authority in limited situations.

State and federal laws were a major area of focus in preparing for a potential SARS outbreak in the United States. The National Association for County Commissioners and Health Officers published a checklist calling on state and local health officials preparing for SARS to ensure that their jurisdiction's quarantine and isolation laws, among other laws, were updated and that any gaps had been addressed [36]. To prevent future outbreaks, the Food and Drug Administration (FDA) issued a legal order banning the importation of civets, a type of animal, associated with the spread of SARS. In part because of the SARS outbreak, the International Health Regulations, a treaty pertaining to disease surveillance and reporting, was revised to clarify and speed the process by which events of international concern are reported by the country in which they are occurring.

An outbreak of monkeypox, a disease with symptoms similar to smallpox, in the United States in the early half of the past decade also illustrated the importance of law in controlling infectious disease outbreaks. Not generally found in the United States, monkeypox sickened more than 80 people in the Midwest who had handled or purchased prairie dogs obtained from an Illinois animal distributor or who were in contact with people who were infected [37]. State and local public health authorities used their legal powers to establish disease surveillance, isolate infected individuals, vaccinate

potentially exposed persons and those with known exposures, euthanize infected animals, and restrict the sale or ownership of the animals. The federal government also acted. The FDA and CDC also issued a joint legal order banning importation and prohibiting movement of the implicated animal species [38]. In some states, however, public health lacked adequate authority to limit or restrict ownership of the animal species associated with the outbreak. In these states, public health's lack of legal authority to take needed actions slowed the response and hindered the ability to use data from surveillance and the epidemiological investigation. This issue was subsequently addressed by the legislatures of many of these states [39].

Many other examples can be cited reflecting the important role of law in detecting and controlling infectious diseases. The recent pandemic of H1N1 influenza involved many legal issues, including the confidentiality of information regarding cases identified early in the event, authority for ongoing surveillance of the epidemic, and implementation of control measures [40]. Although these examples of public health events highlight the legal and privacy issues associated with communicable disease surveillance, it is noteworthy that the law provides the authority for all public health practice. All routine surveillance and case reporting to the state, local, tribal, and federal governments is based on law, either an explicit mandate to report a specific disease or condition or a general legal grant of legal authority to public health officials to protect the public's health. Privacy laws also regulate public health officials' ability to use and disclose information, including routine surveillance and case reporting.

Nonemergencies, such as developments in technology and our understanding of disease, have also raised new important questions at the intersection of disease surveillance and the law. For example, new approaches to assessing the overall burden of HIV in a population or community using the composite viral load of all the people in a geographical area [41] raise interesting legal questions about ideas about surveillance, stigma, and privacy and how we define communities—a set of questions that may be very different from the legal issues associated with surveillance and reporting around individual cases of disease. As information technology tools make it possible to connect large databases containing public and private data (for example, prescription drug monitoring data and Medicaid claims) and raise important questions about consent, use of data for public health surveillance and intervention purposes must be addressed.

Key summary points for public health practitioners

Laws are a key foundation for the infrastructure of the public health system within which infectious disease surveillance takes place. Laws and regulations also play important roles in limiting the use and disclosure of public health information. However, it is important for public health professionals engaged in disease surveillance activities to recognize that legal protection for information is not sufficient alone. There are some simple steps that public health practitioners can take to understand the law related to disease surveillance and to adopt practices that protect the privacy of individuals. These steps include the following:

- Seek out opportunities to meet attorneys and ethicists for advice on public health practice-related issues to your agency.
- Familiarize yourself with your organization's data security and confidentiality policies.
- Learn about the specific laws and regulations that affect practice in your jurisdiction.

Following some basic principles found in many laws can also help practitioners and their partners maintain the public's trust and protect data. These principles include the following:

- Communicate with affected populations about the purpose of the data collection, how the data will be used, and with whom it will be shared.
- If possible, provide an opportunity for the individual to exercise a choice about participation in the data collection through a consent process or an opportunity to opt out.
- If the data collection is mandatory, disclose the legal authority for the collection.
- Disclose the minimum amount of information necessary to achieve the intended purpose.
- Release only aggregate data only whenever possible and withhold data from public release in areas with a small population or a small number of cases.
- Assess and minimize the potential for re-identification in de-identified or partially de-identified data that is released to the public.

- When storing or transmitting data sets, separate identifiers to minimize the possibility of accidental release.
- Consider the ethical implications of releasing or using data. Although it may be legal to release data, it does not mean it is the right thing to do.

Organizations, such as state and local health departments and their partners, can also take steps to ensure that practitioners involved in disease surveillance understand their legal authorities and obligations. For example, leaders of public health organizations should become familiar with the extent of their authority. Staff should receive training on privacy, confidentiality, and security of data on a regular basis. In addition, organizations should update their policies to reflect changes in the law, technology, and practices and to address new situations.

STUDY QUESTIONS

1. How does the balance of power between the states and the federal government affect surveillance of infectious diseases?
2. Consider a recent infectious disease outbreak. What role did the law play in surveillance at the national level? At the state or local level? What role did the law play in using that surveillance information to make public health decisions?
3. You are engaged in an HIV surveillance project and you are scheduled to present your findings at a national conference in a week. Your data demonstrate that your state overall has very little HIV, except in two urban, low-income communities. If you describe the communities and the affected population, it will be very clear where they are located, almost down to the street level. Are there other ways to share the data?
4. There is an ongoing outbreak of salmonella in your jurisdiction. The health officer determines it is appropriate to issue a warning to the public about the likely source. One person has died. If the person's age and county are released, it would not be difficult for the deceased to be identified through obituaries published in the local paper. Should this information be released with the warning, and why or why not?
5. Your state is designing a new data system to manage surveillance data. What factors should be considered in creating and managing the new system?

References

1. Centers for Disease Control and Prevention. Public health surveillance slide set. Available at http://www.cdc.gov/ncphi/disss/nndss/phs/overview.htim (accessed March 24, 2014).

2. Teutsch S, Churchill RE. *Principles and Practice of Public Health Surveillance.* New York: Oxford University Press; 2000.

3. Goodman RA, Buehler JW, Koplan JP. The epidemiologic field investigation: Science and judgment in public health practice. *Am J Epidemiol* 1990;**132**:9–16.

4. Gregg MB. Conducting a field investigation. In: Greg MB, ed. *Field Epidemiology.* New York: Oxford University Press; 2001:62–77.

5. O'Connor J. Informational privacy protections: Do state laws offer public health leaders the flexibility they need? (Dissertation). Chapel Hill, NC. 2009. Available at http://www.sph.unc.edu/images/stories/academic_programs/hpaa/documents/oconnor.pdf (accessed March 24, 2014).

6. Gostin L. Health care information and the protection of personal privacy: Ethical and legal considerations. *Ann Intern Med* 1997;**127**(8 Pt 2):683–690.

7. Myers J, Frieden TR, Bherwani KM, Henning KJ. Privacy and public health at risk: Public health confidentiality in the digital age. *Am J Public Health* 2008;**98**:793–801.

8. 45 CFR 164.514 (2009).

9. Rothstein MA. Is deidentification sufficient to protect health privacy in research? *Am J Bioeth* 2010;**10**(9): 3–11.

10. Broome CV, Horton HH, Tress D, Lucido SJ, Koo D. Statutory basis for public health reporting beyond specific diseases. *J Urban Health* 2003;**80**(2 Suppl 1):114–122.

11. U.S. Constitution, amendment X.

12. Jajosky R, Rey A, Park M, Aranas A, Macdonald S, Ferland L. Findings from the Council of State and Territorial Epidemiologists' 2008 assessment of state reportable and nationally notifiable conditions in the United States and conditions for the future. *J Public Health Manag Pract* 2011;**17**(3):255–264.

13. O'Connor J, Matthews G. Informational privacy, public health, and state laws. *Am J Public Health* 2011;**101**(10): 1845–1850.

14. Horton H, Misrahi JJ, Matthews GW, Kocher PL. Critical biological agents: Disease reporting as a tool for bioterrorism preparedness. *J Law Med Ethics* 2002;**30**:262–266.

15. 5 USC 552a (2009).

16. 5 USC 552a(a)(5) (2009).

17. 5 USC 552a(e) (2009).

18. 5 USC 552a(b) (2009).

19. 45 CFR 160; 45 CFR 164 (2009).

20. Office for Civil Rights. Summary of the HIPAA privacy rule. (2003). Available at http://www.hhs.gov/ocr/privacy/hipaa/understanding/summary/index.html (accessed March 24, 2014).

21. 45 CFR 160.102.

22. 45 CFR 164.512(b).

23. 45 CFR 164.501.

24. 45 CFR 164.512(a).

25. 45 CFR 164.512(j).

26. 45 CFR 164.502(b).

27. 42 USC 241(d), 42 USC 242m(d).

28. 42 USC 242m(d).

29. 42 USC 241(d).

30. 20 USC 1232g; 34 CFR 99.

31. 20 USC 1232g(b)(1)(I).

32. Rooker LS. Letter to Alabama Department of Education re: Disclosure of immunization record. February 25, 2004. Available at http://www2.ed.gov/policy/gen/guid/fpco/ferpa/library/alhippaa.html (accessed March 24, 2014).

33. 5 USC 552 as amended by Public Law No. 104-231, 110 Stat. 3048.

34. 5 USC 552(b)6.

35. 5 USC 552(b)3.

36. Hopkins RS, Misegades L, Ransom J, Lipson L, Brink EW. SARS preparedness checklist for state and local health officials. *Emerg Infect Dis [serial online]* 2004;**10**(2). Available at http://wwwnc.cdc.gov/eid/article/10/2/03-0729.htm (accessed March 24, 2014).

37. Centers for Disease Control and Prevention. Update: Multistate outbreak of monkeypox—Illinois, Indiana, Missouri, Ohio, and Wisconsin, 2003. *MMWR Morb Mortal Wkly Rep* 2003;**52**(27):642–646.

38. Department of Health and Human Services Food and Drug Administration. Control of communicable diseases; restrictions on African rodents, prairie dogs, and certain other animals. Rule by Food and Drug Administration on September 8, 2008.

39. Madigan E. Monkeypox outbreak reveals gaps in state laws. Stateline. June 25, 2003. State headlines. Available at http://www.pewstates.org/projects/stateline (accessed March 24, 2014).

40. Association of State and Territorial Health Officials. *Assessing Policy Barriers to Effective Public Health Response in the H1N1 Influenza Pandemic.* Arlington, VA: ASTHO; 2010.

41. National Alliance of State and Territorial AIDS Directors. Guidance on community viral load. October 13, 2011. Available at http://www.nastad.org/Docs/101303_Community%20Viral%20Load%201-Pager%20-%2010.13.11.pdf (accessed March 24, 2014).

CHAPTER 3

National, state, and local public health surveillance systems

Ruth A. Jajosky[1] and Jennifer Ward[2]

[1] Centers for Disease Control and Prevention, Atlanta, GA, USA
[2] Tennessee Department of Health, Nashville, TN, USA

Organization and roles of public health infectious disease surveillance infrastructure in the United States and steps in the surveillance process

State and local public health organization and roles

Organization of state, territorial, and local public health entities is varied across the United States. Each state and territory has a department of health (DOH) with legal responsibility for protection of the public's health, including surveillance, investigation, and control of infectious diseases. States and territories may be further subdivided into regions and local health departments. Regions may consist of individual counties (common in metropolitan areas) or a collection of counties or other geographic subdivisions. In some states, particularly in the Northeast, local or regional areas may be further divided into local boards of health. Local jurisdictions may have additional authorities granted to them by state law. Jurisdictions divided in this way are often referred to as "home rule" states. Some large metropolitan areas (such as New York City) function in the same capacity as a state or territorial DOH and are independent to some extent from the state in which they are located. In some cases, they may even share surveillance data with federal public health authorities directly rather than through the state DOH in which they are located.

Several models for surveillance, investigation, and control responsibilities exist; and some public health jurisdictions have a combination of models. Models can typically be classified into three primary categories: centralized, decentralized, and a combination of both. In centralized models, the state or territorial public health entity coordinates surveillance, investigation, and control efforts at the local, regional and state/territorial levels. In decentralized models, primary investigation and control responsibilities are delegated to local and regional levels with the state serving a coordination and strategic role. Some public health jurisdictions have a combined model. For example, metropolitan areas within the state may carry primary responsibility for surveillance and control whereas these activities in more rural areas may be centralized by the state or territorial authority.

Disease reporting in the United States is mandated by law or regulation only at the local, state, or territorial levels [1,2]. Each state and territory determines which conditions to include on their reportable disease lists; these conditions are designated *reportable* conditions. Each state and territory also designates who (i.e., healthcare providers, laboratories) is required to report these conditions, what information should be reported, how to report, and how quickly disease information must be reported to public health authorities. The list of reportable conditions varies across states and from

Concepts and Methods in Infectious Disease Surveillance, First Edition. Edited by Nkuchia M. M'ikanatha and John K. Iskander.
Published 2014 by John Wiley & Sons, Ltd.

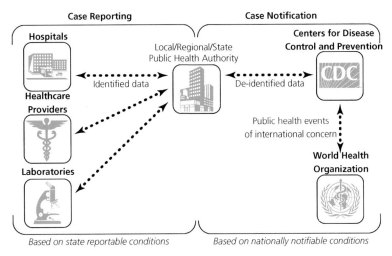

Figure 3.1 Public health surveillance data flow for state reportable and nationally notifiable diseases.

year to year. The term *case reporting* refers to healthcare entities (i.e., healthcare providers, laboratories, and hospitals) identifying reportable conditions and submitting information about these conditions to a local, county, state, or territorial public health agency (Figure 3.1). Individual case reporting requires patient information such as name, address, and phone number. Healthcare entities report suspected or confirmed diagnoses, laboratory tests and results, or information about outbreaks to public health using case morbidity report forms. These report forms can usually be either mailed, faxed, phoned, or submitted electronically. Following submission of the report, public health staff conducts follow-up investigations to confirm the cases based upon the criteria in the surveillance case definition (defined later in this chapter) for the reported disease and identify information needed for prevention and control.

Public health surveillance data are primarily collected at the local public health level where prevention and control activities occur. Then, data are reported in a hierarchical fashion to the regional, state, or territorial health departments. If a condition is considered important at the national level, it is defined as *nationally notifiable* and the reporting hierarchy continues from the state or territorial department to the federal Centers for Disease Control and Prevention (CDC) (see Figure 3.1 and the section "State-reportable and national notifiable condition surveillance" in this chapter). Table 3.1 lists how each level of public health uses infectious disease

surveillance data [3]. Under this system, CDC is not the primary party responsible for public health surveillance; instead, this is the responsibility of local, state, and territorial public health authorities. CDC provides assistance or consultative services to local, state, and territorial health departments in performing and evaluating surveillance as well as in planning and implementing disease control and prevention. For example, CDC plays an important role in developing guidelines (e.g., surveillance system evaluation guidelines) to help assess the adequacy of existing systems [7–12].

CDC surveillance systems receive data collected by local, county, state, and territorial public health officials. Data reported to CDC may include information about laboratory tests and results; the healthcare provider's diagnosis; vaccine history; signs and symptoms recorded by the healthcare entity; as well as demographic data, geographic information, risk factor information, and information about which criteria in the national surveillance case definition was met. No direct personal identifier, such as name, is sent to CDC. Data that are shared with CDC are a subset of the data collected and used by local or state level, including data collected during public health investigations to determine if public health intervention is appropriate and to further make the determination if a suspected case meets the surveillance case definition(s).

Public health surveillance case definitions may include combinations of clinical, epidemiologic, and

Table 3.1 Potential uses of infectious disease surveillance data by level of the public health system.

Intended uses	Public health system level of use	Example
Identify individual cases or clusters in a jurisdiction to prompt intervention or prevention activities.	Local, state (national)	Meningococcal disease occurring in a college student living in a dormitory requires not only immediate treatment for the patient but also identification of close contacts so that antibiotic prophylaxis can be administered to those potentially exposed.
Identify multistate disease outbreaks or clusters.	State, national	In 2011, a multistate listeriosis outbreak was associated with contaminated cantaloupes that had been distributed from a farm in Colorado and associated with infections in 139 people from 28 states [4].
Monitor trends to assess the public health impact of the condition under surveillance.	State, national (local)	After the licensure of the varicella vaccine in the United States, public health monitored the impact of the vaccine to document the decline in disease incidence and to identify whether disease was occurring in fully vaccinated persons.
Demonstrate the need for public health intervention programs and resources, as well as allocate resources.	State, national (local)	Surveillance data may identify demographic groups with higher disease incidence than others, which may merit targeted intervention, such as the targeted tuberculosis program for foreign-born residents who have immigrated from countries with high tuberculosis rates [5].
Formulate hypotheses for further study.	National (state)	Surveillance data may suggest an outbreak-specific or previously unknown risk factor associated with a disease, but public health needs to perform a study to ascertain the associations (e.g., Turkish pine nuts and salmonellosis) [6].

Note: A public health system level appearing in parenthesis represents secondary use of the data for that purpose.
Source: Adapted from Jajosky RA, Groseclose SL. Evaluation of reporting timeliness of public health surveillance systems for infectious diseases. *BMC Public Health* 2004; 4:29;1–9. Available from http://www.biomedcentral.com/1471-2458/4/29.

laboratory criteria used to define what a "case" of disease is for surveillance purposes. These definitions enable public health to classify and enumerate cases consistently across reporting jurisdictions. National case definitions are used by states and territories to guide what data are sent to CDC in a case notification, to ensure CDC aggregates data across reporting jurisdictions consistently. States and territories may adopt national surveillance case definitions for use within their jurisdictions or may develop additional case definitions for surveillance or outbreak purposes. Surveillance case definitions are not intended to guide healthcare providers in making medical decisions about individual patients [13].

Surveillance process roles and responsibilities

The primary purpose of public health surveillance for infectious diseases is to identify problems amenable to public health action aimed at controlling or preventing disease spread. When a potential case of infectious disease is identified through surveillance activities, the response will vary depending on the disease as well as

other factors. For example, whether further investigation into the suspected case is undertaken depends on many factors, including but not limited to likelihood of transmission, availability of effective interventions, severity of the disease and public health impact, local and state priorities, and available resources. Once the decision is made to perform a public health investigation, additional data are usually collected. An investigation may be as simple as a phone call to the physician who provided the case report, or it may involve other actions such as performing an inspection at a facility that may be the site of exposure, as well as extensive interviews with multiple individuals.

Public health investigation processes vary across jurisdictions. Typically, a laboratory report or a report of a suspected case of disease is identified, either through passive or active surveillance systems, and triggers the investigation process. Note, however, that not all reports of suspected cases trigger further investigation. Public health staff conducting the investigation will collect clinical, epidemiologic and laboratory data from multiple sources and combine them to confirm the case and determine which public health actions are needed.

The investigation may be completed by a single person (such as a public health nurse) or by a multidisciplinary team (common with outbreak investigations), which may consist of a public health physician and nurse, an epidemiologist, an environmentalist, a laboratorian, a veterinarian, or another specialist. If the investigation is part of an emergency response effort, law enforcement, emergency management officials, and other partners outside core public health may be involved in the investigation. During an investigation, data may also be exchanged across jurisdictional boundaries (such as across states). Other entities (such as CDC, U.S. Food and Drug Administration, or United States Department of Agriculture for a multistate foodborne outbreak) may also need to be engaged, depending on the type of investigation.

Control of disease spread is achieved through public health actions. Public health actions resulting from information gained during the investigation usually go beyond what an individual physician can provide to his or her patients presenting in a clinical setting. Examples of public health actions include identifying the source of infection (e.g., an infected person transmitting disease or a contaminated food vehicle); identifying persons who were in contact with the index case or any infected person who may need vaccines or antiinfectives to prevent them from developing the infection; closure of facilities implicated in disease spread; or isolation of sick individuals or, in rare circumstances, quarantining those exposed to an infected person.

Analysis and use of surveillance data

Monitoring surveillance data enables public health authorities to detect sudden changes in disease occurrence and distribution, identify changes in agents or host factors, and detect changes in healthcare practices [1]. An example of a change in healthcare practice is the increasing use of nonculture-based testing (e.g., enzyme immunoassay for campylobacter) to verify the etiologic organism responsible for an infection. It is important to understand how changes in testing practices affect surveillance and laboratory criteria for surveillance case confirmation. Public health officials need to review new laboratory testing methods to help guide analysis and interpretation of data.

The primary use of surveillance data at the local and state public health level is to identify cases or outbreaks in order to implement immediate disease control and prevention activities. CDC works collaboratively with states to identify and control multistate disease outbreaks. Surveillance data are also used by states and CDC to monitor disease trends, demonstrate the need for public health interventions such as vaccines and vaccine policy, evaluate public health activities, and identify future research priorities. See Table 3.1 for a description of how surveillance data are used by all levels of public health.

CDC routinely aggregates and analyzes data across reporting jurisdictions and shares the analytical results with the data providers [1,14–16]. Analyses of public health surveillance data on nationally notifiable conditions enables public health authorities to monitor disease trends, assess the effectiveness of prevention and control measures, identify high-risk populations or geographical areas, allocate resources appropriately, formulate prevention and control strategies, and develop public health policies [1,2,17].

One example of an analysis CDC performs weekly on aggregated provisional data reported to CDC's National Notifiable Diseases Surveillance System (NNDSS) represents the application of the historical limits aberration detection algorithm, run at the national level and published as Figure I in the CDC's *Morbidity and Mortality Weekly Report* (*MMWR*) [18]. This method compares the number of cases reported in the current 4-week period for a specific disease with the historical mean for that disease. The historical mean is based on the cases reported for 15 4-week periods comprised of the previous, comparable, and subsequent 4-week periods for the past 5 years. This analysis assists epidemiologists in identifying departures from past disease reporting patterns, which may require further investigation. CDC subject matter experts also monitor the provisional surveillance data on a weekly basis, comparing current case counts with incidence for the same time period in past years in order to detect changes in reporting patterns which may merit further study or investigation.

State reportable and national notifiable condition surveillance

Many reportable conditions are designated by the Council of State and Territorial Epidemiologists (CSTE) as being *nationally notifiable* [1,19]. CSTE is an organization that represents the collective public health interests of state and territorial epidemiologists. Figure 3.1 illustrates

Table 3.2 Case reporting and case notification.

	Data sender	Data receiver	Required or voluntary	Contains personal identifiers
Case reporting	Healthcare providers, laboratories, and other entities required to report	Local, state, and territorial public health authorities	Required by local, state, and territorial laws and regulations	Yes
Case notification	Local, state, and territorial public health authorities	CDC	Voluntary	No

the components of surveillance data flow that relate to public health case reporting within states and territories and those that relate to case notification from state or territorial health departments to CDC for Nationally Notifiable Conditions (NNC). Annual changes to the list of infectious (and noninfectious) NNC, as well as new and revised national surveillance case definitions, are decided upon and implemented through CSTE.

The official CSTE NNC list classifies the conditions according to the time frames in which CDC should be notified [19]. Three categories of time frames for case notification exist; these include immediate extremely urgent, immediate urgent and standard notification. Data on each of these three notification categories use the same electronic submission protocol, although they differ in terms of the recommended timeliness for each category of case notification [20]. In addition, the protocol for the two immediate notification categories includes a step requesting an initial voice notification to CDC's Emergency Operations Center in order to facilitate timely communication about details and circumstances of the event between subject matter experts in the state or territory and CDC. A subset of NNC case notifications may be notified to the World Health Organization (WHO) as per the International Health Regulations (IHR) (2005) because of the potential for a public health emergency of international concern (see Figure 3.1) [21]. In the United States, the CDC notifies the Department of Health and Human Services, which submits events under IHR to the WHO.

When proposing revisions to the list of NNC, CDC, and CSTE collaboratively consider the goals, purposes, and objectives of surveillance, as well as factors such as incidence (how frequently new cases of the condition occur in the population); severity of the condition, such as the case-fatality rate; communicability (how readily the disease is spread); preventability; impact on the population or community; and need for public health action. The CSTE recommends that all states and territories enact laws or regulations making NNC reportable in jurisdictions [22]. State and territorial health departments voluntarily submit data about NNC to CDC. The term *case notification* refers to the submission of electronic data by states and territories to CDC about nationally notifiable disease cases (see Figure 3.1 and Table 3.2). This differs from *case reporting*, which represents reporting of identifiable information from health care, laboratories, and other reporting entities to local/state/territorial public health in accordance with reporting laws and regulations (see Figure 3.1 and Table 3.2). State health departments usually submit electronic data in a standardized format to CDC to facilitate data aggregation and analysis across reporting jurisdictions.

CDC administers NNDSS in collaboration with CSTE. The NNDSS is a collection of state-based surveillance systems that primarily includes infectious diseases. Fifty-seven reporting jurisdictions—including 50 U.S. states; New York City; Washington, DC; and five U.S. territories—report provisional data, primarily at the individual case level, each week to CDC's NNDSS. These provisional data are published weekly in CDC's *MMWR* Table I (Summary of provisional cases of selected notifiable diseases, United States), Table II (Provisional cases of selected notifiable diseases, United States), and Figure I [18]. Finalized NNDSS data are published each year in the *MMWR: Summary of Notifiable Diseases, United States* [1]. The NNDSS represents the only source of national statistics on infectious diseases that are nationally notifiable. The NNDSS data are shared with CDC subject-matter experts responsible for the prevention and control of the NNC.

Historically, CDC's NNDSS has compiled data across several surveillance systems that utilize a variety of methods for collection, management, and submission of data to CDC. However, the NNDSS has defined a core set of data elements that are standardized across most NNCs. In addition, the NNDSS has created standardized disease-specific data elements. The original purpose of standardization was to facilitate CDC's ability to aggregate and analyze data across public health reporting jurisdictions. Now, with the increasing adoption of electronic systems (e.g., electronic health records), there is a need for public health and the healthcare communities to use the same data standards, whenever possible, to optimize sharing of data across both partners to improve individual and population health.

In 1999, CDC initiated the National Electronic Disease Surveillance System (NEDSS) as a new approach to the collection and management of surveillance data to support public health surveillance for infectious diseases. NEDSS arose from the interest public health had in developing efficient, integrated, and interoperable surveillance systems at the local and state levels, which would facilitate the sharing of data across jurisdictions and the electronic transfer of information needed by public health from clinical and laboratory information systems in the healthcare sector in order to reduce the burden on healthcare providers [23]. NEDSS is an initiative focused on promoting and facilitating the adoption of standards, policies, practices, and tools, as well as the provision of technical assistance and funding to support sharing of information across entities throughout the public health investigation workflow. Though NEDSS is not a surveillance information system, there is a surveillance information system component. Public health reporting jurisdictions commonly refer to their integrated surveillance systems for infectious diseases as NEDSS systems.

There are numerous challenges related to the implementation of integrated and interoperable surveillance systems. Only a few challenges are presented here. First, these systems require that public health staff possess a variety of different technical skills (e.g., epidemiology, informatics, information technology, messaging and vocabulary expertise, and project management) [24] and use different technical terminology to collaborate and communicate effectively with each other to address public health needs. Second, health department staff frequently experience competing priorities with their surveillance activities, and surveillance programs have experienced reductions in the resources needed to support surveillance. Additionally, there have been few incentives available to healthcare entities and laboratories to work with public health to fully implement the vision of electronic disease surveillance. However, legislation to promote meaningful use of electronic health records has taken a step in the direction of providing financial incentives to hospitals submitting electronic data on reportable laboratory results to public health agencies [25,26].

Methods used for surveillance

There are many different types of surveillance conducted at the state, local, and federal level. Surveillance methods will not be discussed in detail in this chapter. However, some examples of common types of surveillance conducted at the state, local, and territorial levels are summarized.

Active versus passive surveillance

The majority of reportable disease surveillance is conducted through passive surveillance methods. Passive surveillance means that public health agencies inform healthcare providers and other entities of their reporting requirements, but they do not usually conduct intensive efforts to solicit all cases; instead, the public health agency waits for the healthcare entities to submit case reports. Because passive surveillance is often incomplete, public health agencies may use hospital discharge data, laboratory testing records, mortality data, or other sources of information as checks on completeness of reporting and to identify additional cases. This is called active surveillance. Active surveillance usually includes intensive activities on the part of the public health agency to identify all cases of a specific reportable disease or group of diseases. For example, a local public health department may audit hospital laboratory logs on a monthly basis to identify patients with positive tests for enteric pathogens. Because it can be very labor intensive, active surveillance is usually conducted for a subset of reportable conditions, in a defined geographic locale and for a defined period of time. Examples of active population-based surveillance include the Foodborne Diseases Active Surveillance Network (FoodNet) [27] and Active Bacterial Core (ABC) surveillance [28], which are part of the Emerging Infections Program (EIP).

Active surveillance may be conducted on a routine basis or in response to an outbreak (defined as an increase in the number of cases observed versus what is expected during a specific period of time). When an outbreak is suspected or identified, another type of surveillance known as enhanced passive surveillance may also be initiated. In enhanced passive surveillance methods, public health may improve communication with the healthcare community, schools, daycare centers, and other facilities and request that all suspected cases be reported to public health. Enhanced passive surveillance still relies on others to report cases to public health [29].

Laboratory-based surveillance

Case-based surveillance is supplemented through laboratory-based surveillance activities. As opposed to case-based surveillance, the focus is on laboratory results themselves, independent of whether or not an individual's result is associated with a "case" of illness meeting the surveillance case definition. Laboratory-based surveillance is conducted by state public health laboratories as well as the healthcare community (e.g., hospital, private medical office, and commercial laboratories).

State public health laboratories (SPHL) or other clinical laboratories may participate in several types of laboratory-based surveillance, some of which are covered in other areas of this text. These surveillance initiatives are often focused on defining characteristics of pathogens isolated (e.g., subtype, serotype, antimicrobial resistance profile, and genotype). The SPHL may conduct specialized testing and submit results to a larger national database for identification of clusters of illness across geographic boundaries. Examples include PULSENet for enteric pathogens [30] and the National Respiratory and Enteric Virus Surveillance System for influenza [31].

Other surveillance

Other surveillance methods supplement the existing approaches discussed above. They may include, but are not limited to, sentinel, enhanced, syndromic, and envi-ronmental surveillance. (Syndromic and environmental surveillance are discussed in other chapters.)

State and local public health entities participate in sentinel surveillance activities. With sentinel methods, surveillance is conducted in a sample of reporting entities, such as healthcare providers or hospitals, or in a specific population known to be an early indicator of disease activity (e.g., pediatric). However, because the goal of sentinel surveillance is not to identify every case, it is not necessarily representative of the underlying population of interest; and results should be interpreted accordingly. State and local public health authorities participate in sentinel surveillance for influenza, for example. In the Sentinel Provider Network for influenza surveillance, a sample of representative providers is chosen to participate. Providers report weekly counts of influenza-like illness by predefined age groups and submit laboratory isolates for subtyping during the influenza season. The data are entered by providers into a web-based system managed by CDC. Outreach, recruitment of participating providers, and specimen transport are often handled by the local or state public health entity.

Resources

Funding for public health activities, including personnel, is derived from a variety of sources. States provide funding for surveillance activities, and funding is also provided by federal grants and cooperative agreements [24]. For example, the Epidemiology and Laboratory Capacity and the Public Health Emergency Preparedness Cooperative Agreements are the primary sources of funding for infectious disease surveillance systems in the United States [32,33]. Distinct CDC programs may also provide programmatic funding to local, state, and territorial public health to support surveillance activities. Examples include CDC programs for HIV/AIDS, tuberculosis, and sexually transmitted diseases. As a result, the public health surveillance infrastructure in the United States is heavily reliant on the availability of federal funding to support surveillance activities. With state and local surveillance budgets decreasing in the past decade, this dependency on federal funding sources has become even greater.

Although the number of personnel available to conduct surveillance activities is heavily affected by funding, other factors also play a part. With the emphasis in the last decade on electronic data exchange for surveillance, the skill sets needed to conduct surveillance have changed. Epidemiologists are now expected to possess skills in informatics and management of complex relational datasets [34]. The CDC and CSTE applied epidemiology competencies recognize the need for public health staff to be trained in informatics principles in order to improve public health practice [34]. Expertise in informatics (a professional discipline distinct from information technology) is necessary for the efficient functioning of public health surveillance information systems. Informaticians, epidemiologists, and information technology staff must work together to achieve a cohesive, holistic approach to public health information systems. Information technology staff must be skilled in the use of tools for data manipulation, exchange, and standards. Data standards are mentioned later in this chapter.

Electronic methods and other recent innovations

For the past decade, efforts have shifted to focus on automation of many parts of the surveillance process to increase timeliness and completeness of reporting, improve sustainability of systems (particularly during outbreaks or other public health emergencies), and decrease the burden on entities responsible for providing and managing surveillance data. These initiatives include integration of surveillance systems, electronic reporting of laboratory and case reports, standards-based case notification, and syndromic surveillance. Syndromic surveillance is discussed in detail in another chapter of this book.

Integrated and interoperable surveillance systems

Public health operated for many decades (and still does to some extent) using stand-alone, case-based information systems for collection of surveillance data that do not allow information sharing between systems and do not permit the ability to track the occurrences of different diseases in a specific person over time. One of the primary objectives of NEDSS is to promote person-based surveillance and integrated and interoperable surveillance systems. In an integrated person-based system,

information is collected to create a public health record for a given person for different diseases over time. This enables public health to track public health conditions associated with a person over time, allowing analyses of public health events and comorbidities, as well as more robust public health interventions. An interoperable system can exchange information with other systems. For example, data are shared between surveillance systems or between other public health or clinical systems, such as an electronic health record or outbreak management system. Achieving the goal of establishing a public health record for an individual over time does not require one monolithic system that supports all needs; this can, instead, be achieved through integration and/or interoperability of systems.

Standards-based public health surveillance

With the adoption of more integrated and interoperable systems, a need has arisen for vocabulary (data elements and coding formats) and messaging standards. In general, standards can be defined as rules, definitions, guidelines, specifications or characteristics for repeated processes or procedures. In the context of public health surveillance, for example, standards allow two systems to record information in the same manner, allowing data to have the same meaning from one system to another. This includes standardization of data elements (also known as concepts), values for coded data elements (also known as vocabulary), as well as standards for the structure of information and transport of information from one system to another. Some examples of standards used in the healthcare sector are as follows:

- Health Level 7 (HL7) Clinical Document Architecture (CDA) as the standard for messaging electronic health information contained in a public health case report from healthcare entities to local and state public health [35].
- HL7 version 2.5 as the standard for submitting case notifications from state health departments to CDC [36].
- Logical Observation Identifiers Names and Codes (LOINC) as the standard for transmitting laboratory test names and the Systematized Nomenclature of Medicine (SNOMED) as the standard for test results [37,38].

Standards continue to evolve and develop as electronic data exchange between partners and systems occurs. The information that follows below is presented according to the data flow in Figure 3.1, from case ascertainment sources for surveillance data to case notifications sent to CDC.

Electronic laboratory results reporting

For over a decade, public health has focused on automation of reporting of laboratory results to public health from clinical laboratories and healthcare providers. Paper-based submission of laboratory results to public health for reportable conditions results in delays in receipt of information, incomplete ascertainment of possible cases, and missing information on individual reports. All of these aspects are improved through automation of the process [39–43]. A more complete discussion of electronic laboratory reporting (ELR) is included in another chapter. Recent initiatives have invested significant financial resources into moving this work forward, primarily healthcare reform initiatives for widespread adoption of electronic health records (EHRs) in the healthcare community and the meaningful use of electronic health records [25,26]. Meaningful use of EHRs is being implemented in stages. Stage 1 contains ELR as one of the key uses of EHRs to support public health functions. Future stages will likely include other public health functions.

Another area involving automation of laboratory reporting includes sharing of information collected from laboratory-based surveillance methods with CDC subject matter experts and with other public health laboratories. For example, the Public Health Laboratory Interoperabilty Project (PHLIP) defines standards for data sharing of laboratory-based surveillance data for influenza and other pathogens [44].

Electronic public health case reporting

Another area of automation involves reporting of case or morbidity data known as public health case reporting (PHCR) [45,46]. PHCR in this context can refer to reporting of suspect cases from healthcare providers to public health, as well as sharing of case data between public health departments and different systems (e.g., from one state to another). Successful pilot implementations have occurred [47,48].

Standards-based case notification to CDC

Since the early 1990s, case notification data have been transmitted to CDC for surveillance of NNC using the National Electronic Telecommunications System for Surveillance format. In 2008, CDC began transitioning case notification data to an HL7 standard based on version 2.5. The transition to the new format (HL7) is not currently complete.

Conclusion

Public health agencies collect infectious disease surveillance data in order to target and implement public health intervention and prevention activities where they are most needed. While infectious disease surveillance data are primarily collected at the local, regional, and state levels, all levels of public health, including the federal level (and international level, when appropriate) work collaboratively to protect the population's health. Federal public health agencies provide technical assistance, consultative guidance, and resources needed by local, regional, state, and territorial public health agencies in order to perform their work.

Each state and territory defines their own list of reportable infectious diseases and conditions as well as a list of who is required to report, such as physicians, laboratories, hospitals, and others. These lists are defined based on the health priorities of individual jurisdictions, as well as consideration of which conditions are nationally notifiable. Not all nationally notifiable conditions are reportable in each jurisdiction. In addition, reports of nationally notifiable conditions are voluntarily sent to CDC (without personal identifiers) by local and state health public health departments.

The public health surveillance infrastructure in the United States is undergoing a major transition from case-based, stand-alone electronic and paper-based systems to electronic systems that can track multiple diseases and instances of the same disease in an individual. Public health is working with the healthcare system to automate case ascertainment to reduce the burden associated with manual reporting methods. Although transition to automated processes requires an up-front investment, increases in completeness and timeliness of information combined with decreased burden on individual healthcare providers and public health workers should make the system more sustainable.

Public health has limited resources to implement innovations in the surveillance process aimed at providing more complete and timely data to use for intervention and prevention purposes. Hence, it is becoming increasingly important for public health to focus on the most critical information needed, to share resources, to learn from each other, and to be efficient in the way innovations are implemented.

References

1. Centers for Disease Control and Prevention. Summary of notifiable diseases—United States 2010. *MMWR Morb Mortal Wkly Rep* 2012;**59**(53):1–110. Available at http://www.cdc.gov/mmwr/PDF/wk/mm5953.pdf (accessed March 24, 2014).

2. Jajosky R, Rey A, Park M, et al. Findings from the Council of State and Territorial Epidemiologists' 2008 assessment of state reportable and nationally notifiable conditions in the United States and considerations for the future. *J Public Health Manage Pract* 2011;**17**(3):255–264.

3. Jajosky RA, Groseclose SL. Evaluation of reporting timeliness of public health surveillance systems for infectious diseases. *BMC Public Health* 2004;**4**(29):1–9. Available at http://www.biomedcentral.com/1471-2458/4/29 (accessed March 25, 2014).

4. Centers for Disease Control and Prevention. Investigation Update: Multistate outbreak of listeriosis linked to whole cantaloupes from Jensen Farms, Colorado. November 2, 2011. Available at http://www.cdc.gov/listeria/outbreaks/cantaloupes-jensen-farms/110211/index.html (accessed March 25, 2014).

5. Centers for Disease Control and Prevention. Targeted tuberculin testing and interpreting tuberculin skin test results. December 2011. Available at http://www.cdc.gov/tb/publications/factsheets/testing/skintestresults.htm (accessed March 24, 2014).

6. Centers for Disease Control and Prevention. Investigation update: Multistate outbreak of human *Salmonella* Enteritidis infections linked to Turkish pine nuts. 2011. Available at http://www.cdc.gov/salmonella/pinenuts-enteriditis/111711/index.html (accessed March 24, 2014).

7. Centers for Disease Control and Prevention. Guidelines for evaluating surveillance systems. *MMWR Morb Mortal Wkly Rep* 1988;**37**(S-5):1–18. Available at http://www.cdc.gov/mmwr/preview/mmwrhtml/00001769.htm (accessed March 25, 2014).

8. Centers for Disease Control and Prevention. Updated guidelines for evaluating public health surveillance systems: Recommendations from the guidelines working group. *MMWR Morb Mortal Wkly Rep* 2001;**50**(RR13):1–35. Available at http://www.cdc.gov/mmwr/preview/mmwrhtml/rr5013a1.htm (accessed March 25, 2014).

9. Centers for Disease Control and Prevention. Framework for evaluating public health surveillance systems for early detection of outbreaks. *MMWR Morb Mortal Wkly Rep* 2004;**53**(RR-5):1–11. Available at http://www.cdc.gov/mmwr/preview/mmwrhtml/rr5305a1.htm (accessed March 25, 2014).

10. Centers for Disease Control and Prevention. Chapter 18: Surveillance indicators. *Manual for the Surveillance of Vaccine-Preventable Diseases*, 5th ed. Atlanta, GA: Centers for Disease Control and Prevention; 2011. Available at http://www.cdc.gov/vaccines/pubs/surv-manual/chpt18-surv-indicators.html (accessed March 24, 2014).

11. Centers for Disease Control and Prevention. Monitoring tuberculosis programs—National tuberculosis indicator project, United States, 2002–2008. *MMWR Morb Mortal Wkly Rep* 2010;**59**(10):295–298. Available at http://www.cdc.gov/mmwr/preview/mmwrhtml/mm5910a3.htm?s_cid=mm5910a3_e (accessed March 25, 2014).

12. Centers for Disease Control and Prevention. Tuberculosis program evaluation resources. 2012. Available at http://www.cdc.gov/tb/programs/Evaluation/Default.htm (accessed March 25, 2014).

13. Centers for Disease Control and Prevention. Case definitions for public health surveillance. *MMWR Morb Mortal Wkly Rep* 1990;**39**(RR-13):1–43. Available at http://www.cdc.gov/mmwr/preview/mmwrhtml/00025629.htm (accessed March 25, 2014).

14. Centers for Disease Control and Prevention. Reported tuberculosis in the United States. 2009. Available at http://www.cdc.gov/tb/statistics/reports/2009/pdf/report2009.pdf (accessed March 25, 2014).

15. Centers for Disease Control and Prevention. Sexually transmitted disease surveillance. 2009. Available at http://www.cdc.gov/std/stats09/toc.htm (accessed March 25, 2014).

16. Centers for Disease Control and Prevention. Diagnoses of HIV infection and AIDS in the United States and Dependent Areas. 2009. HIV Surveillance Report Vol. 21. Available at http://www.cdc.gov/hiv/surveillance/resources/reports/2009report/index.htm (accessed March 25, 2014).

17. Thacker SB. Historical development. In: Teutsch SM, Churchill RE, eds. *Principles and Practice of Public Health*

Surveillance, 2nd ed. New York: Oxford University Press; 2000:1–16.

18. Centers for Disease Control and Prevention. Notifiable diseases. *MMWR Morb Mortal Wkly Rep* 2011;**60**(32):1102–1115. Table I, Table II, and Figure I. Available at http://www.cdc.gov/mmwr/preview/mmwrhtml/mm6032md.htm?s_cid=mm6032md_w (accessed March 25, 2014).

19. Council of State and Territorial Epidemiologists. CSTE list of nationally notifiable conditions. 2013. Available at http://c.ymcdn.com/sites/www.cste.org/resource/resmgr/CSTENotifiableConditionListA.pdf (accessed March 25, 2014).

20. Council of State and Territorial Epidemiologists. Position statement 09-SI-04: Process statement for immediately nationally notifiable conditions. 2009. Available at http://c.ymcdn.com/sites/www.cste.org/resource/resmgr/PS/09-SI-04.pdf (accessed March 25, 2014).

21. World Health Organization. *International Health Regulations*, 2nd ed. Geneva, Switzerland: World Health Organization; 2005. Available at http://whqlibdoc.who.int/publications/2008/9789241580410_eng.pdf (accessed March 25, 2014).

22. Council of State and Territorial Epidemiologists. Position statement 10-SI-02: Modification of the process for recommending conditions for national surveillance. 2010. Available at http://c.ymcdn.com/sites/www.cste.org/resource/resmgr/PS/10-SI-02.pdf (accessed March 25, 2014).

23. Centers for Disease Control and Prevention National Electronic Disease Surveillance System Working Group. National Electronic Disease Surveillance System (NEDSS): A standards-based approach to connect public health and clinical medicine. *J Public Health Manage Pract* 2001;**7**(6): 43–50.

24. Turner K. 2010 CSTE NEDSS assessment summary results. NEDSS Stakeholder Meeting. 2010. Available at http://www.phconnect.org/group/nedssforum/forum/topics/2010-cste-nedss-assessment (accessed March 25, 2014).

25. Department of Health and Human Services, Office of the National Coordinator for Health Information Technology. Electronic health records and meaningful use. Available at http://healthit.hhs.gov/portal/server.pt?open=512&objID=2996&mode=2 (accessed March 25, 2014).

26. Blumenthal D, Tavenner M. The "meaningful use" regulation for electronic health records. *N Engl J Med* 2010; **363**:501–504. Available at http://www.nejm.org/doi/full/10.1056/NEJMp1006114 (accessed March 25, 2014).

27. Centers for Disease Control and Prevention. Foodborne diseases active surveillance network (FoodNet). 2011. Available at http://www.cdc.gov/foodnet/ (accessed March 25, 2014).

28. Centers for Disease Control and Prevention. Active Bacterial Core (ABC) surveillance. 2011. Available at http://www.cdc.gov/abcs/index.html (accessed March 25, 2014).

29. M'ikanantha NM, Lynfield R, Julian KG, et al. Infectious disease surveillance: A cornerstone for prevention and control. In: M'ikanantha NM, Lynfield R, Van Beneden C, et al., eds. *Infectious Disease Surveillance*, 1st ed. Oxford, UK: Blackwell Publishing; 2007:11.

30. Centers for Disease Control and Prevention. PulseNet. 2011. Available at http://www.cdc.gov/pulsenet/ (accessed March 25, 2014).

31. Centers for Disease Control and Prevention. National respiratory and enteric virus surveillance. 2011. Available at http://www.cdc.gov/surveillance/nrevss/ (accessed March 25, 2014).

32. Centers for Disease Control and Prevention. Epidemiology and laboratory capacity for infectious diseases. 2013. Available at http://www.cdc.gov/ncezid/dpei/epidemiology-laboratory-capacity.html (accessed March 25, 2014).

33. Centers for Disease Control and Prevention. Funding, guidance, and technical assistance to states, localities, and territories: Public health emergency preparedness cooperative agreement. 2011. Available at http://www.cdc.gov/phpr/coopagreement.htm (accessed March 25, 2014).

34. Centers for Disease Control and Prevention/Council of State and Territorial Epidemiologists. Competencies for applied epidemiologists in governmental public health agencies. 2008. Available at http://www.cdc.gov/AppliedEpiCompetencies/downloads/Applied_Epi_Comps.pdf (accessed March 25, 2014).

35. Health Level 7. Clinical Document Architecture standard description. 2007–2014. Available at http://www.hl7.org/implement/standards/cda.cfm (accessed March 25, 2014).

36. Health Level 7. Standard description version 2.5. 2007–2014. Available at http://www.hl7.org/implement/standards/v2messages.cfm (accessed March 25, 2014).

37. Regenstrief Institute. Logical observation identifiers names and codes (LOINC). 1994–2014. Available at http://loinc.org/ (accessed March 25, 2014).

38. College of American Pathologists. SNOMED terminology solutions. 2014. Available at http://www.cap.org/apps/cap.portal?_nfpb=true&_pageLabel=snomed_page (accessed March 25, 2014).

39. Overhage JM, Grannis S, McDonald CJ. A comparison of the completeness and timeliness of automated electronic laboratory reporting and spontaneous reporting of notifiable conditions. *Am J Public Health* 2008;**98**(2): 344–350.

40. Nguyen TQ, Thorpe L, Makki HA, Mostashari F. Benefits and barriers to electronic laboratory results reporting for notifiable diseases: The New York City Department of Health and Mental Hygiene experience. *Am J Public Health* 2007;**97**:S142–S145.

41. Effler P, Ching-Lee M, Bogard A, et al. Statewide system of electronic notifiable disease reporting from clinical laboratories: Comparing automated reporting with conventional methods. *JAMA* 1999;**282**:1845–1850.

42. Backer HD, Bissell SR, Vugia DJ. Disease reporting from an automated laboratory-based reporting system to a state

health department via local county health departments. *Public Health Rep* 2001;**116**:257–265.

43. Panackal AA, M'ikanatha NM, Tsui FC, et al. Automatic electronic laboratory-based reporting of notifiable infectious diseases at a large health system. *Emerg Infect Dis* 2002; **8**:685–691.

44. Association of Public Health Laboratories. The public health laboratory interoperability project: Ensuring quality CDC-public health laboratory communication. Available at http://www.aphl.org/aphlprograms/informatics/resources/Documents/INF_2013May30_PHLIP-Overview.pdf (accessed March 25, 2014).

45. Department of Health and Human Services. Standards and certification for public health case reporting. 2014. Available at http://www.hitsp.org/InteroperabilitySet _Details.aspx?MasterIS=true&InteroperabilityId=364&P

refixAlpha=1&APrefix=IS&PrefixNumeric=11 (accessed March 25, 2014).

46. PhConnect Collaboration for Public Health. Public health case reporting community. Available at http://www.phconnect .org/group/phcasereporting (accessed March 25, 2014).

47. Klompas M, Lazarus R, Daniel J, et al. Electronic medical record support for public health (ESP): Automated detection and reporting of statutory notifiable diseases to public health authorities. *Adv Dis Surveill* 2007;**3**(3): 1–5.

48. Klompas M, Lazarus R, Hou X, et al. Automated detection and reporting of notifiable diseases using electronic medical records versus passive surveillance—Massachusetts, June 2006–July 2007. *MMWR Morb Mortal Wkly Rep* 2008;**57**(14):373–376. Available at http://www.cdc.gov/mmwr/preview/mmwrhtml/mm5714a4.htm (accessed March 25, 2014).

CHAPTER 4

Quarantine and the role of surveillance in nineteenth-century public health

David S. Barnes

University of Pennsylvania, Philadelphia, PA, USA

Overview

Public health, as a science and as a domain of public policy, was born out of infectious disease surveillance. From plague in Venice in 1486 to typhus in Upper Silesia in 1848 to H1N1 influenza in Mexico City in 2009, epidemics have continually galvanized research and provoked policy responses. Disease surveillance is one of the few weapons in the public health arsenal of 150 years ago that is still relied upon today. However, disease-specific etiologies and the identification of microbial pathogens in the laboratory, which are essential to infectious disease surveillance today, played no role prior to 1880. This chapter explores the debates and controversies that marked infectious disease surveillance in the years just before the Bacteriological Revolution (roughly 1880–1900), when the germ theory of disease transformed medical knowledge and public health policy. The institution of maritime quarantine was especially controversial, and debates about its operation provide a revealing glimpse of the important role played by surveillance in nineteenth-century public health. Notwithstanding advances in microbiology and laboratory techniques, careful observation and correlation of disease patterns remain essential to epidemiology and public health.

Introduction

In the mid-nineteenth century, diseases were understood as dynamic and variable processes with an array of causes operating at various levels, rather than as distinct biological entities with specific microbial causes. Historians have generally dismissed the practice of quarantine as unscientific and ineffective, because in their portrayal it was based on an erroneous belief that diseases like plague, yellow fever, and cholera were contagious—that is, transmitted by direct person-to-person contact [1–5]. In fact, contagion was not the premise on which quarantine was based; many physicians and health officials who vehemently opposed the belief in contagion nevertheless advocated quarantine. Moreover, quarantine was based on rigorous observation of disease outbreaks and their systematic—even scientific—correlation with a wide range of events and circumstances.

In the centuries following the establishment of the first permanent board of health in Venice in 1486, maritime quarantine was the foundation of public health policy (Box 4.1). By the nineteenth century, every major seaport in the Western world had a quarantine station, or "lazaretto," where incoming ships, passengers, and cargo were inspected, and where they were detained for varying periods of time if signs of danger were detected. These stations owed their existence to imported epidemics, and were designed to prevent any transmissible disease from entering and gaining a foothold in the port city. In the United States, recurring and deadly visitations of yellow fever which spread among populations from Boston to New Orleans between 1793 and 1878 prompted a tightening of quarantine regulations in many ports and sparked lively debates about the contagiousness and prevention of the disease. Three

Concepts and Methods in Infectious Disease Surveillance, First Edition. Edited by Nkuchia M. M'ikanatha and John K. Iskander.
© 2015 John Wiley & Sons, Ltd. Published 2015 by John Wiley & Sons, Ltd.

Box 4.1 Timeline: milestones in the history of quarantine and in the nineteenth-century debate over quarantine in the United States.

1348	First official quarantine established in Venice during the Black Death.
1486	First permanent health board established in Venice.
1793	Yellow fever epidemic kills 5000 in Philadelphia and causes tens of thousands more to flee the city.
1794	Permanent board of health established in Philadelphia.
1799	After further devastating yellow fever outbreaks, Philadelphia's Board of Health opens new Lazaretto on Tinicum Island, 12 miles downriver from the city.
1853	Yellow fever epidemic in New Orleans kills nearly 8000.
1857–1860	Annual National Quarantine and Sanitary Conventions assemble the leading health authorities from American port cities.
1870	Yellow fever epidemic at Philadelphia's Lazaretto.
1872	American Public Health Association founded by delegates from the National Quarantine and Sanitary Conventions.
1878	Yellow fever epidemic claims 20,000 lives in New Orleans, Memphis, and the Lower Mississippi Valley.
1892	Cholera epidemic in Hamburg places U.S. seaports on high alert. In response, New York City establishes the first municipal bacteriology laboratory. Ellis Island federal immigration station opens.
1895	Philadelphia's Lazaretto station is closed as part of the gradual assumption of quarantine authority by the federal government.

examples from these debates in the decades immediately preceding the Bacteriological Revolution illustrate the anecdotal but systematic method that generated useful public health knowledge at a time when viruses and vectors were not part of the discussion.

Debating quarantine and yellow fever, 1850–1880

When Philadelphia, the nation's capital and largest city, was ravaged four times by yellow fever in the 1790s, medical careers and personal reputations were staked on one vital question: Was the disease contagious? Partisans of contagion fought for a strict quarantine, while their opponents blamed the epidemics on the filthy condition of the city's wharfside neighborhoods and argued for thorough cleansing and sanitation. After decades of variability in local laws and uneven enforcement, a quest for uniformity and scientific rationality in quarantine regulations prompted the creation of the National Quarantine and Sanitary Convention, which met yearly from 1857 until the outbreak of the U.S. Civil War in 1861.

Contagionists were in a distinct minority, and delegate after delegate denounced the nation's unruly patchwork of quarantine regulations as burdensome

and ineffective. However, the convention was not prepared to recommend the outright abolition of quarantine, despite one delegate's contention that detaining ships at the entrance to New York harbor made as much sense as building "an immense Fire Department at the High Bridge" to protect the city against fire [6]. Even ardent anticontagionists allowed that prudence sometimes required the inspection and detention of certain vessels, cargoes, or passengers. The efficient and judicious implementation of quarantine, and the circumstances under which it was warranted, were the delicate matters that occupied most of the delegates' attention. They spent hours upon hours relating their own observations of yellow fever outbreaks and their interpretations of accounts in the medical literature. The answers they sought, the delegates seemed to agree, lay in the details of each outbreak [6].

Brooklyn's 1856 yellow fever epidemic earned especially detailed consideration. Some blamed quarantine itself for causing that outbreak by concentrating contaminated cargo in dockside warehouses. They claimed that every case of yellow fever could be traced to the neighborhood immediately surrounding those warehouses. Others disputed this contention, and identified victims who never went near that neighborhood [6]. Just as infectious disease surveillance today depends on careful case and contact tracing (e.g., tuberculosis and

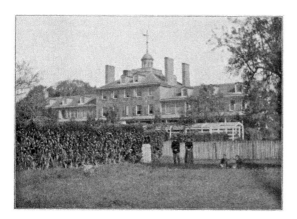

Figure 4.1 Main Building of Philadelphia's Lazaretto quarantine station (ca. late 1880s). The Lazaretto station was built in 1799, 12 miles downriver from the Port of Philadelphia, in response to a series of devastating yellow fever epidemics in the city in the 1790s. Source: Photo from Henry Leffmann, *Under the Yellow Flag* (Philadelphia, 1896).

sexually transmitted infections), this debate in the late 1850s rested on the daily movements of cases and contacts, day by day and street by street.

A similar method can be found in studies of other outbreaks during that era. Yellow fever had revisited Philadelphia only once in 50 years when the brig *Home* arrived at the Lazaretto quarantine station [Figure 4.1] from Jamaica on June 29, 1870. One Lazaretto employee with 60 years' experience on the water called it the filthiest vessel he had ever seen; the captain had died on the voyage after experiencing the classic symptoms of yellow fever. Over the next 6 weeks, the disease struck 29 people, of whom 18 died. Most of the victims were employees or neighbors of the quarantine station, including the Lazaretto physician, quarantine master, and head nurse. Philadelphia's Board of Health, which oversaw the Lazaretto station, commissioned a detailed report on the epidemic from the eminent Dr. René La Roche, author of a widely cited 1400-page textbook on yellow fever [7].

The devoutly anticontagionist La Roche reviewed evidence from dozens of yellow fever outbreaks (including the 1856 Brooklyn epidemic) that might shed light on the circumstances of the disease's transmission. For example, he cited the seven crew members who fell ill aboard the American naval steamer *Water Witch* during its passage from the southern coast of Cuba to Philadelphia in 1860. To prove that the disease was not trans-

mitted to the victims by contagion but rather originated aboard the *Water Witch* itself, La Roche evaluated the movements of the *Water Witch* during its passage from the southern coast of Cuba to Philadelphia in 1860. There was no yellow fever in Cienfuegos, Cuba, or among the ships docked there at the time, La Roche reported, nor on the Isle of Pines, "the healthiest spot in all Cuba, where ... yellow fever seldom if ever originates." He added that none of the stricken sailors was among the crew members who went ashore at either place. Furthermore, all of the cases occurred on the vessel's foredeck, near the galley:

> This part is small—much too small for the number of men confined in it, considering especially the climate of the region where the vessel was cruising, and the additional heat issuing from the galley. It is, besides, low, imperfectly ventilated, and near the pumps and hatches, from which issued a highly offensive smell proceeding from the hold. [7]

In La Roche's view, the lesson of the *Water Witch* outbreak was clear: Yellow fever was not transmitted from person to person, but rather originated in a particular local configuration of heat, humidity, filth, and lack of ventilation. He concluded that "the poison originated on board" [7].

After reviewing a number of similar examples, La Roche went on to reconstruct a painstaking daily accounting of the movements and symptoms of all 29 victims of the 1870 Lazaretto epidemic. Every one of them, he contended, was near and downwind of the brig *Home* shortly before the onset of symptoms. The vessel was moved several times, and those movements matched the patients' locations on the relevant dates as well as the prevailing wind direction. La Roche included a carefully annotated map [Figure 4.2] to illustrate his conclusion: The filthy *Home* generated the poison, which was carried by the prevailing breezes to the Lazaretto staff and neighbors on land [7]. Again, detailed case tracing—a form of surveillance—provided the crucial evidence.

The same method produced an opposite conclusion in 1878, when yellow fever invaded New Orleans with vicious fury. The catastrophe led Samuel Choppin, president of Louisiana's state Board of Health, to reexamine the history of yellow fever outbreaks in North America. In every case, Choppin reported to the annual meeting of the American Public Health Association (APHA), there was evidence of contact between a vessel from a

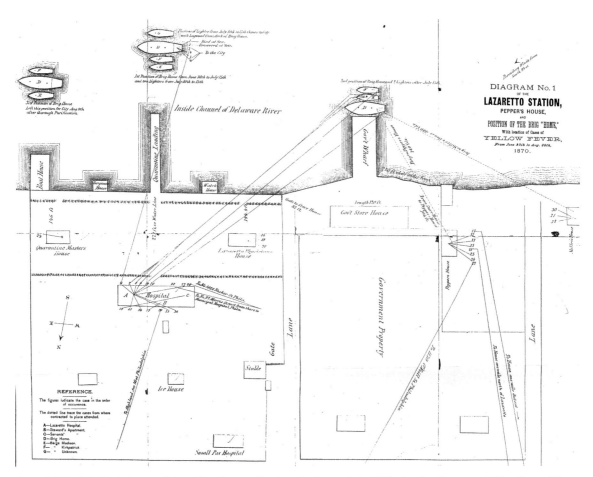

Figure 4.2 René La Roche's map of the yellow fever epidemic at the Lazaretto in 1870, showing the sequential locations of the brig *Home* (thought to have caused the outbreak) and the location of each patient at the time of the onset of symptoms. In La Roche's view, the map showed that each patient was immediately downwind of the infected vessel shortly before becoming ill and contracted the disease from the ship's foul air rather than through contagion. Source: *Remarks on the Origin and Mode of Progression of Yellow Fever in Philadelphia* (Philadelphia: E.C. Markley, 1871).

Caribbean port and the patient or patients at the origin of the epidemic. For example, Choppin had been the house surgeon at the Charity Hospital in New Orleans in 1853 when a newly arrived Irish immigrant named McGuigan, the first of approximately 9000 fatalities in that epidemic, was brought there in the full throes of yellow fever. Choppin reconstructed McGuigan's movements since arriving in New Orleans and the movements of three different ships between the mouth of the Mississippi River and the docks of New Orleans in an attempt to prove that the disease originated in a vessel that had recently arrived from Jamaica [8].

Summary

Choppin told the APHA that his study thoroughly refuted La Roche's insistent anticontagionism and proved yellow fever to be an imported disease, rather than a locally generated disease. He recommended an extreme version of quarantine—"absolute non-intercourse" every April through October between the United States and all Caribbean ports where yellow fever was "indigenous" [8]. Choppin's polemical tone, however, disguises the methodological common ground he shared with La Roche and with the quarantine convention delegates of the 1850s. All sought the truth about yellow fever—and by extension, about public health in general—from the accumulation of everyday stories of sick individuals and their movements, carefully tracked in time alongside the movements of ships and their cargo, the weather, and other local variables.

Choppin explicitly advocated an etiology of yellow fever based on "living germs, probably animalcular"; but the only pathogenic microbe that had been identified by 1878 was the bacillus responsible for anthrax. Etiology was not the basis of his argument. In the absence of a specific agent, Choppin and his opponents relied on surveillance—that methodical, meticulous science of cumulative anecdote, based on case and contact tracing in every apparent outbreak. It was an observational rather than an experimental science, and field based instead of laboratory based; but it was rigorous and systematic in its accumulation and analysis of evidence. From smallpox and cholera to lung cancer, there are many historical examples of epidemiological breakthroughs and effective preventive interventions that took place in the absence of specific etiological knowledge. They depended on the essence of epidemiology and public health—surveillance.

References

1. Shryock RH. *The Development of Modern Medicine*. Philadelphia: University of Pennsylvania Press; 1936.
2. McGrew RE. *Encyclopedia of Medical History*. New York: McGraw-Hill; 1985.
3. Musto D. Quarantine and the problem of AIDS. *Milbank Q* 1986;**64**:97–117.
4. Rosenberg CE. Commentary: Epidemiology in context. *Int J Epidemiol* 2009;**38**(1):28–30.
5. Virginia Foundation for the Humanities. Body Politics: A History of Health Care. BackStory with the American History Guys (radio program), October 1, 2009. [Internet] http://backstoryradio.org/shows/body-politics-a-history-of-health-care/
6. National Quarantine and Sanitary Convention. *Proceedings and Debates of the Third National Quarantine and Sanitary Convention*. New York: E. Jones & Co.; 1859.
7. La Roche R. *Remarks on the Origin and Mode of Progression of Yellow Fever in Philadelphia Based on the Occurrence of the Disease in That City and at the Lazaretto, in the Months of July, August, and September, 1870*. Philadelphia: E.C. Markley & Son; 1871.
8. Choppin S. History of the importation of yellow fever into the United States, from 1693 to 1878. *Public Health Pap Rep* 1879;**4**:190–206.

SECTION II
Specific surveillance systems

CHAPTER 5

Surveillance for vaccine-preventable diseases and immunization

Daniel C. Payne

Centers for Disease Control and Prevention, Atlanta, GA, USA

Introduction

Vaccine-preventable disease (VPD) surveillance is grounded in a firm understanding of the pathogenesis, clinical course, epidemiological risk factors, and molecular characterization of the disease agent targeted for vaccination. Therefore, VPD surveillance begins well before the vaccine is even developed, approved, and widely administered. The clinical, epidemiological, and laboratory characteristics of the disease agent are the foundations for developing valid, scientifically accurate assessments of the VPD in populations during the widespread use of the vaccine.

Critical functions of VPD surveillance activities are those that evaluate vaccine policy, including understanding pathogen epidemiology, vaccine impact, vaccine coverage, safety, and effectiveness. A lab component could monitor for molecular changes, whether influenced by the vaccination program (e.g., when the pathogen genetically adapts to post-vaccine selective pressures) or not (e.g., through antigenic drift). Continued monitoring over time is important and may lead to unexpected findings. Communicating these results through peer-reviewed publications, scientific conferences and symposiums, reports to governmental and industry oversight boards, domestic and international networks, and healthcare providers ensures that the scientific and regulatory communities accumulate a common knowledge of these findings, and can therefore tailor assessments and recommendations appropriately.

In this chapter, we will describe the factors required for understanding VPD and the lessons learned from previous studies. Then, we will review the components of a thorough VPD surveillance portfolio, and learn the importance of continued monitoring and communication of findings. For these objectives, we will use the example of the U.S. rotavirus vaccination program.

Step one: understanding the background: burden and risk factors of VPD illness and transmission processes of the target pathogen

An accurate quantitation of the burden of rotavirus illness represents more than simply an introduction to this particular pathogen. These "burden of disease" estimates are the scientific results that led to the understanding that this pathogen contributes substantially to childhood mortality and morbidity and impacts healthcare systems worldwide. Pre-vaccine era epidemiologic data formed the basis for creating meaningful surveillance systems that would come to fruition years later, when vaccines would be developed and introduced, and that would enable public health communities to assess the performance and impact of vaccines upon this VPD.

During the pre-vaccine era, rotavirus infected nearly every unvaccinated child before their fifth birthday. In the absence of vaccine, multiple rotavirus infections may occur during infancy and childhood. Rotavirus

Concepts and Methods in Infectious Disease Surveillance, First Edition. Edited by Nkuchia M. M'ikanatha and John K. Iskander.
Published 2014 by John Wiley & Sons, Ltd.

causes severe diarrhea and vomiting (acute gastroenteritis [AGE]), which can lead to dehydration, electrolyte depletion, complications of viremia, shock, and death. Nearly one-half million children around the world die of rotavirus infections each year, meaning that it is a significant source of mortality and morbidity among children globally [1].

Even in the United States and other developed countries, where rotavirus infections were much less likely to cause death, this virus was responsible for 40–50% of hospitalizations because of acute gastroenteritis during the winter months in the era before vaccines were introduced. Hundreds of thousands of emergency department (ED) and outpatient visits were a result of rotavirus as well, costing approximately $1 billion each year [2].

Meticulous studies describing how the virus infects humans and observations of when the most severe infections occurred were keys to determining when and how an effective vaccine would be developed and introduced. First rotavirus infections are most likely to result in moderate–severe cases of rotavirus gastroenteritis but subsequent infections are progressively milder. Velazquez et al. [3] found that the adjusted efficacy of a child's first natural rotavirus infection in protecting against subsequent natural rotavirus-associated diarrhea was 77%. This protection increased to 83% after two natural infections and to 92% after three natural infections. A 3-year study compared rotavirus-infected neonates with uninfected neonates. A similar proportion of neonatally infected and uninfected infants had rotavirus infections during the follow-up period. Symptoms among those neonatally infected, however, were less frequent and less severe leading to the conclusion that neonatal rotavirus infection protects against clinically severe disease during reinfection [4]. A similar finding was reported among a sample of Indian neonates infected in healthcare settings, most of whom had asymptomatic infections, resulting in a protective effect against rotavirus gastroenteritis lasting throughout the 2-year follow-up period, with protection concentrated in the first year of life [5].

The rationale for developing and implementing a vaccination program against rotavirus derived from observations that control measures, such as clean-water initiatives and improvements to personal hygiene, led to dramatic declines in bacterial and parasitic gastroenteritis infections across the world, but rates of rotavirus infection and illness among children in industrialized and less-developed countries remained similar [6–11]. Hygienic measures were unlikely to lead to corresponding declines in rotavirus burden [12]. Because first infections have been shown to induce strong immunity against severe rotavirus reinfections [3] and because vaccination mimics such first infections without causing illness, vaccination was identified as the optimal strategy for decreasing the burden associated with severe and fatal rotavirus diarrhea.

Any changes that may be later attributed to vaccination effects require knowledge of the pre-licensure (i.e., baseline) rates and trends in the target disease as a reference. Baseline data gives public health practitioners the grounding needed to quantitate the extent of observations (whether these are changes in hospital stays attributed to the VPD, mortality rates in a given age group, or other relevant measurements) after the vaccine is being used widely and helps delineate whether any post-licensure changes are likely due to the vaccine or are part of another underlying trend. Efforts to obtain baseline data are necessary before a vaccine is licensed and introduced [13].

Through an understanding of these epidemiological dynamics, VPD surveillance systems would later be able to track the correct clinical settings, clinical characteristics, transmission patterns, and the most likely ages of potential severe infections. This data, in turn, allows accurate assessments of the impact and performance of vaccines in childhood populations.

Step two: understanding the vaccines

VPD surveillance activities should be tailored to an understanding of the vaccines to be assessed and the mechanisms of immunologic protection, as well as the studied and approved parameters by which the vaccines are administered.

During the pre-licensure clinical trial studies that are conducted prior to a vaccine's approval for widespread use, extensive data is collected regarding the vaccine's performance in controlled environments, its safety, and other factors that may influence when and how the vaccine is administered. These other factors may include assessments of the ideal age for vaccination and how many vaccine doses are needed to induce an acceptable level of immunity. Early phases of clinical trial (Phase II) may even indicate the best anatomic location for an intramuscular vaccine, dose-ranging studies, or whether an adjuvant improves the immunologic response against a particular antigen in the vaccine.

Using our example of rotavirus vaccines, very large pre-licensure clinical trials indicated that rotavirus vaccines are safe and are not associated with severe vaccine adverse events [14–16]. Rotavirus vaccines are orally administered, live-attenuated vaccines designed for infant immunization in order to avoid the most severe rotavirus infections expected to occur in the first months of life. Following licensure by the Food and Drug Administration (FDA), in February, 2006, a pentavalent (five-strain containing) human-bovine reassortant rotavirus vaccine (RotaTeq™, Merck and Co.) was recommended by the U.S. Advisory Committee on Immunization Practices (ACIP) for routine vaccination of U.S. infants with a 3-dose series administered at ages 2, 4, and 6 months [17]. In June 2008, ACIP updated its recommendations to include the use of a monovalent (single-strain) human attenuated rotavirus vaccine (Rotarix™, GlaxoSmithKline Biologicals) as a 2-dose series administered at ages 2 and 4 months [18].

These findings and recommendations brought several implications to the VPD surveillance for these vaccines. Rotavirus vaccines were tested and approved for very specific age ranges in anticipation that this would reduce the likelihood that the vaccines would be associated with a particular vaccine adverse event (intussusception [IS]—a rare telescoping of the intestine that can lead to serious complications and death) that disproportionately occurs at specific ages. So, assessing rotavirus epidemiologic trends and vaccine safety concerns is clearly linked to age at vaccination. Additionally, the approved number of vaccine doses, which differs between the two rotavirus vaccines, should be taken into consideration. Finally, the fact that the vaccine is live attenuated should be considered: This may influence whether vaccine virus is shed by the recipient, if exposure to this shed virus influences indirect protection among children who did not receive vaccine, and whether the vaccine virus undergoes viral reassortment [19].

Step three: identify the data sources for disease surveillance and their availability, strengths, and weaknesses

Understanding the characteristics of a particular pathogen, the illness it causes, and the qualities of the vaccines are critical to development of accurate and comprehensive VPD surveillance. Equally important is the comprehension of data sources, their availability, potential biases, and what perspectives they could provide into the world of VPD surveillance.

Many VPDs that are uncommon or do not require laboratory confirmation are made nationally notifiable, either before or after vaccine licensure. The Nationally Notifiable Diseases Surveillance System (NNDSS) is a nationwide collaboration that enables all levels of public health (local, state, territorial, federal, international) to share health information to monitor, control, and prevent the occurrence and spread of state-reportable and nationally notifiable infectious and some noninfectious diseases and conditions. The costly and time-consuming process of creating a completely novel surveillance system is prohibitive in most settings. Typically, existing data sources are assessed for their availability and utility in evaluating the impact of vaccines on epidemiologic trends for a particular pathogen. Sometimes, existing data that is routinely collected is used in a different way for the new function of VPD surveillance.

There is no single perfect data source for assessing any VPD. Meaningful surveillance is achieved by the much broader approach of employing diverse datasets. The true impact of a vaccine or the accurate assessment of disease trends in a population is more likely the result of evaluating many datasets having different strengths and weaknesses. Only by understanding these strengths and weaknesses can a public health practitioner give the appropriate consideration to the findings derived from these data.

National inpatient datasets collect hospital data for large numbers of children, providing powerful tools for estimating whether or not changes in the occurrence of a VPD illness have occurred over time. However, these data may be collected for reasons other than VPD surveillance, such as to track healthcare utilization and expenditures over time by a managed-care organization. Therefore, they may not provide the perfect fit to the VPD surveillance and, instead, may provide just one perspective on epidemiologic trends.

Within our rotavirus VPD surveillance context, an important component of VPD surveillance includes assessing hospitalization trends for certain AGE diagnoses using the Nationwide Inpatient Sample (NIS), a sample of 20% of all U.S. hospital admissions [20]. Knowing that rotavirus causes diarrhea and vomiting, we would be interested in evaluating the proportions of children who are admitted to U.S. hospitals in a given year whose hospital records were given discharge diagnosis codes for AGE. These codes are commonly in the format of the *International Classification of Diseases—9th Revision—Clinical Modification (ICD-9-CM)*, and there are several codes which represent AGE symptoms [6]. One would wish to select the appropriate codes, which conform to the prior understanding of the potential clinical outcomes from the VPD, and observe them for the ages when the most-severe outcomes would be likely (children under age 5 years, for rotavirus). By knowing how often and in what proportions these codes occur in the time period before vaccine was introduced (pre-licensure period) versus the period after vaccines were introduced (post-licensure period), judgments can be made as to whether hospitalizations for the VPD decreased in the post-licensure period.

As important as it is to distinguish the relative impact of a vaccine upon disease burden using a large, administrative dataset, we would not be completely certain that these associations were directly because of the direct impact of vaccine alone. This type of VPD surveillance analysis would not necessarily tell us if the children having the AGE codes were laboratory-confirmed rotavirus cases. Therefore, we could not be absolutely certain that the decreases were actually occurring in the AGE cases directly because of rotavirus. And, we would not necessarily be certain that vaccination was the most plausible reason for the observed declines. In the absence of vaccination data, the reasons for any decline could be because of factors unrelated to vaccine, (e.g., historical changes in the pathogen's occurrence, sometimes called secular trends). Nonetheless, a finding of a decrease in the vaccine's target disease would be an indication that requires follow-up and confirmation from other data sources.

Step four: assessing the performance: conducting post-marketing VPD surveillance and assessing vaccine effectiveness

The most critical question to be asked during the introduction of a vaccine is how well it prevents the illness or symptoms for which it was intended. The principal efforts to assess this question in large populations are Phase III and Phase IV trials. In a Phase III clinical trial, the vaccine is typically administered to large numbers of people who have met certain inclusionary and exclusionary criteria and are then randomly selected to receive either the vaccine or a placebo. Vaccination status is recorded, but remains known only to members of a data safety monitoring board (DSMB) which oversees the ethical conduct of the trial. The Phase III clinical trial is meant to confirm how well the vaccine performs in an environment strictly controlled for potential biases, to monitor undesired side effects, and to collect any other information needed to improve the study vaccine's safety and performance.

During the Phase III trials, which are normally required to obtain licensure from the FDA prior to a vaccine's introduction, a vaccine's efficacy is studied. Outcome data are measured as the proportionate reduction in the disease attack rate between vaccinated and unvaccinated cohorts, measured in terms of relative risk. Phase III trials represent the "best case scenario" of vaccine protection, although they are a costly method of measurement.

Once the Phase III trials show adequate protection and safety, the vaccine may be licensed by the FDA and then approved for use by scientific deliberating bodies, such as the U.S. Advisory Committee on Immunization Practices. When the vaccine is used in routine clinical practice, Phase IV trials (called post-licensure studies or post-marketing studies) are initiated. These are the evaluations conducted during the course of VPD surveillance that delineate additional performance information in settings where strict controls on who receives the vaccine are not present. Persons having different underlying health status, differing adherence to the vaccination regimen, recognized or unrecognized complicating factors, and study biases are frequently included. Often, measuring vaccine performance in the broader population yields slightly lower protective results compared to Phase III clinical trials because of these "real-world" features.

During these post-licensure Phase IV studies, it is not the vaccine's efficacy but its effectiveness that is assessed. These evaluations are conducted under natural, field conditions and must employ epidemiologic techniques to control biases among the sample. The retrospective case control analysis (using the odds ratio) is methodologically most familiar, but other methods to assess vaccine effectiveness may be used, including cohort or coverage designs. Benefits and risks from the vaccination program as a whole can be assessed using Phase IV studies, which are not restricted solely to measuring vaccine effectiveness.

VPD surveillance data can often be used both to evaluate trends in targeted pathogens and disease outcomes and to assess the effectiveness of vaccines. The most elemental vaccine effectiveness evaluation simply calculates the incidence ratio of a disease outcome relative to vaccination status, but adjusting for other variables such as age and socioeconomic indicators are also desirable for controlling biases. Whenever possible, public health practitioners should look for opportunities to not only document VPD epidemiologic trends but also to directly assess vaccine performance using these vaccine effectiveness methods.

The diverse surveillance techniques employed by a well-rounded, post-licensure VPD surveillance portfolio may include active surveillance, passive surveillance, and surveillance using administrative datasets. Active VPD surveillance normally involves the labor-intensive review of patient admission records to gauge individuals who may fit surveillance case definitions for the target disease. Eligible subjects are enrolled and further data and biological specimens are directly obtained. This is a powerful VPD surveillance tool, with potential for obtaining large quantities of high quality epidemiologic, clinical, vaccination and laboratory data. These data are sometimes linked by personal identifiers in order to determine differences in risk factors (including vaccine exposure) by disease status, and personal data protections are of utmost importance.

When the VPD surveillance system depends upon voluntary submission of disease status data or biological specimens for disease detection, this is termed "passive surveillance." When laboratories that test clinical specimens for healthcare providers then voluntarily share these specimens or results (stripped of personal identifiers) with a third party (often a public health agency) for analysis, this exemplifies passive surveillance [21]. Although less expensive and less labor-intensive, passive VPD surveillance is sometimes unable to link the disease status with other exposure or risk factors, including important variables such as vaccination status and age.

Administrative datasets may be created by research institutions, managed-care organizations, or national healthcare utilization repositories. They are not specifically created for VPD surveillance and may contain coded data (using ICD-9 CM or other coding systems) on health events. They often do not provide laboratory confirmation of specific diseases, unlike passive and active VPD surveillance. Sometimes the data-hosting organization limits accessibility to the full dataset, or specific variables, for proprietary or data protection rationales. Nonetheless, administrative datasets offer huge sample sizes, which allow for powerful inferences within the confines of any data limitations.

Ideally, VPD surveillance produces findings that are disseminated to interested partners in a proactive, transparent manner. Communicating results of VPD surveillance through peer-reviewed publication; scientific conferences and symposiums; reports to governmental and industry oversight boards, domestic and international networks, and healthcare providers ensures that the scientific and regulatory communities accumulate a common knowledge of these findings and can therefore tailor future policies and assessments appropriately. While transparently disclosing methods and results breeds trust, public health practitioners are also held to the standard of observing appropriate legal and ethical protections for their data. Finding a suitable median between scientific expectations of transparency and the legal protection of sensitive data is essential to the acceptance (and therefore the future success) of any VPD surveillance portfolio.

Step five: preparing for the unexpected and continuing the evaluation

Randomized clinical trials cannot assess everything that might be discovered during the post-licensure period. For example, what if the sample size is too small to detect an uncommon adverse event possibly associated with the vaccine; what are the effects of a population-wide vaccination program on individuals who are not vaccinated; or even what is the impact of inclusion of a substance that was not originally intended to be in the vaccine? Each of these questions has emerged during the course of our chapter's example, rotavirus vaccines, during VPD surveillance.

What if the sample size is too small to detect an uncommon adverse event possibly associated with the vaccine?

Rotavirus vaccine clinical trials for the purpose of assessing the risk of IS, which had been an unexpected finding in a previous vaccine (now removed from the market by its manufacturer), were some of the largest vaccine trials ever conducted. These clinical trials enrolled >70,000 children in various countries and found no increased risk of intussusception among those who were vaccinated compared with those who were not. However, once millions of children had received these vaccines, post-licensure surveillance for intussusception detected a modest increased risk of rare intussusception events during the days following vaccination. After several years of continued vaccinations, these uncommon occurrences combined to a sample size that was able to be statistically tested and a slightly increased risk of the adverse event was observed among vaccinees within 7 days of vaccine receipt in areas of the United States, Australia, and Mexico.

By the time these analyses were conducted, strong evidence of benefits gained from the vaccination programs had accumulated as well. A quantitative risk:benefit comparison was then possible, using the data compiled from many surveillance data sources in different regions over time, allowing vaccine policy makers to make an educated judgment that continuation of the U.S. vaccination program held benefits that far outweighed any risk from this adverse event [22].

What are the effects of a population-wide vaccination program on individuals who are not vaccinated?

After the first year of widespread rotavirus vaccination coverage in 2008, very large and consistent decreases in rotavirus hospitalizations were noted around the country. Many of the decreases in childhood hospitalizations resulting from rotavirus were 90% or more, compared with the pre-licensure, baseline period. Because of the tremendous impact in reducing severe disease, combined with good vaccine effectiveness findings, it was reasonable to suppose that the finding was because of the new vaccination program. The data were intriguing for other reasons as well. Once the hospitalization data was stratified by age groups, public health practitioners were surprised to find that large reductions had occurred among children who were too old to have been eligible for vaccination. Further analysis of the

VPD surveillance data indicated that not only were there large hospitalization reductions directly attributable to vaccine, but also that older children were receiving indirect protection as well. These older children included siblings and community contacts of immunized infants, who now had less chance for community and household exposure to rotavirus [23]. This evidence of indirect protection from rotavirus vaccines on the population level—sometimes referred to as "herd immunity"—had not been investigated during the clinical trials and was only observable through post-licensure VPD surveillance stratified by age, once vaccine coverage became sufficiently high.

What is the impact of inclusion of a substance that was not originally intended to be in the vaccine?

In 2010, after millions of children had received rotavirus vaccines worldwide, researchers using novel laboratory techniques found that U.S.-licensed rotavirus vaccines contained DNA or DNA fragments from *Porcine circovirus* (PCV), a virus common among pigs but not believed to cause illness in humans. Previous findings of extraneous viruses in live, attenuated vaccines have been rare and had often arisen through inadvertent introductions of viruses or viral materials (not related to the target disease) during vaccine production, often via incomplete inactivation during the attenuation process. It may not have been technologically possible to detect PCV during the early stages of vaccine development. Nonetheless, this was an unexpected finding.

As PCV was not known to cause illness in humans, traditional VPD surveillance was not relevant in assessing the impact of this finding. For instance, the impact was not to be measured by any increase in hospitalizations or costs averted. Indeed, it was reported that even the vaccine lots produced for administration to children during the randomized clinical trials contained this substance, so inherent in any assessment of vaccine adverse events between vaccinated and unvaccinated children was that any sizable effect from PCV could have been observed from these data. Instead, any potential impact from this finding was qualitative; in particular, whether healthcare providers or mothers of soon-to-be vaccinated infants would accept the vaccine knowing that it contained an unintended substance. To answer this question, formal qualitative methods were employed, including a focus group study to explore perceptions about rotavirus disease, vaccination against rotavirus, and attitudes about the detection of PCV material in rotavirus vaccines [24].

Conclusion

Vaccines, and surveillance for VPD, have lifecycles that begin with careful study and understanding of the epidemiology of the disease targeted for vaccination, including its healthcare and economic burdens, as well as risk factors for repeated or severe infections. Study of vaccine candidates in clinical trials prior to their licensure and usage helps to build knowledge of how well vaccines work under controlled conditions. Following licensure of a vaccine, VPD surveillance involves tracking vaccine coverage, vaccine safety, and vaccine impact on the targeted disease(s). Sources of active, passive, and administrative surveillance data to be compared with baseline data identified prior to the availability of a vaccine should be sought. Because post-licensure surveillance occurs under less-controlled conditions than occur in vaccine trials, systems and data sources must be able to monitor both prespecified events and novel adverse events or other concerns. Using the example of currently licensed rotavirus vaccines, surveillance systems have been able to provide robust analyses regarding a known adverse event of concern (e.g., IS), a potentially adverse unforeseen event (e.g., PCV), and an unexpected beneficial effect (indirect protection of populations not targeted to receive vaccine).

STUDY QUESTIONS

1. Why does surveillance for a VPD need to begin even before a vaccine is available?
2. Other than how well a particular vaccine works, what important information is provided by Phase III clinical trials? How does this information affect subsequent surveillance efforts following vaccine licensing and recommendation?
3. What is the difference between vaccine efficacy and vaccine effectiveness? Is one typically expected to be higher than another; and, if so, why?
4. Besides vaccine effectiveness, what are other important types of information about a vaccine's "real-world" performance that need to be monitored epidemiologically following licensure?

References

1. Tate JE, Burton AH, Boschi-Pinto C, Steele AD, Duque J, Parashar UD. 2008 estimate of worldwide rotavirus-associated mortality in children younger than 5 years before the introduction of universal rotavirus vaccination programmes: A systematic review and meta-analysis. *Lancet Infect Dis* 2012;**12(2)**:136–141. doi:10.1016/S1473-3099(11)70253-5.
2. Widdowson MA, Meltzer MI, Zhang X, Bresee JS, Parashar UD, Glass RI. Cost-effectiveness and potential impact of rotavirus vaccination in the United States. *Pediatrics* 2007;**119**(4):684–697.
3. Velazquez FR, Matson DO, Calva JJ, et al. Rotavirus infection in infants as protection against subsequent infections. *N Engl J Med* 1996;**335**:1022–1028.
4. Bishop RF, Barnes GL, Cipriani E, Lund LS. Clinical immunity after neonatal rotavirus infection. A prospective longitudinal study in young children. *N Engl J Med* 1983;**309**:72–76.
5. Bhan MK, Lew JF, Sazawal S, Das BK, Gentsch JR, Glass RI. Protection conferred by neonatal rotavirus infection against subsequent rotavirus diarrhea. *J Infect Dis* 1993;**168**:282–287.
6. Gurwith M, Wenman W, Gurwith D, Brunton J, Feltham S, Greenberg H. Diarrhea among infants and young children in Canada: A longitudinal study in three northern communities. *J Infect Dis* 1983;**147**:685–692.
7. Black RE, Lopez de Romana G, Brown KH, Bravo N, Grados Bazalar O, Kanashiro HC. Incidence and etiology of infantile diarrhea and major routes of transmission in Huascar, Peru. *Am J Epidemiol* 1989;**129**:785–799.
8. Williams CJ, Lobanov A, Pebody RG. Estimated mortality and hospital admission due to rotavirus infection in the WHO European region. *Epidemiol Infect* 2009;**12**:1–10.
9. Ramani S, Sowmyanarayanan TV, Gladstone BP, et al. Rotavirus infection in the neonatal nurseries of a tertiary care hospital in India. *Pediatr Infect Dis J* 2008;**27**:719–723.
10. Ramani S, Kang G. Burden of disease & molecular epidemiology of group A rotavirus infections in India. *Indian J Med Res* 2007;**125**:619–632.
11. Bodhidatta L, Lan NT, Hien BT, et al. Rotavirus disease in young children from Hanoi, Vietnam. *Pediatr Infect Dis J* 2007;**26**:325–328.
12. Mrukowicz J, Szajewska H, Vesikari T. Options for the prevention of rotavirus disease other than vaccination. *J Pediatr Gastroenterol Nutr* 2008;**46**(Suppl 2):S32–S37.
13. Tate JE, Haynes A, Payne DC, Cortese MM, Lopman BA, Patel MM, Parashar UD. Trends in national rotavirus activity before and after introduction of rotavirus vaccine into the National Immunization Program in the United States, 2000–2012. *Pediatr Infect Dis J* 2013;**32**:741–744.
14. Vesikari T, Matson DO, Dennehy P, et al. Safety and efficacy of a pentavalent human-bovine (WC3) reassortant rotavirus vaccine. *N Engl J Med* 2006;**354**(1):23–33.

15. Ruiz-Palacios GM, Perez-Schael I, Velazquez FR, et al. Safety and efficacy of an attenuated vaccine against severe rotavirus gastroenteritis. *N Engl J Med* 2006;**354**(1):11–22.

16. Vesikari T, Karvonen A, Prymula R, et al. Efficacy of human rotavirus vaccine against rotavirus gastroenteritis during the first 2 years of life in European infants: Randomised, double-blind controlled study. *Lancet* 2007;**370**(9601): 1757–1763.

17. Parashar UD, Alexander JP, Glass RI, Centers for Disease Control and Prevention. Prevention of rotavirus gastroenteritis among infants and children: Recommendations of the Advisory Committee on Immunization Practices (ACIP). *MMWR Recomm Rep* 2006;**55**(RR-12):1–13.

18. Cortese MM, Parashar UD, Centers for Disease Control and Prevention. Prevention of rotavirus gastroenteritis among infants and children: Recommendations of the Advisory Committee on Immunization Practices (ACIP). *MMWR Recomm Rep* 2009;**58**(RR-2):1–25.

19. Boom JA, Sahni L, Payne DC, et al. Symptomatic infection and detection of vaccine and vaccine-reassortant rotavirus strains in 5 children: A case series. *J Infect Dis* 2012;**206**: 1275–1279.

20. Healthcare Cost and Utilization Project (HCUP). HCUP NIS Database documentation. November 2011. Agency for Healthcare Research and Quality, Rockville, MD. Available at http://www.hcup-us.ahrq.gov/nisoverview.jsp (accessed March 31, 2014).

21. Tate JE, Mutuc JD, Panozzo CA, et al. Sustained decline in rotavirus detections in the United States following the introduction of rotavirus vaccine in 2006. *Pediatr Infect Dis J* 2011;**30**(1 Suppl):S30–S34.

22. Cortese MM. Summary of intussusception risk and benefits of rotavirus vaccination in the United States. Centers for Disease Control and Prevention Advisory Committee on Immunization Practices. June 20, 2013. Available at http://www.cdc.gov/vaccines/acip/meetings/downloads/slides-jun-2013/06-Rotavirus-Cortese.pdf (accessed March 31, 2014).

23. Payne DC, Staat MA, Edwards KM, et al. Direct and indirect effects of rotavirus vaccination upon childhood hospitalizations in 3 US counties, 2006–2009. *Clin Infect Dis* 2011;**53**(3):245–253.

24. Payne DC, Humiston S, Opel D, et al. A multi-center, qualitative assessment of pediatrician and maternal perspectives on rotavirus vaccines and the detection of *Porcine circovirus*. *BMC Pediatr* 2011;**11**:83.

CHAPTER 6

Surveillance for seasonal and novel influenza viruses

Bruno Christian Ciancio and Piotr Kramarz

European Centre for Disease Prevention and Control, Stockholm, Sweden

Introduction

Influenza is a vaccine-preventable viral infection that causes systemic and respiratory symptoms. Infected patients present with a wide range of clinical severity. The virus is spread primarily through airborne transmission via droplets and droplet nuclei. Epidemics in humans occur worldwide with marked winter seasonality in temperate regions and a more stable background activity in the tropics [1]. The virus undergoes frequent genetic changes through mutation or reassortment. These may result in minor or major antigenic changes known as *drifts* or *shifts*, respectively. Antigenic changes may alter the effectiveness of the influenza vaccine, and therefore vaccines are reformulated annually. Furthermore, major virus antigenic changes may result in influenza pandemics, essentially an epidemic of worldwide proportions. Influenza pandemics are rare events which occur when a novel influenza virus strain emerges and is (1) pathogenic for humans, (2) easily transmissible, and (3) antigenically unique (i.e., pre-existing immunity in the population is low). Because of pandemics' unpredictability, their potential to cause more severe illness and to affect wider portions of the population, and the difficulties in rapidly producing and deploying an effective vaccine, pandemics are considered major public health threats. Substantial and constant efforts are made by public health authorities to maintain an adequate level of preparedness to effectively respond to influenza pandemics and reduce their impact.

Influenza poses many challenges to surveillance because of its changing nature, its ability to rapidly spread worldwide and affect large portions of the population, the nonspecificity of its clinical symptoms, and the wide range of possible severity and complications. As a consequence, public health surveillance of influenza is often based on collection, integration, and analysis of information from multiple sources and systems. Although each surveillance system has specific objectives, it is only by combining data from multiple systems that it is possible to have an understanding of the burden of disease. Precise estimates of the global burden of influenza are also missing because of the absence of surveillance systems in many low- and middle-income countries. Based on extrapolations of U.S. surveillance data, the World Health Organization (WHO) estimates an annual influenza burden of up to 1 billion infections, 3–5 million cases of severe disease, and 300,000–500,000 deaths [1]. This chapter describes the primary objectives of influenza surveillance and the methods applied to achieve these objectives.

Clinical, epidemiological, and virological characteristics and implications for surveillance

Clinical manifestations of influenza include combinations of systemic and respiratory symptoms. Typically patients with influenza report abrupt onset of fever,

Concepts and Methods in Infectious Disease Surveillance, First Edition. Edited by Nkuchia M. M'ikanatha and John K. Iskander.
© 2015 John Wiley & Sons, Ltd. Published 2015 by John Wiley & Sons, Ltd.

myalgia, headache, malaise, and anorexia. Respiratory manifestations include dry cough, pharyngeal pain, nasal obstruction, and discharge. Symptoms last for 2–7 days (although cough can persist for weeks) with a wide range of possible clinical severities and complications. Influenza cannot be distinguished from other respiratory infections based on clinical criteria alone [2]. Based on their cause, complications from influenza can be classified into three main categories: (1) directly related to the viral infection (e.g., acute respiratory failure), (2) secondary bacterial infections (e.g., bacterial pneumonia), and (3) exacerbation of pre-existing conditions (e.g., chronic obstructive pulmonary disease, myocardial infarction, stroke). Because clinical symptoms and possible complications of influenza are nonspecific, and because the incidence of disease in the population can be very high during epidemic periods, most influenza infections are not confirmed by laboratory testing. In addition, influenza can cause mild symptoms, and many patients do not consult a physician. This implies that assumptions need to be made when interpreting surveillance data.

There are three types of influenza viruses—A, B, and C— of which only types A and B cause widespread outbreaks in humans. Influenza A viruses are classified into subtypes based on antigenic differences between their two surface glycoproteins, hemagglutinin and neuraminidase. Seventeen hemagglutinin subtypes (H1–H17) and nine neuraminidase subtypes (N1–N9) have been identified. Viruses of all hemagglutinin and neuraminidase subtypes have been recovered from aquatic birds, but only three hemagglutinin subtypes (H1, H2, and H3) and two neuraminidase subtypes (N1 and N2) have established stable lineages in the human population since 1918. Only one subtype of hemagglutinin and one of neuraminidase are recognized for influenza B viruses [3]. The internationally accepted naming convention for influenza viruses contains the following elements: the type (e.g., A, B, C), geographical origin (e.g., Perth, Victoria), strain number (e.g., 361), year of isolation (e.g., 2011), for influenza A the hemagglutinin and neuraminidase antigen description (e.g., H1N1), and for nonhuman origin viruses the host of origin (e.g., swine) [4].

Because the influenza virus undergoes frequent antigenic changes, the vaccine has to be reformulated annually and separately for the two hemispheres. This requires global collaborations to ensure efficient monitoring of strains of viruses circulating in each season and consolidated mechanisms to provide timely recommendations to vaccine producers. Often in the Northern and Southern Hemispheres, annual influenza epidemics occur following certain geographical patterns of spread, thus offering early warning surveillance systems opportunities for informing public health action.

The burden of influenza can be estimated by means of various measures, including numbers of infections, physician office visits, hospitalizations, complications, deaths, and composite burden of disease measures like disability-adjusted life years (DALYs). DALYs estimates account for both premature mortality (years of life lost) and time spent with reduced health (years lived with disability) [5]. Various factors influence the burden of disease including the virulence of the circulating strains, the characteristics of the affected population (level of natural immunity and vaccination coverage, age structure, prevalence of individuals with chronic conditions, proportion living in long-term care facilities) and the setting in which infection occurs (level of access to and quality of healthcare systems) [6]. Use of DALYs to estimate the burden of influenza underestimates the real burden of disease because this measure does not fully account for the whole spectrum of consequences of infection, as is the case for many other infectious diseases [7].

Possible surveillance schemes

Virologic surveillance

Virologic surveillance of influenza has the main objective of monitoring virus strain circulation globally in order:

1. to inform the process of vaccine strain selection twice yearly and provide virus seeds for vaccine production;
2. to rapidly identify novel viruses that may pose a pandemic threat; and
3. to monitor levels of antiviral resistance.

In combination with epidemiological and clinical surveillance, laboratory surveillance contributes to identifying when and where influenza epidemics are occurring and to understanding the relation between virus strain circulation and clinical severity.

Laboratory diagnosis of influenza

The most important diagnostic tests for surveillance purposes are reverse transcriptase polymerase chain reaction (RT-PCR) and viral culture. Because of its high sensitivity and specificity, RT-PCR is the preferred test for virus detection and initial characterization by type and subtypes. Results are usually available within less than one day. A subset of positive specimens can be placed in culture for further genetic and antigenic characterization. Although performed less frequently than molecular detection methods, virus isolation through culture provides critical information for surveillance. This includes identification of novel strains that would be classified as unsubtypable by RT-PCR, antigenic characterization evaluating virus relatedness with the recommended vaccine strains, and antiviral resistance testing.

Commercial rapid influenza diagnostic tests are also available and provide results in 10–30 minutes, but they have limited value for surveillance because of their low sensitivity compared with RT-PCR and culture. Preferred respiratory samples for influenza testing include nasopharyngeal or nasal swab or nasal wash or aspirate. Samples should be collected within the first 4–5 days of illness as virus shedding decreases rapidly thereafter, compromising the sensitivity of the tests (i.e., increasing the number of false negative results).

In order to increase representativeness, specimens for virological surveillance should be collected from various sources year round and from patients with a range of clinical severities. Settings where specimens for virological testing can be collected include primary care physicians' offices, hospitals, nursing homes, occupational settings, and outbreak investigation settings such as schools. It is important to ensure a variety of sources as theoretically some strains can be linked to clinical severity. Because of the potential risk of zoonotic infections and/or emergence of reassorted human/animal viruses, specimens should also be taken from subjects in specific occupational categories, including veterinarians, and in settings where food animals such as poultry and swine are in contact with humans. Even in temperate regions, influenza viruses circulate year round and novel strains can emerge at any time and virological surveillance must be performed year round. At the beginning of each season, the number of specimens collected for laboratory testing must be increased in order to verify vaccine-virus match and to inform the vaccine strain selection process for the following influenza season.

WHO global influenza surveillance network

At the global level, virologic surveillance is coordinated by WHO through its Global Influenza Surveillance and Response System (GISRS) [8]. The network was established in 1952 and comprises six WHO Collaborating Centres (CCs), four Essential Regulatory Laboratories (ERLs), and 137 National Influenza Centres (NICs) in 107 WHO Member States (Figure 6.1).

Although NICs' laboratories represent the first level of the GISRS, their functions, as well as virus detection and characterization capacities, vary depending on the country. In some countries these are the only laboratory facilities in place for influenza virus detection, whereas in others they are part of larger networks of laboratories. According to WHO, NICs should be able to undertake initial identification of virus type and subtype [9]. At the national level one or more NICs receive specimens collected from patients with suspected influenza. Specimens may come directly from primary care physicians, hospitals, and other health institutions or through networks of subnational laboratories. NICs usually receive a combination of specimens, some of which have been collected as part of well-defined surveillance schemes (e.g., from sentinel physicians swabbing patients presenting with an influenza-like illness during the influenza surveillance period).

Vaccine strain selection

Influenza strains to be included in seasonal influenza vaccines are selected during WHO consultations, which occur twice a year (in February for Northern Hemisphere and in September in the Southern Hemisphere). The two influenza A strains currently circulating in humans, A(H3N2) and A(H1N1), and an influenza B strain are recommended for vaccine inclusion. Advisors from WHO CCs and ERLs take part, and consultations are observed by multiple experts from WHO CCs, WHO ERLs, WHO H5 Reference Laboratories, NICs, and other institutions. The process relies on the number, quality, timeliness of collection, and geographical representation of analyzed isolates [10–12].

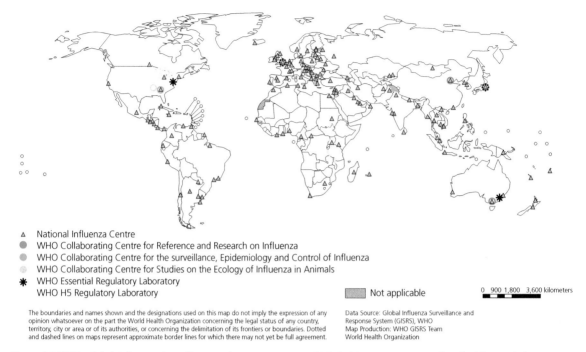

△   National Influenza Centre
●   WHO Collaborating Centre for Reference and Research on Influenza
●   WHO Collaborating Centre for the surveillance, Epidemiology and Control of Influenza
◉   WHO Collaborating Centre for Studies on the Ecology of Influenza in Animals
✳   WHO Essential Regulatory Laboratory
    WHO H5 Regulatory Laboratory

Not applicable

0   900 1,800   3,600 kilometers

The boundaries and names shown and the designations used on this map do not imply the expression of any opinion whatsoever on the part the World Health Organization concerning the legal status of any country, territory, city or area or of its authorities, or concerning the delimitation of its frontiers or boundaries. Dotted and dashed lines on maps represent approximate border lines for which there may not yet be full agreement.

Data Source: Global Influenza Surveillance and Response System (GISRS), WHO
Map Production: WHO GISRS Team
World Health Organization

Figure 6.1 WHO Global Influenza Surveillance and Response System (GIRS), 2013. Source: Reproduced with permission from WHO.

Antiviral resistance

Only two antiviral drug classes are licensed for chemoprophylaxis and treatment of influenza—the adamantanes (amantadine and rimantadine) and the neuraminidase inhibitors (oseltamivir and zanamivir). Amantadine has been in use since the mid-1960s, whereas the neuraminidase inhibitors (zanamivir and oseltamivir) became available in the late 1990s [13,14]. Antivirals shorten duration of illness, reduce the risk of severe complications, and prevent transmission or reduce disease severity when administered as chemoprophylaxis pre- or postexposure [15]. Antiviral resistant strains arise through selection pressure in individual patients during treatment. Strains selected under the pressure of antiviral treatment may result in treatment failure; however, they usually do not transmit further (because of impaired virus fitness) and have limited public health implications. On the other hand, primarily resistant viruses have emerged in the past decade and in some cases have completely replaced the susceptible

strains. This happened for A(H3N2) viruses resistant to adamantanes since 2003 [16,17], seasonal A(H1N1) resistant to oseltamivir since 2007 [18,19], and 2009 pandemic A(H1N1)pdm09 viruses resistant to adamantanes [13]. Antiviral resistance can be tested by genotypic identification of mutations that are known to be associated with drug resistance or analysis of the drug concentration that inhibits neuraminidase activity by 50%.

Surveillance of antiviral resistance has direct implications for the clinical management of patients. Antivirals are most effective if administered within 48 hours from onset of symptom. This short window of opportunity does not allow routine performance of antiviral resistance testing to guide treatment. Clinicians therefore choose among the few available antiviral classes based on updated antiviral resistance prevalence data combined with local data on the relative prevalence of each virus type and subtype [15]. It is therefore important that information on subtype circulation and levels of antiviral resistance is readily available at subnational levels as differences in distribution of subtypes may exist in different parts of a country.

Outpatient sentinel surveillance

One of the most important objectives of influenza surveillance is to detect rapidly when and where the influenza season is starting and which virus types and subtypes are circulating and to monitor the geographical progression of seasonal epidemics. This information is used to guide public health interventions at the local, national, and global levels. Examples of interventions may include activating hospital preparedness plans and recommendations for use of antivirals without waiting for the results of laboratory tests. Other measures may be aimed at strengthening ongoing vaccination campaigns and promoting hand-hygiene practices to reduce transmission. Indications of the geographical spread and progression of the annual epidemics allow mobilization of local and national resources and better coordination of efforts to manage demands on the healthcare system, including increased use of intensive care facilities. At an international level, alert mechanisms can be established so that neighboring countries are rapidly informed that the influenza season has started. This information, along with an initial indication of the characteristics of the epidemic in terms of severity, population attack rates, predominant virus types and subtypes, and antigenic and genetic characteristics of viruses and their relatedness to vaccine strains allows countries to prepare accordingly. Surveillance systems based on primary healthcare services are often used to provide this information.

System based on sentinel physicians

In Europe a multinational surveillance network now known as the European Influenza Surveillance Network (EISN) has been operational since 1996; it is currently operated by the European Centre for Disease Prevention and Control (ECDC) for the European Union (EU) and from the WHO Regional Office for Europe for the remaining countries of the European Region of WHO. EISN data is based on sentinel primary care physicians who report numbers of cases of influenza-like illness (ILI) or acute respiratory infections (ARI) observed in their practices during a predefined surveillance period, usually between International Organization for Standardization (ISO) weeks 40 of one year and 20 of the

following year. In the EU, ILI is defined as sudden onset of symptoms and at least one of the following four systemic symptoms: fever or feverishness, malaise, headache, and myalgia, and at least one of the three respiratory symptoms (cough, sore throat, shortness of breath) [20]. Weekly aggregate data on ILI or ARI are transmitted with limited epidemiological information, usually age groups and sex. In some cases, presence of risk factors for severe influenza and vaccination status are also collected and reported. Data collected through sentinel networks are analyzed at national and international levels and used for the production of weekly bulletins [21,22].

Sentinel physicians are usually general practitioners and pediatricians who represent 1–5% of primary care physicians, depending on the size of the country. The denominator for calculating weekly incidences is the number of individuals registered with the sentinel physicians or the population under their catchment area. In the absence of reliable denominators, some countries monitor the proportion of weekly consultations for ILI or ARI over the total number of weekly consultations. Aggregated data are transferred to the national level and then to ECDC and WHO using a single online entry form. It is therefore possible to monitor trends of ILI and/or ARI incidence in the community and detect when such incidence increases above certain thresholds. Statistically defined thresholds can be calculated to define epidemic periods using time series analysis techniques such as the moving average method [23].

Integration of clinical, epidemiological, and virological surveillance

A proportion of sentinel physicians are also asked to collect nasopharyngeal swabs from a subset of patients with ILI. Ideally, patients are selected using a systematic approach to increase representativeness. For example, all ILI cases presenting on a certain day of the week or the first ILI case presenting on predefined days of the week are selected. Swabs are sent to local or national reference laboratories for virus testing, usually using RT-PCR. This allows calculation of the proportion of reported potential cases that are positive for influenza each week. The proportion of samples testing positive for influenza gives an indication of the influenza virus circulation in the community compared to other respiratory infections. Integrated systems allow for the monitoring of the distribution of virus types and sub-types and collection of representative samples and/or isolates for genetic and antigenic characterization. If specimens are collected systematically and if the sampling fraction is known (i.e., the proportion of all observed ILI and/or ARI cases that are positive for influenza), such integrated systems give important information for understanding the burden of disease. Sentinel integrated systems have also been used to monitor the effectiveness of the seasonal vaccines. A proper integration between clinical and virological surveillance is difficult to achieve as it requires that a sufficient number of sentinel physicians are recruited each year, that they are distributed in a geographically representative way, that they are committed to adhere to the surveillance protocol throughout the surveillance period, that a system is in place to ensure rapid transfer of specimens to the reference laboratories, and that there is sufficient laboratory capacity to test specimens collected.

Use of qualitative indicators

A number of qualitative indicators are used to describe influenza activity by intensity, trend, geographic spread, and impact. Intensity and trend can be directly derived from the outpatient ILI incidence and can give an indication of the proportion of the population experiencing ILI in a given week and whether such proportion is increasing, decreasing, or stable compared to the previous week (Figure 6.2). Geographic spread describes the extent of virus circulation in a given country or region. It ranges from no activity to widespread activity. Impact refers to the degree of disruption of healthcare services as a result of acute respiratory disease and can range from low (no increased demand) to severe (i.e., shortages of hospital and/or intensive care beds).

The specific indicators selected for use ultimately represent the judgment of national and or local surveillance authorities, taking into account additional sources of information such as absenteeism rates from schools or workplaces. Reporting of qualitative indicators may be the only option for countries with limited resources. Furthermore, if routine surveillance systems are disrupted because of catastrophic events or increased demand for clinical assistance, which may occur during a severe pandemic, a reporting system for qualitative indicators could be of great value. There is some evidence that qualitative indicators correlate well with

quantitative data [24]. WHO currently encourages reporting of these indicators (along with quantitative epidemiological data if available) through the FluID system [25], which is currently in its piloting phase.

Indirect indicators of influenza circulation

Recently, nontraditional approaches to influenza surveillance have proliferated due to pressure to provide more timely information utilizing electronic information sources. These approaches are usually based on the information-seeking behavior (usually through the Internet) and on healthcare utilization. These methods often utilize syndromic surveillance principles [26]. The rationale for several of the indirect systems is that influenza is the only virus that causes such a rapid, recurrent, and pronounced increase in absenteeism rate and demands for health assistance and information.

For example, analysis of weekly over-the-counter drug sales of selected medications likely to be used for treatment of ILI (e.g., cough suppressants, expectorants, nasal decongestants) were used to forecast ILI incidence to detect the onset of influenza season and forecast its trend with a good correlation between forecasted and observed ILI incidence [27]. However, over-the-counter drug sales could be triggered by increased interest (unrelated to illness) in a specific drug. Numbers of ambulance calls and after-hours calls for service from general practitioners (where reasons for calls and final diagnoses are recorded in electronic databases) also correlated with the onset and peak of ILI activity [28]. It has also been shown that school absenteeism precedes the recognition of the outbreak of some infectious diseases [29] and that student absenteeism increases during peak influenza activity. School absenteeism data correlate well with levels of less severe illness and therefore may provide evidence of an epidemic earlier than other surveillance systems. Work absenteeism data may also be valuable [30,31].

There have been attempts to use the Internet as a tool for indirect surveillance of influenza. An example is a study where search queries submitted to a Swedish medical website, Vårdguiden.se (www.vardguiden.se), were analyzed [32]. Google.org has developed a tool called Google.org Flu Trends that uses an automated method of identifying influenza-related search queries using the Google search engine. Studies have shown very good correlation between data generated by

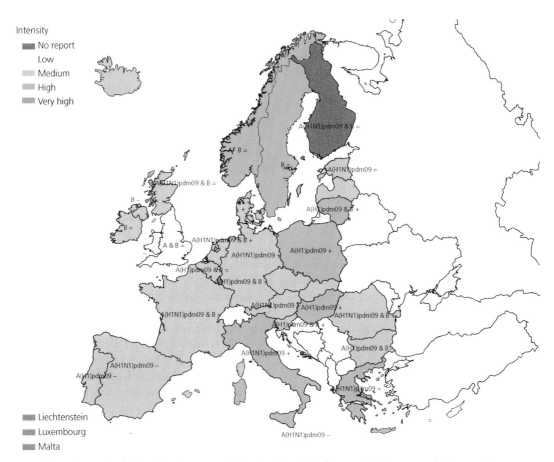

Intensity
- No report
- Low
- Medium
- High
- Very high

- Liechtenstein
- Luxembourg
- Malta

* A type/subtype is reported as dominant when at least ten samples have been detected as influenza positive in the country and of those > 40 % are positive for the type/subtype.

Legend:

No report	Intensity level was not reported	+	Increasing clinical activity
Low	No influenza activity or influenza at baseline levels	−	Decreasing clinical activity
Medium	Usual levels of influenza activity	=	Stable clinical activity
High	Higher than usual levels of influenza activity	**A & B**	Type A and B
Very high	Particularly severe levels of influenza activity	**A(H1)pdm09**	Type A, Subtype (H1)pdm09
		A(H1)pdm09 & B	Type B and Type A, Subtype (H1)pdm09
		A(H1N1)pdm 09	Type A, Subtype (H1N1)pdm09
		A(H1N1)pdm 09 & B	Type B and Type A, Subtype (H1N1)pdm09
		B	Type B

Figure 6.2 Influenza intensity, trends, and dominating strain in European Union countries, week 5, 2011. Source: European Centre for Disease Prevention and Control.

Google.org Flu Trends and the ILI trends reported from traditional surveillance systems [33–35]. However, more recent analyses have shown potential limitations of this approach [36]. Finally, monitoring of telephone consultations can also be used as an indirect measure of influenza activity as in the example of NHS Direct, a telephone helpline run by the National Health Service (NHS) in England [37–39].

Surveillance of severe influenza cases

Surveillance of severe influenza illness is challenging because most cases remain undiagnosed. This happens because influenza causes a wide range of nonspecific clinical symptoms that do not necessarily prompt virological testing. In addition, most of the influenza burden on the healthcare system is because of complications such as secondary bacterial infections and exacerbations of pre-existing chronic diseases, and often influenza is not suspected as an underlying cause. Even if suspected, the virus could have been already cleared from the respiratory secretions when the testing is performed, making diagnostic confirmation impossible.

Surveillance of severe influenza has the following main objectives:

1. Estimate the burden of disease to support resource allocation decisions.
2. Determine incidence of severe illness in order to compare with previous seasons, and refine mitigation strategies accordingly.
3. Determine risk factors for severe illness to guide vaccination and antiviral treatment strategies.
4. Understand the clinical spectrum of illness, including the role and microbiological features of secondary bacterial infections in order to guide clinical management.

It is very difficult for a single surveillance system to meet all of the above objectives. In the United States, surveillance of influenza-confirmed hospitalizations is mostly conducted within the Emerging Infections Program (EIP) complemented with data provided by the Influenza Hospitalization Surveillance Project (IHSP), a separate network started during the 2009 A(H1N1) pandemic. The EIP collects data on hospitalized children and adults in 60 counties covering 12 metropolitan areas of 10 states. Once a laboratory test is positive for influenza, additional information is actively sought by reviewing hospital laboratory and admission databases, as well as infection control logs. Incidence rates are calculated and published weekly during the influenza season using population estimates from the National Center for Health Statistics database. Rates calculated through this system represent an underestimate of the true rates of severe influenza cases, firstly because the EIP is not nationally representative, and secondly because (as previously discussed) influenza may not be diagnosed. Assuming that the number of reporting sites and testing practices remain stable over time, however, EIP allows comparisons of rates by seasons and by age groups (Figure 6.3) [40]. Because additional information is collected on hospitalized, confirmed cases, this system allows evaluation of risk factors for severity (including possible new risk factors such as morbid obesity) and quantification of the proportion of otherwise healthy individuals experiencing severe illness [41].

Conducting active population-based surveillance of hospitalized influenza cases is labor and resource intensive, which represents a major limitation for establishing similar systems in low- and middle-income countries. More advanced technologies that allow automatic exploration and extraction of data from electronic clinical and laboratory databases may decrease resource requirements for such systems.

Sentinel SARI surveillance

The objective of monitoring of severe acute respiratory infections (SARI) through networks of sentinel hospitals is to detect and interpret trends of severe influenza over time. This is important as it allows early influenza severity assessment. Furthermore, virus isolates from patients with severe illness contribute to providing a representative pool of viruses for antigenic and genetic characterization. During the surveillance period, sentinel hospitals report the total number of SARI cases admitted by week, and incidence rates are calculated using the population under the hospital catchment area or the total number of all-cause weekly admissions that have been screened for SARI. Laboratory specimens are collected from a subset of patients for confirmation of the infecting pathogen.

The selection of sentinel hospitals should be based on predefined criteria. The most important criteria to be assessed is the feasibility for a given hospital to perform SARI surveillance. Feasibility is related to the degree of commitment and motivation of hospital administrators

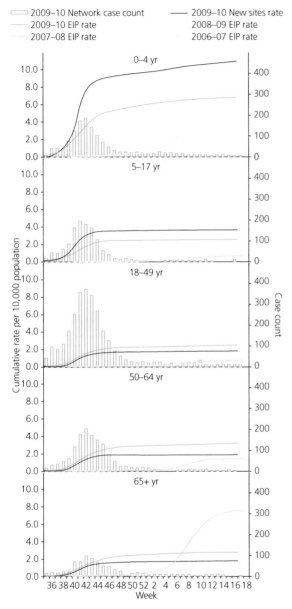

Figure 6.3 EIP influenza laboratory-confirmed cumulative hospitalization rates, 2009–2010 and the previous three seasons. *The 2008–2009 EIP rate ended as of April 14, 2009, because of the onset of the 2009 H1N1 season. Source: Centers for Disease Control and Prevention.

and staff, organizational and logistical factors, and volume of weekly admissions.

Protocols for SARI surveillance have been developed by CDC and the Pan American Health Organization (PAHO) [42] and more recently by the WHO Regional Office for Europe [43]. Case definitions for SARI vary depending on the desired sensitivity of the system. The case definition proposed by CDC and PAHO in 2006 for persons ≥5 years old is:

- sudden onset of fever over 38°C, AND
- cough or sore throat, AND
- shortness of breath or difficulty breathing, AND
- need for hospital admission.

Any child <5 years old clinically suspected of having pneumonia or severe/very severe pneumonia and requiring hospital admission meets the case definition.

SARI surveillance overestimates the true incidence of severe influenza as infections caused by other viruses are included in the numerator. SARI data must be interpreted taking into account information from integrated virological surveillance systems.

Influenza-related mortality monitoring

The U.S. CDC estimates that during 1976–2007, annual influenza-associated deaths from respiratory and circulatory causes (including pneumonia and influenza causes) ranged from 3,349 in 1986–1987 to 48,614 in 2003–2004 [44]. Only a small proportion of all deaths caused by influenza are classified as influenza related on death certificates. Therefore estimating influenza related mortality requires application of statistical methods to surveillance and vital statistics data [45]. Although influenza-specific codes exist in *International Classification of Diseases, 10th Revision* (ICD-10), most often influenza-related deaths are reported using the ICD-10 codes for pneumonia, respiratory, cardiovascular, or cerebrovascular diseases. This can be demonstrated by retrospectively comparing trends in influenza activity with trends of reported causes of deaths. Influenza peaks coincide with peaks in the rates of pneumonia and influenza deaths, respiratory and circulatory deaths, and all-cause deaths [46]. As processing of death certification takes months to years, depending on the country [4] mortality surveillance based only on death certificates is not useful for the rapid assessment of an influenza epidemic or pandemic severity. Detection of excess mortality in real time can be done by establishing specific monitoring systems that overcome these delays. Because of the need to ensure timeliness, real-time monitoring of mortality is often confined to sentinel sites representing a smaller proportion of the population. In order to detect and quantify excess mortality signals, statistical methods are applied to historical data to define baseline mortality and excess mortality thresholds [47,48].

The 122 Cities Mortality Reporting System coordinated by the U.S. CDC monitors the total number of death certificates processed and the number of those for which pneumonia or influenza is listed as the underlying or contributing cause of death in 122 U.S. cities. These data are used to define a baseline and epidemic threshold for mortality because of pneumonia and influenza (P & I) and provide a means to compare P & I mortality from year to year. An example of an all-cause mortality monitoring system in Europe is the "European monitoring of excess mortality for public health action" (EuroMOMO), which collects, analyzes, and disseminates mortality data from up to 19 countries on a weekly basis [49].

Animal influenza surveillance

Influenza is in essence a zoonotic virus that infects a variety of wild and domesticated animals including pigs, birds, horses, and marine mammals [50,51]. Surveillance of influenza viruses in animal populations is extremely important both for animal and human health. The objectives of the global surveillance of animal influenza viruses include (1) detection of outbreaks of influenza among animals, (2) monitoring changes in animal influenza viruses, and (3) providing early identification of viruses with human pandemic potential.

Animal influenza surveillance data can be collected as part of passive or active surveillance systems. Passive systems rely on identification and reporting of clinical cases from farmers and local veterinarians. The quality of data is therefore affected by factors such as local disease awareness and availability of diagnostic and veterinary services. Active systems imply searching for cases in a systematic way (e.g., collecting specimens from live animal markets at regular intervals or from a fixed proportion of chickens at slaughter). Active surveillance is resource intensive, and therefore it must be targeted to specific populations considered at risk. In addition to systematic surveillance, important data on influenza in animals are collected as part of the response to outbreaks and in ad hoc research studies. Depending on the animal species involved, the surveillance systems may be based on veterinary services linked to the food industry or exist as part of wildlife research programs.

Systematic surveillance in animals is performed by laboratories and institutes independent from or affiliated with the World Organisation for Animal Health (OIE), Food and Agriculture Organization (FAO), or WHO.

There are wide differences in the availability, structures, and performance of veterinary influenza surveillance systems. Systems also differ depending on the species under surveillance (e.g., avian versus swine). There are inherent limitations of animal surveillance systems related to the fact that this surveillance is often reactive (e.g., data are collected in response to outbreaks) and passive. As a result, this surveillance may generate incomplete data and may suffer from delays in data availability [52]. Furthermore, there is an overall lack of animal influenza surveillance data, including in countries considered at risk because of the prevalence of outbreaks in animals and the close contact between humans and animals (e.g., Southeast Asia and Africa).

Surveillance during a pandemic

Influenza pandemics are unpredictable events that occur when a novel influenza virus strain emerges that is (1) pathogenic for humans, (2) easily transmissible, and (3) antigenically unique (i.e., pre-existing immunity in the population is low). A virus with these characteristics can spread worldwide rapidly. During a pandemic, countries may experience one or more periods of increased virus circulation exceeding epidemic thresholds for one or more years. Ultimately, when large proportions of the population have acquired protective immunity, the pandemic virus will be replaced by a seasonal virus. There have been four pandemics in the past 100 years (1918–1919, 1957, 1968, and 2009), each with distinct clinical, epidemiological, and virological features.

For the purposes of guiding surveillance efforts at the national level during a pandemic, WHO advises countries to plan for enhanced surveillance comprised of three components: (1) early detection and investigation, (2) comprehensive assessment of the first 100 or so cases, and (3) pandemic monitoring (Table 6.1) [53]. Rapid identification of a potential pandemic influenza strain may allow containment and theoretically even control at the epidemic stage. For this to happen, intense virological surveillance, active surveillance at the

Table 6.1 Summary of the three components of pandemic surveillance.

	Component 1	Component 2	Component 3
	Early detection and investigation	**Comprehensive assessment**	**Monitoring**
Objective	Detect sustained human-to-human transmission of influenza virus with pandemic potential	Characterize the features of the new disease • Virological • Epidemiological • Clinical	Monitor the disease • Geographical spread • Trend • Intensity • Impact
Time frame	Early	Early	Throughout pandemic
Using existing system	Yes: Event-based system	Probably no: Will require preparation	Yes: Seasonal influenza system with modifications
Action at the national level	• Rapid containment for the first affected country • Alert phase for all other countries	• Review and revise pandemic plan • Define high-risk groups to prioritize interventions	• Monitor the situation
Action at the global level	• Change the pandemic phase • Deploy support to affected countries	• Change the vaccine composition • Provide early assessment of severity and subsequent updates	• Monitor the pandemic • Change the pandemic phase (e.g., end of first wave, end of pandemic)

Source: Reproduced with permission from WHO: *Global Surveillance during an Influenza Pandemic*. Version 1. Updated draft April 2009; p.12.

animal–human interface (e.g., settings where close and prolonged contacts between humans and animals occur), and rapid identification and reporting of outbreaks of respiratory infections are necessary. Despite significant progress made in these three areas in recent years, influenza surveillance systems are lacking in many low-income countries.

Once a pandemic virus starts to spread widely, it is essential to rapidly obtain information on clinical, epidemiological, and virological features through intensive investigation of the first reported cases and outbreaks. During this period, information can be obtained by enhancing existing surveillance systems and by performing ad hoc investigations [24]. The information that should be obtained at this stage includes:

1. an understanding of the clinical spectrum of disease and risk factors for severity in order to develop clinical management guidelines and vaccination strategies;
2. knowledge of transmission characteristics, attack rates, case-fatality rates, and case-hospitalization rates to guide community mitigation decisions, and

3. virological characterization to inform development of a vaccine and diagnostic tests and to guide antiviral use.

Once a pandemic is ongoing, this full set of investigations does not need to be performed in each newly affected country. Most of the basic virologic, epidemiological, and clinical features can be determined in the first affected countries and results can be extrapolated to others. Other parameters, however, such as the impact of the pandemic in terms of morbidity and mortality, the duration of a pandemic wave, the occurrence of subsequent waves, and the ability of healthcare systems to cope with demands for assistance may vary substantially among countries. Therefore, all countries should also be able to monitor the progress of the pandemic, including geographical spread, impact on morbidity and mortality, and effectiveness of interventions. Most of the information needed during the monitoring phase can be obtained by routine seasonal influenza surveillance schemes if these are available. Qualitative indicator reporting can be helpful, especially from countries with limited surveillance infrastructures.

In addition to guiding public health interventions, availability of timely and reliable surveillance information facilitates communication with media and delivery of accurate information to the population. The experience with the 2009 A(H1N1) influenza pandemic identified substantial gaps in global epidemiological surveillance for respiratory disease [24]. Strengthening surveillance systems already in place for seasonal influenza can bridge most of these gaps.

Depending on the severity of the pandemic (measured by population attack rates, case hospitalization rates, and case fatality rates) surveillance systems based on reports from primary care physicians, hospitals, and laboratories could be strained at a time when the demand for data is increased. Surveillance plans should therefore be in place to guide operation of surveillance systems during a pandemic to ensure that a minimum set of essential information is collected even if there are disruptions to health services.

Monitoring of vaccination programs

Seasonal influenza vaccination is the single most effective protective measure against influenza infection. Influenza vaccination programs are extremely complex and costly. More than half a billion doses of influenza vaccines are produced annually in two separate vaccine production cycles, one for the Northern Hemisphere and one for the Southern Hemisphere [54]. Because the influenza virus evolves constantly and vaccines are reformulated yearly, both vaccine effectiveness and safety need to be monitored routinely. Vaccination campaigns are also organized annually and require continuous public health efforts to maintain an acceptable level of vaccination coverage in the targeted population.

Vaccination coverage monitoring

Influenza vaccination coverage can be estimated using population surveys (e.g., telephone surveys) or using administrative methods (e.g., immunization registries, analysis of vaccine sales data) [55]. Administrative methods are usually based on routinely collected data and are overseen by public health authorities also responsible for vaccination campaigns. In order to estimate vaccine coverage, the number of vaccine doses administered is divided by the total estimated number of people in the target population, assuming a single-dose schedule. Various data sources can be used, and often multiple sources need to be linked to obtain the final coverage figures. Examples of data sources are vaccination registries, sentinel GP systems, and other primary care registries (providing data on vaccine doses administered) and national and local public health authorities and pharmacies (providing data on vaccine doses distributed).

Population surveys can be conducted to estimate the immunization coverage at either national or subnational levels. The validity of coverage estimates obtained through surveys mostly depends on the population sampled being representative of the target population. Therefore choosing and implementing the sampling method to select the study population is an especially relevant issue when planning a population survey. Extensive guidelines on sampling methods for vaccine coverage are provided by WHO [43]. The two main methods recommended by WHO are (1) the Expanded Program on Immunization (EPI) cluster survey (a modified 2-stage cluster sample) and (2) the lot quality assessment sampling (LQAS) (a type of stratified sampling). Surveys are used to establish baseline information or to provide a comparison with administrative estimates [56]. Although the primary objective of an immunization coverage survey is to provide a vaccine coverage estimate, other information that is usually not available through routine monitoring systems (e.g., reported reasons for nonimmunization in a target group) can be collected simultaneously [18].

Vaccination safety monitoring

Monitoring and assessing influenza vaccine safety are critical elements of influenza vaccination systems. Millions of influenza vaccinations are given each year in Europe and the United States; and, as a result, many infections and deaths are prevented. Some adverse events are detected in the premarketing phase; but, in general, preauthorization studies cannot detect extremely rare adverse events or those which occur late after vaccination. So effective postauthorization monitoring is essential. A comprehensive postmarketing vaccine safety monitoring system is composed of four main components:

1. **Detection of vaccine safety signals** is based on routine spontaneous reporting by healthcare providers or vaccine recipients. Such systems are the mainstay of vaccine safety monitoring and exist in most countries. Receivers of such reports are usually national regulatory agencies (e.g., the FDA). Spontaneous reporting systems may quickly detect vaccine safety signals but are subject to underreporting and biased reporting. Importantly, one cannot prove or disprove an association between a vaccine and an adverse event in these systems. An individual report may be only temporally associated with vaccination (i.e., coincidentally occur following vaccination).Therefore, spontaneous reporting systems can generate hypotheses about adverse events which later have to be tested in formal epidemiological studies.

2. **Verification of vaccine safety signal.** This is usually done by the regulatory authorities. If a signal arises, they call on experts to evaluate it and then may recommend further epidemiological studies. Such assessment often compares what is observed through spontaneous reporting to what can be expected to occur without vaccination, the so-called "background" rate of an event.

3. **Epidemiological studies to test safety signals that have been identified and verified in previous steps.** These are case-control, retrospective cohort, or self-controlled case series studies. For very rare adverse events, extremely large populations need to be studied (e.g., millions of study subjects), and large-linked databases are employed. Such data linkages electronically connect information on vaccination with that on clinical diagnoses. As these analyses primarily use electronic data already collected, they provide results in a timely manner, which is extremely important in reacting to vaccine safety concerns [57].

4. **Risk communication.** Effective risk communication is extremely important to translate the results of vaccine safety studies into messages understandable and acceptable to the general public.

Vaccination effectiveness monitoring

Influenza vaccines are introduced to the market if they meet certain standards of efficacy and safety established by the regulatory agencies. A hemagglutination inhibition (HI) test is performed for each vaccine strain before licensure and predefined criteria are used to assess the level of seroprotection. The efficacy of vaccines can then be evaluated directly by their capacity to reduce disease incidence in vaccinated individuals compared to unvaccinated individuals in the context of randomized clinical trials (RCT) (usually phase III trials). However, because annual vaccination is recommended to large portions of the population, withholding the vaccine in control groups in the context of RCT would be unethical. Post-licensure observational studies are therefore performed to evaluate vaccine effectiveness (how the vaccine works in the field). Different study designs have been used to regularly evaluate influenza vaccine effectiveness [58]. Systems for monitoring effectiveness during the influenza season usually operate concurrently with outpatient sentinel surveillance systems and use data collected as part of existing surveillance systems [59–62]. Vaccine effectiveness is dependent on the degree of relatedness between the vaccine and the circulating strains and on other factors including the characteristics of the target population. For example, vaccine effectiveness can be lower in immunocompromised individuals [63]. As a result, vaccine effectiveness may vary from year to year and requires close monitoring. Estimates of vaccine effectiveness provided rapidly while the epidemic is still ongoing can inform public health measures such as wider use of antivirals if lower vaccine effectiveness is estimated in certain groups. Despite the many challenges posed by the variability of the influenza virus, annual vaccination remains the most effective single preventive measure against seasonal influenza.

Conclusions

Surveillance of influenza is a complex activity that requires substantial public health efforts at local, national, and international levels. These efforts are justified by the importance of surveillance data for disease prevention and control. Global influenza surveillance coordinated by WHO is essential for the annual reformulation of the influenza vaccines, early detection of virus strains with pandemic potential, and monitoring of influenza epidemics in time and place.

Influenza surveillance systems are lacking in many parts of the world especially in low-income countries. This represents a major limitation for understanding the burden of disease in these countries and for the introduction of effective vaccination programs. Should a pandemic start in a country with a poor surveillance system, the chances of early detection are limited, thus hampering the possibility of control or containment of the new virus. Therefore public health investments to fund development of flexible and sustainable influenza surveillance systems in regions of the world where surveillance systems are lacking are warranted. Recent successful initiatives from international and local public health authorities to establish influenza surveillance systems in Africa go in this direction and are showing very promising results [64,65].

Multiple systems exist for detecting, assessing, and monitoring influenza epidemics. A better integration of epidemiological and clinical surveillance with virological surveillance would increase usefulness of each of these systems and ensure an efficient vaccine strain selection process. The 2009 H1N1 pandemic highlighted the difficulties of understanding the burden of severe influenza even in well-resourced countries. Population-based surveillance of severe influenza should be strengthened worldwide in order to improve our understanding of the influenza burden and to rapidly assess seasonal and pandemic severity. Finally, huge efforts are made and resources spent to produce and distribute influenza vaccines annually. Despite these efforts, vaccination coverage among those at risk in many parts of the world remains low. Development of new vaccines that do not require annual reformulation would dramatically improve vaccination coverage and effectiveness, thus reducing the disease burden. Surveillance for influenza, though complex, should be focused on prevention of the most severe influenza-related outcomes through use of available interventions including vaccine.

Acknowledgements

We would like to thank the following: Johan Giesecke, Chief Scientist, European Centre for Disease Prevention and Control; Adrian Vasile Prodan, Data Management & TESSy Helpdesk, Surveillance and Response Support Unit, European Centre for Disease Prevention and Control; Lucia Pastore Celentano, Head of Vaccine Preventable Disease Programme, Office of the Chief Scientist, European Centre for Disease Prevention and Control.

STUDY QUESTIONS

1. What are the main reasons for undertaking laboratory-based virologic surveillance of influenza? What key public health information or actions are shaped by knowledge about which strains of influenza are circulating?

2. What is meant by "severe influenza?" How does its monitoring differ from routine surveillance of influenza illness, and what justifies devoting additional resources to these efforts? Provide an example of a system that is used to monitor severe influenza in a country or region.

3. Provide a brief public health rationale for conducting influenza surveillance in the animal population.

4. When circulation of a pandemic strain virus is confirmed or suspected within a human population, what are some of the initial priorities for public health surveillance?

5. What are some of the aspects of an influenza vaccination program that should be monitored using surveillance? What types of systems are typically used to gather this information?

References

1. Viboud C, Alonso W, Simonsen L. Influenza in tropical regions. *PLoS Med* 2006;**3**(4):e89.
2. Mandell GL, Bennett JE, Dolin R. *Principles and Practice of Infectious Diseases*, Vol. 1 & 2, 5th ed. New York: Churchill Livingstone; 2000.
3. Nicholson K, Wood J, Zambon M. Influenza. *Lancet* 2003;**362**(9397):1733–1745.
4. A revision of the system of nomenclature for influenza viruses: A WHO memorandum. *Bull World Health Organ* 1980;**58**(4):585–591.
5. Salomon JA, Vos T, Hogan DR, et al. Common values in assessing health outcomes from disease and injury: Disability weights measurement study for the Global Burden of Disease Study 2010. *Lancet* 2012;**380**(9859):2129–2143.
6. European Centre for Disease Prevention and Control. Factsheet for professionals on seasonal influenza. Available

at http://www.ecdc.europa.eu/en/healthtopics/seasonal_influenza/basic_facts/Pages/factsheet_professionals_seasonal_influenza.aspx (accessed April 10, 2014.).

7. Kretzschmar M, Mangen MJ, Pinheiro P, et al. New methodology for estimating the burden of infectious diseases in Europe. *PLoS Med* 2012;**9**(4):e1001205.

8. World Health Organization. Global influenza surveillance and response system. Available at http://www.who.int/influenza/gisrs_laboratory/en/ (accessed April 10, 2012).

9. World Health Organization. Terms of reference for National Influenza Centres. Available at http://www.who.int/influenza/gisn_laboratory/national_influenza_centres/terms_of_reference_for_national_influenza_centres.pdf (accessed April 10, 2014).

10. Gerdil C. The annual production cycle for influenza vaccine. *Vaccine* 2003;**21**(16):1776–1779.

11. WHO. Consultation and information meeting on the composition of influenza virus vaccines for the Northern Hemisphere 2012–2013. 2012. Available at http://www.who.int/influenza/vaccines/virus/recommendations/consultation201202/en/index.html (accessed April 24, 2012).

12. European Centre for Disease Prevention and Control. WHO recommendation on influenza virus vaccines for the Northern Hemisphere 2012–2013 season. 2012. Available at http://www.ecdc.europa.eu/en/activities/sciadvice/Lists/ECDC%20Reviews/ECDC_DispForm.aspx?List=512ff74f%2D77d4%2D4ad8%2Db6d6%2Dbf0f23083f30&ID=1256 (accessed April 30, 2012).

13. Hayden F, de Jong M. Emerging influenza antiviral resistance threats. *J Infect Dis* 2011;**203**(1):6–10.

14. Moscona A. Neuraminidase inhibitors for influenza. *N Engl J Med* 2005;**353**(13):1363–1373.

15. Fiore A, Fry A, Shay D, Gubareva L, Bresee J, Uyeki T. Antiviral agents for the treatment and chemoprophylaxis of influenza—Recommendations of the Advisory Committee on Immunization Practices (ACIP). *MMWR Recomm Rep* 2011;**60**(1):1–24.

16. Bright R, Medina M, Xu X, et al. Incidence of adamantane resistance among influenza A (H3N2) viruses isolated worldwide from 1994 to 2005: A cause for concern. *Lancet* 2005;**366**(9492):1175–1181.

17. Bright R, Shay D, Shu B, Cox N, Klimov A. Adamantane resistance among influenza A viruses isolated early during the 2005–2006 influenza season in the United States. *JAMA* 2006;**295**(8):891–894.

18. Ciancio B, Meerhoff T, Kramarz P, et al. Oseltamivir-resistant influenza A(H1N1) viruses detected in Europe during season 2007–8 had epidemiologic and clinical characteristics similar to co-circulating susceptible A(H1N1) viruses. *Euro Surveill* 2009;**14**(46): pii: 19412. Available at http://www.eurosurveillance.org/ViewArticle.aspx?ArticleId=19412 (accessed April 10, 2014).

19. Dharan N, Gubareva L, Meyer J, et al. Infections with oseltamivir-resistant influenza A(H1N1) virus in the United States. *JAMA* 2009;**301**(10):1034–1041.

20. Commission E. Commission Decision of 28 April 2008 amending Decision 2002/253/EC laying down case definitions for reporting communicable diseases to the Community network under Decision No 2119/98/EC of the European Parliament and of the Council. *Off J Eur Union* 2009:64.

21. ECDC. Weekly influenza surveillance overview (WISO). 2012. Available at http://ecdc.europa.eu/en/healthtopics/seasonal_influenza/epidemiological_data/pages/weekly_influenza_surveillance_overview.aspx (accessed April 27, 2012).

22. http://www.euroflu.org/. WHO/Europe influenza surveillance. 2014. Available at http://www.euroflu.org/ (accessed April 27, 2012).

23. Vega T, Lozano JE, Meerhoff T, et al. Influenza surveillance in Europe: Establishing epidemic thresholds by the Moving Epidemic Method. *Influenza Other Respir Viruses* 2012 Aug 16;**7**:546–558. PubMed PMID: 22897919. Epub 2012/08/18. Eng.

24. Briand S, Mounts A, Chamberland M. Challenges of global surveillance during an influenza pandemic. *Public Health* 2011;**125**(5):247–256.

25. WHO. FluID—A global influenza epidemiological data sharing platform: WHO. 2014. Available at http://www.who.int/influenza/surveillance_monitoring/fluid/en/ (accessed April 10, 2014).

26. Elliot A. Syndromic surveillance: The next phase of public health monitoring during the H1N1 influenza pandemic? *Euro Surveill* 2009;**14**(44). PubMed PMID: 19941780. Epub 2009/11/28. eng.

27. Vergu E, Grais RF, Sarter H, et al. Medication sales and syndromic surveillance, France. *Emerg Infect Dis* 2006;**12**(3):416–421.

28. Coory M, Grant K, Kelly H. Influenza-like illness surveillance using a deputising medical service corresponds to surveillance from sentinel general practices. *Euro Surveill* 2009;**14**(44):pii=19387. Available at http://www.eurosurveillance.org/ViewArticle.aspx?ArticleId=19387 (accessed April 10, 2014).

29. Proctor ME, Blair KA, Davis JP. Surveillance data for waterborne illness detection: An assessment following a massive waterborne outbreak of Cryptosporidium infection. *Epidemiol Infect* 1998;**120**(1):43–54.

30. Besculides M, Heffernan R, Mostashari F, Weiss D. Evaluation of school absenteeism data for early outbreak detection, New York City. *BMC Public Health* 2005;**5**:105.

31. Zhao H, Joseph C, Phin N. Outbreaks of influenza and influenza-like illness in schools in England and Wales, 2005/06. *Euro Surveill* 2007;**12**(5):E3–E4.

32. Hulth A, Rydevik G, Linde A. Web queries as a source for syndromic surveillance. *PLoS ONE* 2009;**4**(2):e4378.

33. Ginsberg J, Mohebbi MH, Patel RS, Brammer L, Smolinski MS, Brilliant L. Detecting influenza epidemics using search engine query data. *Nature* 2009;**457**(7232): 1012–1014.

34. Eurosurveillance Editorial Team. Google FLU TRENDS includes 14 European countries. *Euro Surveill* 2009; **14**(40).

35. Google.org. Google flu trends. 2009. Available at http://www.google.org/flutrends (accessed May 17, 2012).

36. Olson DR, Konty KJ, Paladini M, Viboud C, Simonsen L. Reassessing Google Flu Trends data for detection of seasonal and pandemic influenza: A comparative epidemiological study at three geographic scales. *PLoS Comput Biol.* 2013;**9**(10):e1003256.

37. Baker M, Smith GE, Cooper D, et al. Early warning and NHS Direct: A role in community surveillance? *J Public Health Med* 2003;**25**(4):362–368.

38. Cooper DL, Smith GE, Hollyoak VA, Joseph CA, Johnson L, Chaloner R. Use of NHS Direct calls for surveillance of influenza—A second year's experience. *Commun Dis Public Health* 2002;**5**(2):127–131.

39. Cooper DL, Smith GE, O'Brien SJ, Hollyoak VA, Baker M. What can analysis of calls to NHS direct tell us about the epidemiology of gastrointestinal infections in the community? *J Infect* 2003;**46**(2):101–105.

40. Prevention CfDCa. FluView. 2009–2010 influenza season summary. 2014. Available at http://www.cdc.gov/flu/weekly/weeklyarchives2009-2010/09-10summary.htm (accessed April 10, 2014).

41. Prevention CfDCa. FluView. 2011–2012 influenza season week 17 ending April 28, 2012. Influenza-Associated Hospitalisations. 2012. Available at http://www.cdc.gov/flu/weekly/index.htm#HS (accessed April 10, 2014).

42. PAHO-CDC. Generic protocol for influenza surveillance. 2006. Available at http://www.paho.org/english/ad/dpc/cd/flu-snl-gpis.pdf (accessed April 10, 2014).

43. WHO Regional Office for Europe. Guidance for sentinel influenza surveillance in humans. 2011. Available at http://www.euro.who.int/__data/assets/pdf_file/0020/90443/E92738.pdf (accessed April 10, 2014).

44. Thomopson MG, Shay DK, Zhou H, et al. Influenza Div., National Center for Immunization and Respiratory Diseases, CDC. Estimates of deaths associated with seasonal influenza—United States, 1976–2007. *MMWR Morb Mortal Wkly Rep* 2010;**59**(33):1057–1062.

45. Nicoll A, Ciancio BC, Lopez Chavarrias V, et al. Influenza-related deaths-available methods for estimating numbers and detecting patterns for seasonal and pandemic influenza in Europe. *Euro Surveill* 2012;**17**(18):pii=20162. Available at http://www.eurosurveillance.org/ViewArticle.aspx?ArticleId=20162 (accessed Aprili 10, 2014).

46. Thompson WW, Moore MR, Weintraub E, et al. Estimating influenza-associated deaths in the United States. *Am J Public Health* 2009;**99**(S2):S225–S230.

47. Serfling RE. Methods for current statistical analysis of excess pneumonia-influenza deaths. *Public Health Rep* 1963;**78**(6):494–506.

48. Lui KJ, Kendal AP. Impact of influenza epidemics on mortality in the United States from October 1972 to May 1985. *Am J Public Health* 1987;**77**(6):712–716.

49. EuroMOMO website. 2014. Available at http://www.euromomo.eu/ (accessed April 10, 2014).

50. World Health Organization. WHO Manual on Animal Influenza Diagnosis and Surveillance. 2002.

51. Fouchier RA, Osterhaus AD, Brown IH. Animal influenza virus surveillance. *Vaccine* 2003;**21**(16):1754–1757.

52. Butler D. Flu surveillance lacking. *Nature* 2012;**483**(7391): 520–522.

53. WHO. Global surveillance during an influenza pandemic. Version 1, updated draft April 2009. Available at http://www.who.int/csr/disease/swineflu/global_pandemic_influenza_surveillance_apr09.pdf (accessed April 10, 2014).

54. Collin N, de Radiguès X. Vaccine production capacity for seasonal and pandemic (H1N1) 2009 influenza. *Vaccine* 2009;**27**(38):5184–5186.

55. Kroneman M, Paget WJ, Meuwissen LE, Joseph C, Kennedy H. An approach to monitoring influenza vaccination uptake across Europe. *Euro Surveill* 2008;**13**(20). PubMed PMID: 18761972. Epub 2008/09/03. eng.

56. Muller D, Nguyen-Van-Tam JS, Szucs TD. Influenza vaccination coverage rates in the UK: A comparison of two monitoring methods during the 2002–2003 and 2003–2004 seasons. *Public Health* 2006;**120**(11):1074–1080.

57. Eurosurveillance Editorial Team. ECDC in collaboration with the VAESCO consortium to develop a complementary tool for vaccine safety monitoring in Europe. *Euro Surveill* 2009;**14**(39).

58. Valenciano M, Kissling E, Ciancio BC, Moren A. Study designs for timely estimation of influenza vaccine effectiveness using European sentinel practitioner networks. *Vaccine* 2010;**28**(46):7381–7388.

59. Valenciano M, Kissling E, Cohen J-M, et al. Estimates of pandemic influenza vaccine effectiveness in Europe, 2009–2010: Results of Influenza Monitoring Vaccine Effectiveness in Europe (I-MOVE) multicentre case-control study. *PLoS Med* 2011;**8**(1):e1000388.

60. Skowronski DM, Janjua NZ, De Serres G, et al. A sentinel platform to evaluate influenza vaccine effectiveness and new variant circulation, Canada 2010–11 season. *Clin Infect Dis* 2012;**55**:332–342.

61. Belongia EA, Kieke BA, Donahue JG, et al. Effectiveness of inactivated influenza vaccines varied substantially with antigenic Match from the 2004–2005 season to the 2006–2007 season. *J Infect Dis* 2009;**199**(2):159–167.

62. Fielding JE, Grant KA, Tran T, Kelly HA. Moderate influenza vaccine effectiveness in Victoria, Australia, 2011. *Euro Surveill* 2012;**17**(11):pii=20115. Available at http://

www.eurosurveillance.org/ViewArticle.aspx?ArticleId =20115 (accessed April 10, 2014).

63. Osterholm MT, Kelley NS, Sommer A, Belongia EA. Efficacy and effectiveness of influenza vaccines: A systematic review and meta-analysis. *Lancet Infect Dis* 2012;**12**(1): 36–44.

64. Katz MA, Schoub BD, Heraud JM, Breiman RF, Njenga MK, Widdowson MA. Influenza in Africa: Uncovering the epidemiology of a long-overlooked disease. *J Infect Dis* 2012;**206**(Suppl 1):S1–S4.

65. Radin JM, Katz MA, Tempia S, et al. Influenza surveillance in 15 countries in Africa, 2006–2010. *J Infect Dis* 2012; **206**(Suppl 1):S14–S21.

CHAPTER 7

Population-based surveillance for bacterial infections of public health importance

Lee H. Harrison[1] and Gayle Fischer Langley[2]

[1] University of Pittsburgh Graduate School of Public Health and School of Medicine, Pittsburgh, PA, USA
[2] Centers for Disease Control and Prevention, Atlanta, GA, USA

Introduction

The Hungarian physician Ignaz Semmelweis monitored the incidence of Kindbettfieber, or childbed fever, at two divisions of the Vienna Maternity Hospital in the 1840s [1]. Through this surveillance and a series of other observations, he concluded that the higher rates of childbed fever among women delivering their babies in the physicians' division was a result of inadequate hand washing among physicians conducting autopsies before delivering babies. Semmelweis postulated that "during the examination of gravidae, parturients, and puerperae, the hand contaminated by cadaveric particles is brought into contact with the genitals of these individuals, and hence the possibility of absorption...into the vascular system of these individuals is postulated, and by this means the same disease is produced in these puerperae." This statement is remarkable because Semmelweis put forth this hypothesis before the discovery of bacteria; childbed fever is believed to have been caused by streptococcal species [2]. In 1847, Semmelweis established a controversial hand washing policy using chlorinated water that led to a decline in the incidence of childbed fever. Thus, Semmelweis established surveillance for a syndrome caused by a serious invasive bacterial disease, designed an intervention to reduce the incidence, and documented the positive impact of the intervention. The pioneering work of Semmelweis reminds us that surveillance is "information for action" and has as its ultimate goal the reduction of morbidity and mortality. Or, in Semmelweis' words, "My doctrines exist to rid maternity hospitals of their horror, to preserve the wife for her husband and the mother for her child."

The Active Bacterial Core surveillance (ABCs) network and its predecessor have been examples of using surveillance as information for action for over 20 years. ABCs has been used to measure disease burden, to provide data for vaccine composition and recommended-use policies, and to monitor the impact of interventions. ABCs data have been widely disseminated in the peer-reviewed scientific literature, and ABCs exemplify use of data to prevent the diseases targeted by surveillance.

In this chapter, we describe the history of ABCs and its methodology; give examples of how ABCs has been used to make advances in the prevention of three ABCs pathogens: group B *Streptococcus* (GBS), *Streptococcus pneumoniae*, and *Neisseria meningitidis*; and discuss challenges and opportunities.

History of ABCs

In 1986, to address questions about the risk of toxic shock syndrome (TSS) associated with the contraceptive

Concepts and Methods in Infectious Disease Surveillance, First Edition. Edited by Nkuchia M. M'ikanatha and John K. Iskander.
Published 2014 by John Wiley & Sons, Ltd.

sponge, the Centers for Disease Control (CDC) established active surveillance for TSS in Los Angeles County and in Missouri, New Jersey, Oklahoma, Tennessee, and Washington [3,4]. TSS is a serious, toxin-mediated illness caused by *Staphylococcus aureus*. Previously, TSS surveillance in the United States had been passive [5]. At the same time, active surveillance was also established for invasive infections caused by *Haemophilus influenzae, Neisseria meningitidis*, GBS, and *Listeria monocytogenes* in the same geographic areas.

This active surveillance system was used to determine the effectiveness of *H. influenzae* type b polysaccharide [6,7] and conjugate vaccines [8] in young children and to assess the cost-effectiveness of different approaches to preventing GBS disease in newborns [9]. This system was the precursor of ABCs, which started at CDC in 1995 under the Emerging Infections Program (EIP) as part of the agency's strategy to address the worldwide threat of emerging infectious diseases. ABCs was developed to fulfill key components of the strategy, which included conducting surveillance and applied research activities and evaluating public health interventions related to infectious diseases that were viewed as an increasing threat to the public's health [10]. In the 1970s, GBS became the leading cause of serious bacterial infections in neonates [11–13]. In the 1980s, group A *Streptococcus* (GAS)–associated necrotizing fasciitis and TSS were increasingly recognized [14–16]. In the 1990s, multidrug-resistant *Streptococcus pneumoniae* was emerging in the United States [17,18] and vaccines to prevent *S. pneumoniae, H. influenzae, and N. meningitidis*, had recently been developed or were under development. Active, laboratory, population-based surveillance for these five pathogens, which persist as major causes of community-acquired invasive bacterial infections, continues today. Surveillance for invasive methicillin-resistant *Staphylococcus aureus* (MRSA), which had long been recognized as an important healthcare-associated pathogen, began at three ABCs sites in 2001 and later expanded to nine sites because it emerged as an important cause of community-acquired infection [19]. Surveillance for *L. monocytogenes* was transitioned between 1999 and 2003 to the FoodNet component of the EIP, which conducts active surveillance for foodborne pathogens.

ABCs has continuously evolved to address challenging questions posed by the six pathogens (*H. influenzae; GAS, GBS, S. pneumoniae, N. meningitidis*, and MRSA)

and other emerging infections. Through basic surveillance and special studies, ABCs has served as a platform to track the impact of pneumococcal and meningococcal conjugate vaccines on invasive infections [20–22]. Data have been used in developing and assessing the potential impact of GAS, GBS, MRSA and serogroup B meningococcal vaccines [23–26]. ABCs has also been used to develop and evaluate guidelines for the prevention of perinatal GBS disease [27–29]. Trends in antimicrobial resistance, including reductions in penicillin non-susceptible invasive *S. pneumoniae* disease in the era of vaccination [30] and increases in GBS resistance to clindamycin and erythromycin [31], have been tracked through ABCs. ABCs analyses have helped to shed light on risk factors and racial disparities associated with invasive bacterial diseases [32–35]. In addition to surveillance for invasive infections, surveillance for infections caused by *Bordetella pertussis* and other *Bordetella* species and by *Legionella* species were added in 2011. Despite a successful vaccine program, pertussis remains endemic to the United States and outbreaks continue to be recognized. The objective of enhanced pertussis surveillance through the ABCs program is to improve case ascertainment and epidemiologic and laboratory data collection beyond what is obtained through national passive surveillance. From 2000 to 2009, age-adjusted incidence rates of diseases caused by *Legionella* increased 170% from 0.40 to 1.08 per 100,000 persons according to national passive surveillance [36]. Through active legionellosis surveillance, ABCs hopes to improve population-based estimates of disease and to better characterize its clinical course and outcomes.

ABCs sites and infrastructure

ABCs is a collaboration among CDC, state health departments, and academic institutions that are part of the EIP network. Originally established in 1995 at four sites (California, Connecticut, Oregon, and Minnesota), ABCs now operates at ten sites with the additions of Georgia, Maryland and New York (1997), Tennessee (1999), Colorado (2000), and New Mexico (2003). These sites represent wide geographic diversity and approximately reflect the race and urban-to-rural mix of the U.S. population [37]. Currently, the population under surveillance is 19–42 million and varies by pathogen and project. Surveillance for the least common pathogens (*N. meningitidis, H. influenzae*) is conducted over the entire surveillance area, but catchment areas for more common pathogens, including GBS and GAS (catchment area: ~32 million), *S. pneumoniae* (catchment area: ~30 million) and MRSA (catchment area: 19 million), are more restricted. For certain projects that require larger case counts, sites outside of the EIP network may collaborate, using the same study protocol. For the meningococcal vaccine effectiveness study, for example, additional counties outside ABC areas in three states (California, Colorado, and New York) and nine non-ABCs states (Maine, Massachusetts, Michigan, New Hampshire, Pennsylvania, South Carolina, Texas, West Virginia, and Wisconsin) were added to cover approximately 54% of the United States population.

ABCs methods

The ABCs Steering Committee comprised of the principal investigators from each site and representatives from CDC, the Infectious Diseases Society of America (IDSA), the American Society of Microbiology (ASM) and the Council of State and Territorial Epidemiologists (CSTE) set the general scientific direction and track scientific progress of ABCs activities. For the six core pathogens, the objectives are (1) to determine the incidence and epidemiologic characteristics of invasive disease in geographically diverse populations in the United States through active, laboratory, and population-based surveillance; (2) to determine molecular epidemiologic patterns and microbiologic characteristics of isolates collected as part of routine surveillance in order to track antimicrobial resistance; (3) to detect the emergence of new strains with new resistance patterns and/or virulence and contribute to development and evaluation of new vaccines; and (4) to provide an infrastructure for surveillance of other emerging pathogens and for conducting studies aimed at identifying risk factors for disease and evaluating prevention policies.

For routine ABCs surveillance, a case of invasive bacterial disease is defined as isolation of *H. influenzae, N. meningitidis*, GAS, GBS, *S. pneumoniae*, or MRSA from a normally sterile anatomic site in a resident of one of the surveillance areas. A normally sterile site is defined as a portion of the human body in which no microorgan-

isms are found in a healthy state. Every clinical laboratory that routinely processes specimens from residents of a surveillance area is contacted for case identification. At least yearly audits of reporting laboratories are conducted to ensure that all cases are being captured. Once a case patient is confirmed to meet the ABCs case definition, a case report form is completed and an isolate from the first positive culture is collected for most core pathogens (a convenience sample of MRSA isolates is collected). Data collected for the case report form originate from the medical record and include information on patient demographics, clinical course (i.e., length of stay, intensive care admission), outcome (survived or died), infection type, infection site, underlying conditions and vaccination history. Isolates are tested for serotype or serogroup and antimicrobial susceptibility at CDC and other reference laboratories. Aliquots of over 75,000 *S. pneumoniae*, GA, and GBS isolates are currently stored in an isolate bank that is accessible to ABCs partners and external researchers by request [38]. A representative sample of MRSA isolates is deposited at the Network on Antimicrobial Resistance in *Staphylococcus aureus* (NARSA).

Examples of use of ABCs data for specific pathogens

Antimicrobial chemoprophylaxis to prevent early onset GBS

Invasive GBS infection in infants is a serious and often devastating cause of bacteremia, pneumonia, and meningitis. GBS commonly colonizes the genitourinary tract of women and may be transmitted from mother to infant during the perinatal period. Antibiotic prophylaxis during labor was shown to prevent early onset GBS [39], defined as GBS infection occurring in the first week of life. Beginning in 1996, a series of recommendations for prevention of early onset GBS infection using intrapartum prophylaxis were issued by the CDC [29,40,41]. ABCs data on disease burden have been used as a rationale for the national chemoprophylaxis guidelines, to monitor its impact, and to conduct studies that have led to program improvements.

In the early 1990s, the American Academy of Pediatrics (AAP) and the American College of Obstetricians and Gynecologists (ACOG) published separate and somewhat different recommendations for approaches to prevention of early onset GBS infection [42,43]. In 1996, the CDC, along with representatives from ACOG and the American Academy of Pediatrics, published consensus guidelines recommending that all women undergo rectal/vaginal culture for GBS at 35–37 weeks of gestation and that antibiotics be administered to GBS-positive women [40]. An alternative approach of providing antibiotic prophylaxis to women with certain risk factors, such as duration of rupture of membranes ≥ 18 hours, delivery at <37 weeks gestation, intrapartum fever, previous delivery of an infant with invasive GBS infection, or presence of GBS bacteriuria during pregnancy was also deemed acceptable. These two prevention strategies had not been directly compared to each other. To address this issue, a cohort study of 5144 births, including 312 that resulted in early onset GBS infection, was conducted at eight ABCs sites. The incidence of early onset GBS infection was less than half (relative risk of 0.48, 95% confidence interval 0.36–0.60) among infants of women screened by GBS cultures as compared to infants whose mothers were assessed based on risk factors [44]. This finding was incorporated into subsequent guidelines in 2002, when CDC recommended that all women have vaginal/rectal screening for GBS colonization performed at 35–37 weeks' gestation to identify women who should receive intrapartum antibiotic prophylaxis (IAP). Overall, ABCs has documented an approximately 80% reduction in the incidence of early onset GBS infection since implementation of these recommendations, which is remarkable for an intervention that does not involve a vaccine (Figure 7.1).

In a subsequent study conducted at 10 ABCs sites, adherence to the guidelines was assessed by review of the medical records for 254 births that resulted in GBS infection and 7437 births that did not [28]. The rate of screening for GBS during pregnancy increased substantially between 1998–1999 and 2003–2004, from 48% to 85%. Failure to screen mothers for GBS during pregnancy occurred in 13% of the deliveries that resulted in GBS infection. In addition, 61% of mothers delivering term infants with GBS infection had tested negative for GBS during pregnancy. This latter finding suggests that the screening approach, although superior to the risk-factor approach, suffers from a lack of sensitivity for detecting women at risk of having infants with GBS infection. In 2010, the guidelines were further refined

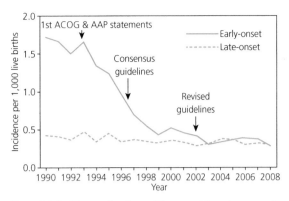

Figure 7.1 Incidence of early- and late-onset invasive group B streptococcal (GBS) disease—Active Bacterial Core surveillance areas, 1990–2008, and activities for prevention of GBS disease (www.cdc.gov/groupbstrep/guidelines/downloads/Figure_1_GBS_Decline.pdf). ACOG: American College of Obstetricians and Gynecologists; AAP: American Academy of Pediatrics. Source: Centers for Disease Control and Prevention.

to provide guidance on appropriate laboratory methods, revised algorithms for women with threatened preterm delivery, an algorithm to enhance appropriate antibiotic selection for women who are allergic to penicillin, and a revised neonatal management algorithm [41]. ABCs continues to monitor antibiotic resistance in invasive GBS isolates.

With the large declines in early onset GBS infection, there is recognition that additional interventions will be required to address the remaining burden of early onset disease and to address late onset disease, which occurs from 7 to 89 days of age and whose incidence has not declined over the past several decades. In that regard, several experimental GBS vaccines are in development. Characterization of ABCs GBS isolates has provided useful information for the formulation of these vaccines [24,45,46]. In addition, ABCs has documented a large and increasing burden of invasive GBS infection in adults, many of whom have underlying medical conditions [46]. It is conceivable that the vaccines that are being developed for infant disease could also be useful for prevention of adult disease. However, whether these vaccines would be sufficiently immunogenic and efficacious in the elderly and persons with chronic medical conditions is not known.

Invasive pneumococcal disease surveillance and vaccine effectiveness studies

S. pneumoniae is a leading cause of pneumonia, bacteremia, meningitis, and otitis media in the United States and globally. Pneumococcal strains can be characterized according to the composition of the polysaccharide capsule; there are currently 93 known serotypes. A 23-valent pneumococcal polysaccharide vaccine was licensed in 1983 and is recommended for adults and children with certain medical conditions. The 23 serotypes covered by this vaccine account for approximately 85% of adult invasive pneumococcal disease. In 2000, a 7-valent pediatric polysaccharide-protein conjugate vaccine (PCV-7) was licensed and recommended for use. The pivotal pre-licensure trial suggested high vaccine efficacy against invasive disease with a primary series at 2, 4, and 6 months of age and a booster dose at 12–15 months [47].

Following licensure of PCV7, ABCs documented dramatic changes in the epidemiology of invasive pneumococcal disease (IPD). First, as expected, there was a large decline in the incidence of IPD in children <5 years old [48,49]. For example, by 2007 the reductions in vaccine serotype IPD in this age group were nearly 100% (Figure 7.2) [48]. Second, the decline in the incidence in this age group was larger than expected based on vaccine coverage in the population. This suggested that

herd protection was playing a role, that is, unimmunized children were protected through reductions in nasopharyngeal carriage of vaccine serotype *S. pneumoniae* among children who had been immunized. Third, there were substantial reductions in vaccine serotype IPD among adults, again suggesting herd protection (Figure 7.3). During 2003, it was estimated that the indirect effects of PCV-7 prevented an additional 20,459 cases of IPD across all age groups beyond the 9140 cases prevented among immunized children [50]. Fourth, although the net impact of the vaccine was extremely favorable, there were increases in some serotypes that were not included in the vaccine, such as serotype 19A [20,49,64] (Figure 7.2 and Figure 7.3). Whether these increases were a result of introduction of PCV-7 or other factors, such as an effect of antibiotic use, has been a matter of debate. Regardless, this indicated the need for a vaccine that included additional serotypes so that disease incidence could be further reduced. A licensed 13-valent pneumococcal conjugate vaccine (PCV13), which includes serotype 19A, replaced PCV7 in the United States in 2010. ABCs data were used to demonstrate both direct effects and herd protection in children and adults for the six new serotypes included in the vaccine within 2 years of introduction [51]. For example, by the last 3 months of 2011, declines in IPD caused by the six new vaccine serotypes had decreased by almost 90% among children under 5 years old and 45–64%

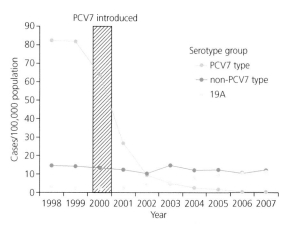

Figure 7.2 Changes in invasive pneumococcal disease incidence by serotype group among children <5 years old, 1998–2007 [20]. Seven-valent pneumococcal conjugate vaccine (PCV7) was introduced in the United States for routine use among young children and infants in the second half of 2000. Source: Reproduced with permission of OUP.

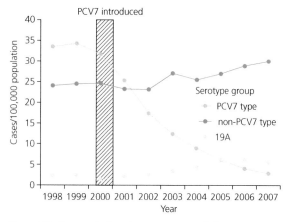

Figure 7.3 Changes in invasive pneumococcal disease incidence by serotype group among adults ≥65 years, 1998–2007 [20]. Seven-valent pneumococcal conjugate vaccine (PCV7) was introduced in the United States for routine use among young children and infants in the second half of 2000. Source: Reproduced with permission of OUP.

among adult age groups. Based on the high burden of IPD in countries with limited resources and the success of pneumococcal conjugate vaccines in the United States and elsewhere, several pediatric pneumococcal conjugate vaccines are being introduced into low- and middle-income countries.

Following licensure of PCV-7, there were several questions that remained unanswered about the vaccine, such as the effectiveness for some of the seven serotypes and whether a dosing schedule that included less than four doses was effective. To address these, ABCs conducted a case-control study of PCV-7 vaccine effectiveness [52]. In this study, high vaccine effectiveness was demonstrated against each of the seven serotypes targeted by the vaccine as well as serotype 6A, which is closely related in structure to vaccine serotype 6B. In addition, schedules that required fewer than four doses were also shown to be effective, including two doses before 7 months of age in combination with a booster dose at 12–16 months of age (the 2 + 1 schedule). These and other ABCs data have been used for the development and guidance of pneumococcal immunization policy, both in the United States and globally. For example, in conjunction with information from immunogenicity studies, these data were used by other countries to establish PCV-7 2 + 1 immunization schedules. The U.S. Advisory Committee on Immunization Practices (ACIP) will be using ABCs IPD data from adults to decide whether the indirect effects of vaccinating children are providing adequate reductions in adult disease to determine whether there would be substantial additional benefit from routine adult vaccination with PCV-13.

Epidemiology and molecular surveillance of meningococcal disease

Invasive meningococcal disease is a major cause of meningitis and other serious bacterial infections, both in the United States and globally [53,54]. Although a quadrivalent polysaccharide vaccine that covers four of the five main meningococcal serogroups (A, C, W-135, and Y—but not B) has been available in the United States since 1981, its use was relatively limited because of the immunologic limitations of polysaccharide vaccines, including poor immunogenicity in infants and lack of induction of immunologic memory [55]. In 2005 and 2010, two new quadrivalent conjugate vaccines, cover-

Table 7.1 Average annual incidence of meningococcal infection, Maryland college students, 1992–1997 [56]. Reproduced with permission of the American Medical Association.

Group	Total cases, no.	Population, no.	Annual incidence per 100,000
4-year college	11	105,623	1.74
On-campus housing*	7	35,974	3.24
Off-campus housing	4	69,649	0.96
General population**	17	196,902	1.44

*$p = 0.05$ for comparison of annual incidence between on-campus versus off-campus housing residents; $p = 0.08$ for comparison of annual incidence between on-campus housing residents and the general population.
**18–22 years old, excluding the 4-year college population.

ing the same serogroups as the polysaccharide vaccine, were licensed in the United States.

ABCs data have been used to guide meningococcal vaccine formulation and policy. For example, studies of meningococcal disease in college students (one a Maryland ABCs site-initiated study and the other a national study coordinated by CDC) demonstrated the increased risk of meningococcal disease in college students and found that 68% of cases in college students were potentially vaccine preventable [56,57]. In the Maryland ABCs study, the incidence of meningococcal disease was higher in 4-year college students residing on campus than those residing off campus (Table 7.1). In the CDC study, freshmen living in dormitories had an increased risk of meningococcal disease compared with other college students. These studies played a role in a recommendation for use of polysaccharide vaccine in college students [58]. Disease burden estimates based on ABCs and national surveillance data were used to formulate meningococcal vaccine policy for adolescents. Once the first quadrivalent conjugate vaccine became available in the United States in 2005, the ACIP recommended routine vaccination at 11–12 years of age and at high school entry for those not previously vaccinated, in addition to routine vaccination for college freshman living in dormitories and other high-risk populations [59]. In June 2007, ACIP revised its recommendation to include routine vaccination of all persons aged 11–18 years at the earliest opportunity [60].

ABCs data have also been used to guide immunization policy since 2005. A case-control study of meningococcal vaccine effectiveness conducted at ABCs sites and other sites throughout the United States indicated an estimated overall effectiveness of 75%, with unexpectedly rapid decline in effectiveness over time [61]. These data and data from the vaccine manufacturer indicating a rapid decline in serum bactericidal antibodies were used by ACIP to recommend a booster dose of vaccine for children who had received the conjugate vaccine at age 11–12 [62,63]. In addition, ABCs and national surveillance data were used in ACIP deliberations to determine that infant immunization was not warranted based on the current epidemiology. The reasons for this decision included the facts that the majority of infections in infants are caused by serogroup B strains, which are not covered by vaccines currently available in the United States, that the rates of disease are at historically low levels, and that a substantial proportion of cases occur before the age that the primary immunization series could be completed. ACIP will continue to use ABCs and other data to support formulation of meningococcal immunization policy.

The collection of case bacterial isolates is a major strength of ABCs. As occurred with pneumococcal vaccine [64], one question that remained following meningococcal vaccine licensure was whether there were increases in infections caused by strains that were not covered by the vaccine. One way in which this can happen is through a mechanism known as capsular switching, by which strains of N. meningitidis exchange DNA that is involved in the production of the polysaccharide capsule. To address this question, two molecular surveillance studies were performed. In the pre-licensure study, 1160 meningococcal isolates from 10 ABCs collected during 2000–2005 demonstrated that capsular switching was common before the introduction of the first quadrivalent meningococcal vaccine in 2005 [65]. This study served as a baseline to which isolates analyzed post-licensure could be compared. In the post-licensure follow-up study, there was no evidence of increased capsular switching [66]. Ongoing molecular analysis of ABCs isolates will be required to continue to address this question.

In a more recent study, the same isolates underwent extensive molecular subtyping to determine whether clonal meningococcal outbreaks that had not previously been recognized could be identified by geotemporal analysis, which identifies cases of disease that cluster temporally and geographically [67]. Thirty-five groups of isolates involving 23 different clones and 111 cases (10.4% of geocoded isolates) that clustered in time and space were identified. This study demonstrated that molecular characterization of isolates, combined with geotemporal analysis, is a useful tool for understanding the spread of virulent meningococcal clones and patterns of transmission in populations.

Challenges and opportunities

A key attribute of surveillance systems should be their ability to continuously evolve to meet public health needs. Over the years, ABCs has added new sites, added new pathogens, and addressed new questions. In the future, there will be opportunities to take advantage of new technologies and opportunities to investigate old and emerging problems in new ways. The challenges will be how to make the best use of these new technologies and how to engage in new activities in an era of tight budgets, without sacrificing data quality.

When ABCs began, most cases were identified by reviewing paper laboratory log sheets and computer printouts; and most case report forms were filled out using paper medical charts. With the increasing use of electronic laboratory reporting (ELR), cases may first be identified through electronic records. Although the availability of ELR may improve timeliness, completeness, and accuracy of reporting, a lag in the adoption of standardized testing and result codes have the potential to adversely affect case identification [68,69]. Sites must continuously work with participating laboratories to make sure submitted data remain complete. Electronic medical records (EMR) are increasingly replacing paper charts as providers take advantage of incentives that increase reimbursements for providing clinical data to public health systems [70]. This has the potential to make reporting more accurate and less labor intensive, but locating appropriate data elements and transferring them into usable formats remains a challenge [71,72].

Currently, with the exception of surveillance for diseases caused by Bordetella and Legionella, the case definition for ABCs pathogens only includes those that are culture proven. Although the ABCs case definition is highly specific, it does not detect culture-negative cases of invasive infection. While culture remains the gold standard for diagnosing invasive infections, the use of culture-independent diagnostics is likely to increase given their potential for improving the rapidity and sensitivity of diagnoses [73,74]. The National Notifiable Disease Surveillance System (NNDSS), a passive surveillance system that covers all of the United States, detects "probable" cases defined by polymerase chain reaction and other culture independent tests in addition to cases "confirmed" by isolation of the organism from a sterile site for meningococcal disease [75]. Although this has not resulted in a substantial increase in cases detected through NNDSS compared to ABCs, this may change in the future if more clinical and state laboratories offer nonculture testing [76]. Validation of culture-independent diagnostics will remain a major consideration in determining whether they are added to the ABCs case definition. Besides being considered the gold standard, a culture-based system allows for the collection of isolates that are used for serotyping or serogrouping and antimicrobial susceptibility testing. While most serotyping and serogrouping is done by serologic methods, molecular testing for these attributes may become more accessible; and molecular approaches to assess drug resistance may become available.

Chronic diseases are the leading causes of morbidity and mortality in the United States. A better understanding of the associations and interactions between chronic diseases and invasive bacterial infections is important for understanding the pathophysiology, modifiable risk factors, health interventions, and prognoses for invasive bacterial infections. ABCs data have been used to analyze the influence of chronic diseases on invasive pneumococcal disease [77] and efforts are underway to analyze the association between obesity and ABCs pathogens.

Assessing public health disparities is an important goal of ABCs. Whereas racial differences are one measure of disparities, it has been difficult to capture other measures of socioeconomic status utilizing information from medical records alone. ABCs analyses have incorporated some geocoding of data to include other parameters, such as poverty and crowded living conditions, in assessing differences in disease incidences [34,78]; but the goal is for this to become a routine part of surveillance methods.

Conclusions

ABCs serves as a model for how surveillance can be used to assess disease burden while monitoring the impact of public health interventions. Throughout its history, ABCs has evolved to meet public health opportunities and challenges posed by new approaches to prevention, new vaccines, and the emergence of important pathogens. ABCs will continue to adapt to changing diagnostic methods, new health information systems, and other unforeseen challenges in the future.

Acknowledgements

The work described in this chapter was supported in part by a grant from the Centers for Disease Control and Prevention and a research career award from the National Institute of Allergy and Infectious Diseases (K24 AI52788 to L.H.H.)

STUDY QUESTIONS

1. What public health problems prompted the establishment of ABCs?
2. What are the main objectives of ABCs? Provide one example of surveillance activities or projects that have fulfilled these objectives.
3. What are the challenges and opportunities associated with identifying cases and obtaining data from ELRs and EMRs, respectively?
4. What are the potential advantages and disadvantages of introducing nonculture-based diagnostics into the ABCs case definition?
5. How have ABCs meningococcal isolates been used to monitor the impact of the program that was started in 2005 to immunize adolescents with quadrivalent meningococcal conjugate vaccine?
6. What are the similarities and differences between ABCs and the surveillance that Ignaz Semmwelweis conducted for childbed fever in the mid-1800s?
7. Briefly describe the ways in which ABCs surveillance for early onset neonatal invasive GBS infection has contributed to the prevention of this disease.
8. Briefly describe the evidence that 7-valent pneumococcal conjugate (PCV-7) vaccine given to children had direct and indirect effects in preventing invasive pneumococcal disease in children and adults.

References

1. Semmelweis IF, Carter KC. *The Etiology, Concept, and Prophylaxis of Childbed Fever.* Madison, WI: University of Wisconsin Press; 1983.

2. Adriaanse AH, Pel M, Bleker OP. Semmelweis: The combat against puerperal fever. *Eur J Obstet Gynecol Reprod Biol* 2000;**90**:153–158.

3. Gaventa S, Reingold AL, Hightower AW, et al. Active surveillance for toxic shock syndrome in the United States, 1986. *Rev Infect Dis* 1989;**11**(Suppl 1):S28–S34.

4. Schwartz B, Gaventa S, Broome CV, et al. Nonmenstrual toxic shock syndrome associated with barrier contraceptives: Report of a case-control study. *Rev Infect Dis* 1989;**11** (Suppl 1):S43–S48; discussion S48–49.

5. Reingold AL, Hargrett NT, Shands KN, et al. Toxic shock syndrome surveillance in the United States, 1980 to 1981. *Ann Intern Med* 1982;**96**:875–880.

6. Harrison LH, Broome CV, Hightower AW, et al. A day care–based study of the efficacy of *Haemophilus* b polysaccharide vaccine. *JAMA* 1988;**260**:1413–1418.

7. Harrison LH, Broome CV, Hightower AW. *Haemophilus influenzae* type b polysaccharide vaccine: An efficacy study. *Haemophilus* Vaccine Efficacy Study Group. *Pediatrics* 1989;**84**: 255–261.

8. Wenger JD, Pierce R, Deaver KA, Plikaytis BD, Facklam RR, Broome CV. Efficacy of *Haemophilus influenzae* type b polysaccharide-diphtheria toxoid conjugate vaccine in US children aged 18–59 months. *Haemophilus Influenzae* Vaccine Efficacy Study Group. *Lancet* 1991;**338**:395–398.

9. Mohle-Boetani JC, Schuchat A, Plikaytis BD, Smith JD, Broome CV. Comparison of prevention strategies for neonatal group B streptococcal infection. A population-based economic analysis. *JAMA* 1993;**270**:1442–1448.

10. Centers for Disease Control and Prevention. Addressing emerging infectious disease threats: A prevention strategy for the United States. *MMWR Morb Mortal Wkly Rep* 1994; **43**:1–15.

11. Anthony BF, Okada DM. The emergence of group B streptococci in infections of the newborn infant. *Annu Rev Med* 1977;**28**:355–369.

12. Howard JB, McCracken GH Jr. The spectrum of group B streptococcal infections in infancy. *Am J Dis Child* 1974;**128**: 815–818.

13. McCracken GH Jr. Group B *streptococci*: The new challenge in neonatal infections. *J Pediatr* 1973;**82**:703–706.

14. Schwartz B, Facklam RR, Breiman RF. Changing epidemiology of group A streptococcal infection in the USA. *Lancet* 1990;**336**:1167–1171.

15. Cone LA, Woodard DR, Schlievert PM, Tomory GS. Clinical and bacteriologic observations of a toxic shock-like syndrome due to *Streptococcus pyogenes*. *N Engl J Med* 1987;**317**: 146–149.

16. Stevens DL, Tanner MH, Winship J, et al. Severe group A streptococcal infections associated with a toxic shock-like syndrome and scarlet fever toxin A. *N Engl J Med* 1989; **321**:1–7.

17. Breiman RF, Butler JC, Tenover FC, Elliott JA, Facklam RR. Emergence of drug-resistant pneumococcal infections in the United States. *JAMA* 1994;**271**:1831–1835.

18. Centers for Disease Control and Prevention. Defining the public health impact of drug-resistant *Streptococcus pneumoniae*: Report of a working group. *MMWR Recomm Rep* 1996;**45**:1–20.

19. Fridkin SK, Hageman JC, Morrison M, et al. Methicillin-resistant *Staphylococcus aureus* disease in three communities. *N Engl J Med* 2005;**352**:1436–1444.

20. Pilishvili T, Lexau C, Farley MM, et al. Sustained reductions in invasive pneumococcal disease in the era of conjugate vaccine. *J Infect Dis* 2010;**201**:32–41.

21. De Serres G, Pilishvili T, Link-Gelles R, et al. Use of surveillance data to estimate the effectiveness of the 7-valent conjugate pneumococcal vaccine in children less than 5 years of age over a 9 year period. *Vaccine* 2012;**30**:4067–4072.

22. MacNeil JR, Cohn AC, Zell ER, et al. Early estimate of the effectiveness of quadrivalent meningococcal conjugate vaccine. *Pediatr Infect Dis J* 2011;**30**:451–455.

23. O'Loughlin RE, Roberson A, Cieslak PR, et al. The epidemiology of invasive group A streptococcal infection and potential vaccine implications: United States, 2000–2004. *Clin Infect Dis* 2007;**45**:853–862.

24. Jordan HT, Farley MM, Craig A, et al. Revisiting the need for vaccine prevention of late-onset neonatal group B streptococcal disease: A multistate, population-based analysis. *Pediatr Infect Dis J* 2008;**27**:1057–1064.

25. Lucero CA, Hageman J, Zell ER, et al. Evaluating the potential public health impact of a *Staphylococcus aureus* vaccine through use of population-based surveillance for invasive methicillin-resistant *S. aureus* disease in the United States. *Vaccine* 2009;**27**:5061–5068.

26. Wang X, Cohn A, Comanducci M, et al. Prevalence and genetic diversity of candidate vaccine antigens among invasive *Neisseria meningitidis* isolates in the United States. *Vaccine* 2011;**29**:4739–4744.

27. Centers for Disease Control and Prevention. Prevention of perinatal group B streptococcal disease: Revised guidelines from CDC, 2010. *MMWR Recomm Rep* 2010;**59**:1–36.

28. Van Dyke MK, Phares CR, Lynfield R, et al. Evaluation of universal antenatal screening for group B streptococcus. *N Engl J Med* 2009;**360**:2626–2636.

29. Schrag S, Gorwitz R, Fultz-Butts K, Schuchat A. Prevention of perinatal group B streptococcal disease. Revised guidelines from CDC. *MMWR Recomm Rep* 2002;**51**:1–22.

30. Hampton LM, Farley MM, Schaffner W, et al. Prevention of antibiotic-nonsusceptible *Streptococcus pneumoniae* with conjugate vaccines. *J Infect Dis* 2011;**205**:401–411.

31. Castor ML, Whitney CG, Como-Sabetti K, et al. Antibiotic resistance patterns in invasive group B streptococcal isolates. *Infect Dis Obstet Gynecol* 2008;**2008**:727505.

32. Factor SH, Levine OS, Harrison LH, et al. Risk factors for pediatric invasive group A streptococcal disease. *Emerg Infect Dis* 2005;**11**:1062–1066.

33. Phares CR, Lynfield R, Farley MM, et al. Epidemiology of invasive group B streptococcal disease in the United States, 1999–2005. *JAMA* 2008;**299**:2056–2065.

34. Burton DC, Flannery B, Bennett NM, et al. Socioeconomic and racial/ethnic disparities in the incidence of bacteremic pneumonia among US adults. *Am J Public Health* 2010;**100**:1904–1911.

35. Harrison LH, Kreiner CJ, Shutt KA, et al. Risk factors for meningococcal disease in students in grades 9–12. *Pediatr Infect Dis J* 2008;**27**:193–199.

36. Centers for Disease Control and Prevention. Legionellosis—United States, 2000–2009. *MMWR Morb Mortal Wkly Rep* 2011;**60**:1083–1086.

37. Pinner RW, Rebmann CA, Schuchat A, Hughes JM. Disease surveillance and the academic, clinical, and public health communities. *Emerg Infect Dis* 2003;**9**:781–787.

38. CDC. CDC Isolates. http://www.cdc.gov/abcs/pathogens/isolatebank/ (accessed August 31, 2012).

39. Boyer KM, Gotoff SP. Prevention of early-onset neonatal group B streptococcal disease with selective intrapartum chemoprophylaxis. *N Engl J Med* 1986;**314**:1665–1669.

40. Prevention of perinatal group B streptococcal disease: A public health perspective. Centers for Disease Control and Prevention. *MMWR Recomm Rep* 1996;**45**:1–24.

41. Verani JR, McGee L, Schrag SJ. Prevention of perinatal group B streptococcal disease: Revised guidelines from CDC, 2010. *MMWR Recomm Rep* 2010;**59**:1–36.

42. Hankins GV, Chalas E. Group B streptococcal infections in pregnancy: ACOG's recommendations. *ACOG Newsl* 1993;**37**:2.

43. American Academy of Pediatrics Committee on Infectious Diseases and Committee on Fetus and Newborn. Guidelines for prevention of group B streptococcal (GBS) infection by chemoprophylaxis. *Pediatrics* 1992;**90**:775–778.

44. Schrag SJ, Zell ER, Lynfield R, et al. A population-based comparison of strategies to prevent early-onset group B streptococcal disease in neonates. *N Engl J Med* 2002;**347**:233–239.

45. Harrison LH, Elliott JA, Dwyer DM, et al. Serotype distribution of invasive group B streptococcal isolates in Maryland: Implications for vaccine formulation. Maryland Emerging Infections Program. *J Infect Dis* 1998;**177**:998–1002.

46. Skoff TH, Farley MM, Petit S, et al. Increasing burden of invasive group B streptococcal disease in nonpregnant adults, 1990–2007. *Clin Infect Dis* 2009;**49**:85–92.

47. Black S, Shinefield H, Fireman B, et al. Efficacy, safety and immunogenicity of heptavalent pneumococcal conjugate vaccine in children. Northern California Kaiser Permanente Vaccine Study Center Group. *Pediatr Infect Dis J* 2000;**19**:187–195.

48. Whitney CG, Farley MM, Hadler J, et al. Decline in invasive pneumococcal disease after the introduction of protein-polysaccharide conjugate vaccine. *N Engl J Med* 2003;**348**:1737–1746.

49. Hsu HE, Shutt KA, Moore MR, et al. Effect of pneumococcal conjugate vaccine on pneumococcal meningitis. *N Engl J Med* 2009;**360**:244–256.

50. Centers for Disease Control and Prevention. Direct and indirect effects of routine vaccination of children with 7-valent pneumococcal conjugate vaccine on incidence of invasive pneumococcal disease—United States, 1998–2003. *MMWR Morb Mortal Wkly Rep* 2005;**54**:893–897.

51. Moore M, Link-Gelles R, Farley M, et al. Impact of 13-Valent Pneumococcal Conjugate Vaccine on Invasive Pneumococcal Disease, U.S, 2010–11. In: Submitted to IDWeek San Diego, California. October 17–21, 2012.

52. Whitney CG, Pilishvili T, Farley MM, et al. Effectiveness of seven-valent pneumococcal conjugate vaccine against invasive pneumococcal disease: A matched case-control study. *Lancet* 2006;**368**:1495–1502.

53. Cohn AC, MacNeil JR, Harrison LH, et al. Changes in *Neisseria meningitidis* disease epidemiology in the United States, 1998–2007: Implications for prevention of meningococcal disease. *Clin Infect Dis* 2010;**50**:184–191.

54. Halperin SA, Bettinger JA, Greenwood B, et al. The changing and dynamic epidemiology of meningococcal disease. *Vaccine* 2011;**30**(2):B26–B36.

55. Granoff DM, Harrison LH, Borrow R. Meningococcal vaccines. In: Plotkin S, Orenstein WA, Offit PA, eds. *Vaccines*, 5th ed. Philadelphia: Saunders Elsevier; 2008:399–434.

56. Harrison LH, Dwyer DM, Maples CT, Billmann L. Risk of meningococcal infection in college students. *JAMA* 1999;**281**:1906–1910.

57. Bruce MG, Rosenstein NE, Capparella JM, Shutt KA, Perkins BA, Collins M. Risk factors for meningococcal disease in college students. *JAMA* 2001;**286**:688–693.

58. Centers for Disease Control and Prevention. Meningococcal disease and college students. Recommendations of the Advisory Committee on Immunization Practices (ACIP). *MMWR Recomm Rep* 2000;**49**:13–20.

59. Bilukha OO, Rosenstein N. Prevention and control of meningococcal disease. Recommendations of the Advisory Committee on Immunization Practices (ACIP). *MMWR Recomm Rep* 2005;**54**:1–21.

60. Centers for Disease Control and Prevention. Revised recommendations of the Advisory Committee on Immunization Practices to Vaccinate all Persons aged 11–18 years with meningococcal conjugate vaccine. *MMWR Morb Mortal Wkly Rep* 2007;**56**:794–795.

61. MacNeil J, Cohn AC, Mair R, Zell ER, Clark TA, Messonnier NE. Interim Analysis of the Effectiveness of Quadrivalent Meningococcal Conjugate Vaccine (MenACWY-D): A Matched Case-Control Study. In: 17th International Pathogenic Neisseria Conference. Banff, Canada. 2010.

62. Centers for Disease Control and Prevention. Updated recommendations for use of meningococcal conjugate vaccines—Advisory Committee on Immunization Practices

(ACIP), 2010. *MMWR Morb Mortal Wkly Rep* 2011;**60**: 72–76.

63. Centers for Disease Control and Prevention. Licensure of a meningococcal conjugate vaccine for children aged 2 through 10 years and updated booster dose guidance for adolescents and other persons at increased risk for meningococcal disease—Advisory Committee on Immunization Practices (ACIP), 2011. *MMWR Morb Mortal Wkly Rep* 2011;**60**:1018–1019.

64. Moore MR, Gertz RE Jr, Woodbury RL, et al. Population snapshot of emergent *Streptococcus pneumoniae* serotype 19A in the United States, 2005. *J Infect Dis* 2008;**197**:1016–1027.

65. Harrison LH, Shutt KA, Schmink SE, et al. Population structure and capsular switching of invasive *Neisseria meningitidis* isolates in the pre-meningococcal conjugate vaccine era—United States, 2000–2005. *J Infect Dis* 2010;**201**:1208–1224.

66. Wang X, Shutt KA, Vuong J, et al. Molecular epidemiology of *Neisseria meningitidis* in the United States before and after quadrivalent meningococcal conjugate vaccine introduction. In: Submitted to the 18th International Pathogenic Neisseria Conference. Würzburg, Germany. 2012.

67. Wiringa AE, Shutt KA, Marsh JW, et al. Geotemporal analysis of *Neisseria meningitidis* clones in the United States: 2000–2005. *PLoS One* 2013;**8**(12):e82048.

68. Overhage JM, Grannis S, McDonald CJ. A comparison of the completeness and timeliness of automated electronic laboratory reporting and spontaneous reporting of notifiable conditions. *Am J Public Health* 2008;**98**: 344–350.

69. Panackal AA, M'Ikanatha NM, Tsui FC, et al. Automatic electronic laboratory-based reporting of notifiable infectious diseases at a large health system. *Emerg Infect Dis* 2002;**8**:685–691.

70. Lenert L, Sundwall DN. Public health surveillance and meaningful use regulations: A crisis of opportunity. *Am J Public Health* 2012;**102**:e1–e7.

71. Apte M, Neidell M, Furuya EY, Caplan D, Glied S, Larson E. Using electronically available inpatient hospital data for research. *Clin Transl Sci* 2011;**4**:338–345.

72. Centers for Disease Control and Prevention. Automated detection and reporting of notifiable diseases using electronic medical records versus passive surveillance—Massachusetts, June 2006–July 2007. *MMWR Morb Mortal Wkly Rep* 2008;**57**:373–376.

73. Bauer M, Reinhart K. Molecular diagnostics of sepsis—Where are we today? *Int J Med Microbiol* 2010;**300**:411–413.

74. Breitkopf C, Hammel D, Scheld HH, Peters G, Becker K. Impact of a molecular approach to improve the microbiological diagnosis of infective heart valve endocarditis. *Circulation* 2005;**111**:1415–1421.

75. Centers for Disease Control and Prevention. 2014 National notifiable infectious conditions. 2014. Available at http://wwwn.cdc.gov/NNDSS/script/ConditionList.aspx?Type=0&Yr=2014 (accessed March 23, 2014).

76. Centers for Disease Control and Prevention. Comparison of meningococcal disease surveillance systems—United States, 2005–2008. *MMWR Morb Mortal Wkly Rep* 2012;**61**: 306–308.

77. Kyaw MH, Rose CE Jr, Fry AM, et al. The influence of chronic illnesses on the incidence of invasive pneumococcal disease in adults. *J Infect Dis* 2005;**192**:377–386.

78. Soto K, Petit S, Hadler JL. Changing disparities in invasive pneumococcal disease by socioeconomic status and race/ethnicity in Connecticut, 1998–2008. *Public Health Rep* 2011;**126**(Suppl 3):81–88.

CHAPTER 8

Surveillance for foodborne diseases

Elaine Scallan[1] and Casey Barton Behravesh[2]

[1] Colorado School of Public Health, Aurora, CO, USA
[2] Centers for Disease Control and Prevention, Atlanta, GA, USA

Introduction

Food may become contaminated by over 250 bacterial, viral, and parasitic pathogens. Many of these agents cause diarrhea and vomiting, but there is no single clinical syndrome common to all foodborne diseases. Most of these agents can also be transmitted by nonfoodborne routes, including contact with animals or contaminated water. Therefore, for a given illness, it is often unclear whether the source of infection is foodborne or not. For example, *Escherichia coli* O157:H7 infections can be acquired by ingesting contaminated food or water or by direct contact with infected animals or persons.

Foodborne diseases are important public health problems worldwide. Diarrheal illness, much of which is foodborne, is a leading cause of mortality in young children. Although diarrheal deaths in developed countries have declined, morbidity remains high. Foodborne diseases can also have an important impact on travel, trade, and development. Prevention of foodborne diseases, therefore, continues to be a challenging and critical public health priority. Surveillance systems for foodborne diseases provide extremely important information for prevention and control.

Foodborne-disease surveillance is typically conducted by local, regional, and national public health authorities who gather reports of diagnosed illnesses. By tracking the number of illnesses over time, surveillance systems can identify demographic, geographic, and temporal trends that can be used by regulators, policy makers, health educators, and others to develop and target interventions aimed at reducing the incidence of disease. Through continued surveillance, the success of these interventions can be evaluated. Surveillance is also crucial for detecting outbreaks of foodborne diseases. Fast and effective outbreak investigations are critical to keeping our food safe. Not only can investigators find and remove unsafe food from the marketplace (e.g., by recalling a contaminated food product) but also investigations provide vital information on what went wrong so that regulatory or other changes can be made to prevent future illnesses.

This chapter describes methods for foodborne-disease surveillance including the advantages and disadvantages of different methods for achieving different public health objectives. The role of surveillance systems in detecting foodborne outbreaks is emphasized.

Objectives of foodborne-disease surveillance

Surveillance is essential to measure, prevent, and control foodborne diseases, as illustrated in Figure 8.1. Information on incidence, trends, and high-risk populations can assist policy makers in prioritizing, monitoring, and

Concepts and Methods in Infectious Disease Surveillance, First Edition. Edited by Nkuchia M. M'ikanatha and John K. Iskander.
Published 2014 by John Wiley & Sons, Ltd.

Epidemiologic and traceback investigations resulted in a recall of 36 million pounds of ground turkey, the largest USDA Class I recall in U.S. history. A Class I recall involves a health hazard situation in which there is a reasonable probability that eating the food will cause health problems or death. Antibiotic resistance profiles of patient and environmental samples matched an identical multidrug-resistant pattern which included several clinically relevant antibiotics. These multidrug-resistant outbreaks highlight the importance of implementing preharvest food safety programs, reducing unnecessary antibiotic usage in animals, and including multidrug-resistant *Salmonella* as an adulterant in food safety legislation.

STUDY QUESTIONS

1. What are the key objectives of foodborne-disease surveillance?
2. Describe each of the different methods for foodborne-disease surveillance.
3. Discuss the differences between active, passive, and sentinel surveillance.
4. Discuss the advantages and disadvantages of each surveillance method for:
   a. examining demographic, geographic, and temporal trends;
   b. evaluating the success of food safety interventions; and
   c. detecting foodborne-disease outbreaks.
5. What series of events must occur between the time when a patient is infected with a foodborne bacteria and the time when public health officials can determine that the patient is part of an outbreak?
6. How are multistate foodborne outbreak investigations conducted? Would these outbreaks have been detected without PulseNet? Why or why not?
7. How can timeliness of surveillance affect response to public health issues, such as outbreak investigations?
8. What are the challenges of investigating outbreaks caused by an ingredient in a food item? How can surveillance systems help? How do positive food samples affect surveillance for outbreak investigations?
9. How did results of antimicrobial testing affect the investigation into the outbreak of *Salmonella* Heidelberg infections?

References

1. Roush S, Birkhead G, Koo D, Cobb A, Fleming D. Mandatory reporting of diseases and conditions by health care professionals and laboratories. *JAMA* 1999;**282**(2): 164–170.
2. Allen CJ, Ferson MJ. Notification of infectious diseases by general practitioners: A quantitative and qualitative study. *Med J Aust* 2000;**172**(7):325–328.
3. Scallan E, Hoekstra RM, Angulo FJ, et al. Foodborne illness acquired in the United States—Major pathogens. *Emerg Infect Dis* 2011;**17**(1):7–15.
4. Thacker S. Historical development. In: Teutsch SM, Churchill RE, eds. *Principles and Practice of Public Health Surveillance*, 2nd ed.New York: Oxford University Press; 2000:1–16.
5. Hutwagner LC, Maloney EK, Bean NH, Slutsker L, Martin SM. Using laboratory-based surveillance data for prevention: An algorithm for detecting *Salmonella* outbreaks. *Emerg Infect Dis* 1997;**3**(3):395–400.
6. Herikstad H, Motarjemi Y, Tauxe RV. Salmonella surveillance: A global survey of public health serotyping. *Epidemiol Infect* 2002;**129**(1):1–8.
7. Tauxe RV. Molecular subtyping and the transformation of public health. *Foodborne Pathog Dis* 2006;**3**(1):4–8.
8. Gerner-Smidt P, Hise K, Kincaid J, et al. PulseNet USA: A five-year update. *Foodborne Pathog Dis* 2006;**3**(1):9–19.
9. Rangel JM, Sparling PH, Crowe C, Griffin PM, Swerdlow DL. Epidemiology of *Escherichia coli* O157:H7 outbreaks, United States, 1982–2002. *Emerg Infect Dis* 2005;**11**(4): 603–609.
10. Anderson AD, Nelson JM, Rossiter S, Angulo FJ. Public health consequences of use of antimicrobial agents in food animals in the United States. *Microb Drug Resist* 2003;**9**(4): 373–379.
11. Food and Drug Administration. National antimicrobial resistance monitoring system. Available at http://www .fda.gov/AnimalVeterinary/SafetyHealth/Antimicrobial Resistance/NationalAntimicrobialResistanceMonitoring System/default.htm (accessed April 4, 2014).
12. Centers for Disease Control and Prevention. Preliminary FoodNet data on the incidence of infection with pathogens transmitted commonly through food—10 states, 2009. *MMWR Morb Mortal Wkly Rep* 2010;**59**(14):418–422.
13. Mounts AW, Holman RC, Clarke MJ, Bresee JS, Glass RI. Trends in hospitalizations associated with gastroenteritis among adults in the United States, 1979–1995. *Epidemiol Infect* 1999;**123**(1):1–8.
14. Wethington H, Bartlett P. The RUsick2 Foodborne Disease Forum for syndromic surveillance. *Emerg Infect Dis* 2004;**10**(3):401–405.
15. Li J, Smith K, Kaehler D, Everstine K, Rounds J, Hedberg C. Evaluation of a statewide foodborne illness complaint surveillance system in Minnesota, 2000 through 2006. *J Food Prot* 2010;**73**(11):2059–2064.

16. Centers for Disease Control and Prevention. Surveillance for foodborne disease outbreaks—United States, 2008. *MMWR Morb Mortal Wkly Rep* 2011;**60**(35):1197–1202.

17. Swaminathan B, Barrett TJ, Hunter SB, Tauxe RV. PulseNet: The molecular subtyping network for foodborne bacterial disease surveillance. *Emerg Infect Dis* 2001;**7**(3):382–389.

18. Centers for Disease Control and Prevention. PulseNet & foodborne disease outbreak detection. 2012. Available at http://www.cdc.gov/features/dsPulseNetFoodborneIllness/ (accessed May 7, 2012).

19. Jackson CR, Fedorka-Cray PJ, Wineland N, et al. Introduction to United States Department of Agriculture VetNet: Status of *Salmonella* and *Campylobacter* databases from 2004 through 2005. *Foodborne Pathog Dis* 2007;**4**(2):241–248.

20. Cavallaro E, Date K, Medus C, et al. *Salmonella* Typhimurium infections associated with peanut products. *N Engl J Med* 2011;**365**(7):601–610.

21. Anderson AD, Nelson MA, Baker NL, Rossiter S, Angulo FJ. Public health consequences of use of antimicrobial agents in agriculture. In: Smulders FJM, Collins JD, eds. *Food Safety Assurance and Veterinary Public Health*. Wageningen: Wageningen Academic; 2005:173–180.

22. Centers for Disease Control and Prevention. Investigation Update: Multistate Outbreak of Human *Salmonella* Heidelberg Infections Linked to Ground Turkey. 2011. Available at http://www.cdc.gov/salmonella/heidelberg/111011/index.html (accessed May 7, 2012).

23. Centers for Disease Control and Prevention. FoodNet population survey. 2012. Available at http://www.cdc.gov/foodnet/studies_pages/pop.htm (accessed May 7, 2012).

Further reading

Centers for Disease Control and Prevention. *Morbidity and Mortality Weekly Report*. Available at www.cdc.gov/mmwr.

Eurosurveillance. Available at www.eurosurveillance.org.

World Health Organization. Weekly Epidemiological Record (WER). Available at http://www.who.int/wer/en/.

CHAPTER 9

Surveillance of healthcare-associated infections

Lennox K. Archibald[1] and Theresa J. McCann[2]

[1] Malcolm Randall Veterans Administration Medical Center, Gainesville, FL, USA
[2] St. George's University, Grenada

Introduction

Each year, approximately 35 million people are hospitalized in the United States, accounting for 170 million inpatient days [1,2]. There are no recent estimates of the numbers of healthcare-associated infections (HAI). However, two decades ago, HAI were estimated to affect more than 2 million hospital patients annually, imposing a financial burden on acute care facilities in excess of $4.5 billion [1]. The mortality attributed to these HAI was estimated at about 100,000 deaths annually. It is likely that the current burden far exceeds these mortality and monetary estimates. The importance of surveillance, prevention, and control of HAI within acute care hospitals is rendered even more compelling by data from the Centers for Disease Control and Prevention (CDC), which indicated that during the 1990s, while the number of general hospital beds have been decreasing across the United States, there has been a concomitant increase in the number of beds in intensive care units (ICU), where patients may be at most risk for HAI [3].

The perennial problem of HAI is compounded by the emergence of antimicrobial resistance among the pathogens that cause these infections. Moreover, there are costs associated with additional inpatient care requirements and protracted duration of hospital stay, expensive agents necessary for treatment of antimicrobial-resistant HAI pathogens, and the toxicities [e.g., renal or hepatic complications] that may be associated with these new agents. There are also costs to the overall community that result from increased prevalence of untreatable infections, increased insurance premiums; and loss of earnings and profits because of job loss and reduced productivity.

Published data from single-center studies have characterized the pathogens commonly associated with HAI in various healthcare settings across the United States and Western Europe, as well as their susceptibility profiles to commonly available antimicrobials. Almost 85% of HAI in the United States are associated with bacterial pathogens, and 33% are thought to be preventable [4]. Because of their documented impact on HAI control and prevention, surveillance of HAI has become a priority in healthcare settings in the United States and in countries across the globe. A key objective in the endeavor to improve patient outcomes includes enhancement of the quality of medical care provided by hospitals through reduction of HAI occurrence, while simultaneously controlling costs. To achieve this objective, surveillance must include monitoring of the quality of care, and monitoring the occurrence, effects, and outcomes of HAI through the estimation of infection rates, using approaches that are strikingly similar to the principles espoused by W. E. Deming for the continuous quality improvement process in manufacturing [5]. These principles include the classification of manufacturing errors as either "special" or "usual" causes. For both manufacturing and healthcare services, the emphasis is on changes at the system rather than the individual level [6].

Concepts and Methods in Infectious Disease Surveillance, First Edition. Edited by Nkuchia M. M'ikanatha and John K. Iskander.
© 2015 John Wiley & Sons, Ltd. Published 2015 by John Wiley & Sons, Ltd.

The estimation of HAI rates in the United States began with surveillance studies of the prevalence and incidence of HAI in individual hospitals conducted in the 1960s [7–9]. The first systematic effort to estimate the magnitude of the problem on a wider scale was made by CDC in a collaborative study of eight community hospitals known as the Comprehensive Hospital Infections Project (CHIP) [7]. Performed in the late 1960s and early 1970s, this study involved very intensive surveillance efforts to detect both hospital- and community-acquired infections. Data from these surveillance efforts suggested that approximately 5% of patients in community hospitals acquired one or more HAI, an estimate that was subsequently widely held to be the national HAI rate.

The purpose and value of HAI surveillance

Microbiology laboratories remain indispensable for carrying out surveillance of infectious diseases primarily because only laboratories can definitely identify and characterize pathogens accurately using standardized testing methodologies.

Methods for HAI surveillance include approaches typically described as either passive or active [10]. In *passive surveillance*, public health officials notify laboratory and hospital staff, physicians, and other relevant sources about infectious disease data that should be reported. These surveillance data sources are expected to voluntarily provide data to the health department or designated reporting center. Although it is less expensive than active surveillance, there is an inherent selection bias in passive HAI surveillance systems—(i.e., the data source is more likely to voluntarily report data indicating the absence rather than presence of HAI, as the latter could put the reporting source in a negative light). In *active surveillance*, public health personnel make contact with laboratory staff regarding specific culture results using standard case definitions. This form of surveillance produces more complete and comprehensive information; however, the data aggregation is more time-consuming and costly compared with passive surveillance [10]. Thus, the validity of infectious disease surveillance data generated by healthcare facilities or microbiology laboratories may vary with the type of surveillance mechanism (i.e., active or passive). Most national surveillance systems for reportable infectious diseases in the United States and Europe are passive. In

contrast, HAI surveillance systems generally tend to be active.

During 1974–1983, CDC carried out the seminal Study on the Efficacy of Nosocomial Infection Control, more commonly known as the SENIC project [4]. One of the objectives of the SENIC project was to derive a precise estimate of the nationwide HAI rate from a statistical sample of U.S. hospitals [11]. The SENIC project was among the first to establish scientifically that HAI surveillance is an essential element of an effective infection control program. With 338 randomly selected general medical and surgical hospitals with 50 beds or more taking part, and examination of over 300,000 patient medical records, the report from the SENIC project estimated that ≥2.1 million HAI occurred among the 37.7 million admissions to the 6449 acute care U.S. hospitals during a 12-month period in 1975 through 1976 [12]. This gave rise to a nationwide overall infection rate of 5.7 HAI per 100 admissions (the infection ratio). Approximately 4.5% of hospitalized patients experienced ~one HAI (the infection percentage). Other key findings of the SENIC project included the following [4]:

1. Hospitals with the lowest HAI rates had both strong surveillance and prevention and control programs.
2. One-third of HAI involving the four major anatomic sites (urinary tract, surgical wounds, respiratory tract, and bloodstream) that would otherwise occur could be prevented by well-organized infection surveillance and control programs.
3. The critical components of an effective HAI preventive program included a balance between surveillance and control efforts; there should be at least one infection control practitioner for and one trained hospital epidemiologist for every 250 hospital beds.
4. HAI rates increased by an average of 3% annually in facilities that had not established infection surveillance and control programs.
5. Different categories of HAI required different control programs, and program effectiveness was not necessarily transferable when applied arbitrarily for control of other classes of HAI.
6. Precise determination of the specific methods and schedules used in performing surveillance was not feasible largely because most of the participating hospitals were performing surveillance for infections at all anatomic sites across all hospital areas. These data suggested that hospital-wide HAI surveillance data

had significant limitations that rendered them invalid for collection of baseline data intended for general comparison.

Subsequently, evidence from other published studies has shown that surveillance activities do, indeed, reduce HAI rates. For example, the collection, calculation, and dissemination of surgeon-specific surgical site infection (SSI) rates to surgeons lowered SSI rates [13–17]. Currently, regulatory and accreditation agencies, such as The Joint Commission (formerly the Joint Commission on Accreditation of Healthcare Organizations [JCAHO]), and the Centers for Medicare and Medicaid Services (CMS) use HAI surveillance data to evaluate the quality of care provided by healthcare institutions. HAI surveillance activities, which enable healthcare facilities to analyze objectively and follow the trends of their own endemic HAI rates over defined time periods, are now an integral component of systemic preventive efforts in healthcare facilities, including acute care hospitals, outpatient clinics, freestanding medical and surgical centers, long-term care facilities, and the home healthcare setting.

The primary purpose of surveillance is to alert clinicians, epidemiologists, and laboratories of the need for targeted prevention activities required to reduce HAI rates. HAI surveillance data help to establish baseline rates that may be used to determine the potential need to change public health policy, to act and intervene in clinical settings, and to assess the effectiveness of microbiology methods, appropriateness of tests, and allocation of resources. Microbiology laboratories might conduct routine surveillance activities for specific microorganisms, special clinical or epidemiologic studies to document trends in incidence or prevalence rates of infections or antimicrobial resistance for certain microorganism-drug combinations, or testing done as part of outbreak investigations. During an outbreak, microbiologic tests may identify the source of the outbreak, trace the spread of the outbreak, or assist in the implementation and evaluation of appropriate control measures. Quantification of baseline (endemic) HAI rates enables hospitals to objectively follow secular trends in these rates, which may be consistent, incremental, or decreasing. If the baseline endemic rate is consistent, any significant variation is usually discernible and may signal that an outbreak is present. As less than 10% of HAI in the United States occur as recog-

nized epidemics [18], HAI surveillance should not be embarked on merely for the detection of outbreaks.

Concept of comparable rates

For surveillance data to be used effectively, infection rates need to be calculated. An infection rate is an expression of the probability of the occurrence of an infection during a certain time interval. The numerator of an infection rate is always the number of infections of a particular type that have been acquired by a specific patient population over a defined time period. For HAI rates to be established as the basis for measuring quality of care, they must be meaningful for comparison either between hospitals or within a single hospital over time.

A *comparable rate* is one that controls for variations in the distribution of major risk factors (e.g., exposure to medical devices, or a surgical procedure) associated with the event. Control for these variables allows the rate to be (1) monitored and analyzed meaningfully within the facility itself or (2) compared with an external standard or benchmark rate. Risk factors are either intrinsic or extrinsic. Intrinsic risk factors includes congenital or hereditary disorders, underlying acquired conditions such as chronic cardiac or pulmonary disease, endocrine disorders, immunosuppression, age and gender, or high severity of illness scores. Extrinsic risk factors include various forms of medical and surgical therapies, procedures or interventions, exposure to antimicrobials or invasive medical devices (e.g. mechanical ventilators, urinary catheters, and chest tubes), receipt of transplanted organs or tissues, duration of hospitalization, or exposure to various healthcare personnel.

There are two types of rate comparisons—intrahospital and interhospital. The primary goals of *intrahospital* comparison are to identify areas within the hospital where HAI are more likely to occur and to measure the efficacy of interventional efforts. Quantification of baseline HAI rates enables hospitals to analyze and follow their HAI trends objectively. Intrahospital monitoring of HAI has the advantage of better control of observer variation, especially for HAI case finding, culturing frequency and technique, and controlling for the case mix of the patient population under study. Unfortunately, sample size comparison within a single facility can be a major problem, especially when monitoring HAI rates associated with surgical procedures. This limitation can be mitigated through participation in a surveillance system that aggregates data from multiple healthcare facilities, thereby enabling *interhospital* comparison of HAI rates.

Interhospital comparison (or comparison to an external standard or benchmark) entails comparing rates with those of other hospitals participating in a multicenter surveillance system. Without external comparisons, hospital infection control departments may not know if the endemic rates in their respective facilities are relatively high or where to focus the limited financial and human resources of the infection control program. Moreover, because only about 10% of HAI occur in recognized epidemics, the endemic infection rate in a facility may be steady and consistent so that variations that signal an outbreak may be absent [18]. An HAI rate found to be relatively high compared with that of other hospitals may suggest a potential problem in the facility of concern. It does not, however, establish by itself that the problem is poor infection control, because it may be a reflection of overzealous or inaccurate case finding, inaccurate aggregation of denominator data, or a reflection of larger numbers of patients requiring invasive medical devices, mechanical ventilation, and antimicrobial usage.

HAI comparisons should be used only as initial guides for setting priorities for further investigation. To be successful, multicenter HAI surveillance and monitoring systems must satisfy three requirements [6]: (1) the purpose must be clear; (2) the system must use standardized HAI definitions, data fields, and protocols; and (3) an aggregating institution must be identified to standardize definitions and protocols, receive the data, assess them for quality, and interpret and disseminate the data to those who need to know [6,19,20]. The CDC has been the central aggregating institution for active HAI surveillance in the United States since the 1960s.

National Healthcare Safety Network

In 1970, CDC helped establish the National Nosocomial Infections Surveillance (NNIS) system, for many years the only source of national data on the epidemiology of HAI in the United States, the pathogens that cause these infections, and their respective antimicrobial susceptibility profiles [21]. Participating hospitals collected and reported to CDC their HAI data on patients using standardized protocols, called surveillance components: for adult and pediatric ICU, high-risk nursery, and surgical patients [21].

In 2004, the NNIS system was combined with two other national healthcare surveillance systems—the National Surveillance System for Healthcare Workers and the Dialysis Surveillance Network—into a single Internet-based system known as the National Healthcare Safety Network (NHSN) [22]. NHSN comprises four surveillance components, each associated with HAI control and prevention: patient safety, healthcare-personnel safety, biovigilance, and electronic surveillance [10]. In June 2007, NHSN released its first report on device-associated infections [23]. Data collected and reported by facilities participating in NHSN include risk-adjusted HAI data, adherence to clinical practices and procedures known to prevent HAI, and incidence and prevalence of multidrug-resistant, healthcare pathogens within the respective facilities. Identities of all NHSN facilities are held confidential in accordance with Sections 304, 306, and 308(d) of the Public Health Service Act. This assurance of hospital confidentiality enhances the likelihood that accurate reporting of infections occurs.

NHSN hospitals collect and report data on all sites of healthcare-associated infection in ICU patients [23]. In addition, ICU-specific denominator data are collected. Thus, site-specific and ICU-specific infection rates may be calculated and risk-adjusted using as the denominator the number of patients at risk, patient days, or days of device use (e.g., days of indwelling urinary catheters mechanical ventilation [Table 9.1]). Graphs with examples of risk-adjusted rates are shown in Figure 9.1.

Table 9.1 Definition of device-associated rates.

Device	Rate
Central line–associated BSI rate	(No. of central line–associated BSIs / No. of central-line days) × 1000
Urinary catheter–associated UTI rate	(No. of urinary catheter–associated UTIs / No. of urinary-catheter days) × 1000
Ventilator-associated pneumonia rate	(No. ventilator-associated pneumonia / No. of ventilator days) × 1000

BSI: Bloodstream infection; UTI: Urinary tract infection.

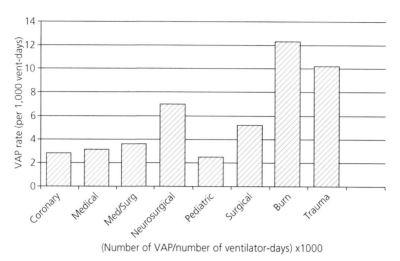

(Number of VAP/number of ventilator-days) x1000

Figure 9.1 Ventilator-associated pneumonia (VAP) rates by type of intensive care unit. Source: 2006 NHSN Annual Report, posted at http://www.cdc.gov/nhsn/dataStat.html.

Because the NHSN allows for uniform collection and analysis of data, several states, including California, Colorado, Illinois, Missouri, New York, Oklahoma, Pennsylvania, South Carolina, Tennessee, Vermont, Virginia, and West Virginia, require their facilities to report directly to the network. Currently, only 21 states require public reporting of hospital data on surgical site infections, and even when disclosure is mandated the information is often not easily accessible to patients.

Questions to address before instituting HAI surveillance

There are a number of factors to consider when contemplating participation in an aggregated national database for purposes of interhospital comparison [10,20]. The questions below are derived from the principles of epidemiology and more than 20 years of published HAI data from healthcare facilities participating in CDC's NNIS and NHSN systems and should be used to guide decisions on whether to participate in an aggregated national survey.

Are the data collected across institutions with attention to the principles of epidemiology?

The definitions of HAI, along with other data fields, and the populations monitored must be standardized and practical to be useful both to the hospital and the aggregating institutions. The surveillance definitions of HAI usually comprise clinical and laboratory parameters. For example, in hospitals that report infections to CDC, laboratory-confirmed bloodstream infections must meet at least one of three criteria that consist of clinical and microbiological features (Table 9.2) [24].

The importance of integrating clinical medicine, epidemiology, and medical microbiology is exemplified by the construct of HAI surveillance case definitions. If a surveillance definition involves only laboratory parameters, one may not know whether a patient actually acquired a clinically significant infection. One may not know if a patient really acquired an HAI, because nearly all laboratory tests have false-negative and false-positive results. Conversely, if only clinical or epidemiologic parameters are used (e.g., a doctor's note, clinical opinion, or diagnosis), there may be too much subjective variation for the event to be useful in comparisons across institutions.

Finding or establishing events in hospitals (known as case finding), such as documenting mortality or a laboratory-confirmed bloodstream infection from an official line listing, occasionally can be straightforward. In general, however, healthcare workers must be trained so that they are able to reliably and accurately determine if a patient's record indicates an existing HAI. Medical record abstractors have consistently performed poorly on HAI case-finding when compared with infection control practitioners [25]. Limited financial and human resources, including lack of trained personnel, make it nearly impossible to monitor all hospitalized

Table 9.2 Laboratory-confirmed bloodstream infections.

Definition:	The term "laboratory-confirmed bloodstream infection" may be used for all patients and must meet one of the following three criteria:
Criterion 1:	Patient has a recognized pathogen cultured from **one** or more blood cultures *and* the organism cultured from the blood is **not** related to an infection at another site.
Criterion 2:	Patient has the following: at least one of the following signs or symptoms: fever (>38°C), chills, or hypotension *and* signs and symptoms and positive laboratory results are **not** related to an infection at another site *and* at least **one** of the following: a. Common skin contaminant (e.g., diphtheroids, *Bacillus* sp., *Propionibacterium* sp., coagulase-negative staphylococci, or micrococci) is cultured from **two** or more blood cultures drawn on **separate** occasions. b. Common skin contaminant (e.g., diphtheroids, *Bacillus* sp., *Propionibacterium* sp., coagulase-negative staphylococci, or micrococci) is cultured from at least one blood culture from a patient with an intravascular line; and the physician institutes appropriate antimicrobial therapy.
Criterion 3:	Patient ≤ 1 year of age has at least **one** of the following signs or symptoms: fever (>38°C, rectal), hypothermia (<37°C, rectal), apnea, or bradycardia *and* signs and symptoms and positive laboratory results are **not** related to an infection at another site *and* at least **one** of the following: a. Common skin contaminant (e.g., diphtheroids, *Bacillus* spp., *Propionibacterium* spp., coagulase-negative staphylococci, or micrococci) is cultured from two or more blood cultures drawn on separate occasions b. Common skin contaminant (e.g., diphtheroids, *Bacillus* spp., *Propionibacterium* spp., coagulase-negative staphylococci, or micrococci) is cultured from at least one blood culture from a patient with an intravascular line, and physician institutes appropriate antimicrobial therapy.

Source: Modified from Centers for Disease Control and Prevention, National Healthcare Safety Network, July 2013, http://www.cdc.gov/nhsn/pdfs/pscmanual/4psc_clabscurrent.pdf.

patients. Therefore, each hospital must know or be able to identify what group of patients (e.g., adult or pediatric ICU patients versus hospital-wide inpatients) to target or monitor. Just as important, the length of time that the hospital monitors the group must be defined and standardized.

Experience in the NNIS and NHSN surveillance systems has confirmed that targeted surveillance is better than hospital-wide surveillance for three main reasons. First, case finding is more accurate if targeted in a specific area, such as a surgical ICU or another specialized critical care unit. Second, targeting a specialized unit is more efficient for the infection control practitioner and for allocation of resources necessary for patient care. And third, risk adjustment is much more feasible for data aggregated in targeted critical care

units. The ICU, high-risk nursery, and surgical-patient components were developed in the NNIS and NHSN systems primarily to address limitations in the hospital-wide component of the NNIS system, and surveillance efforts are targeted using standardized surveillance methods and more specific denominators, such as device days.

While the mean total number of general medical and surgical beds has decreased over the past few decades, the mean total number of ICU beds in participating hospitals has increased significantly [3]. With the increase in patients requiring critical care comes an accompanying increase in medical device use, severity of illness among patients, and antimicrobia use. In facilities with suboptimal infection control practices, procedures, and polices, these risk factors lead to increased

HAI rates as the proportion of ICU to general beds increases. Thus, ICUs remain areas within acute care facilities that should be targeted for surveillance and comparison of HAI rates.

How are numerator and denominator data chosen for the determination of rates?

A crude overall HAI rate is the combined total number of HAI at all sites (e.g., total number of urinary tract infections, pneumonias, surgical wound infections, bloodstream infections) divided by a measure of the population at risk (e.g., the number of admissions, discharges, patient days). The use of crude HAI rates to characterize a hospital's HAI problem has been seriously questioned or rejected [26,27]. In order to use infection rates as a basis for measuring quality of care, rates must be valid to begin with, and meaningful for comparison, either from one hospital to another or within a hospital over time [20]. Various published reports have addressed the importance of adjusting surveillance data for risk factors (e.g., medical-device use, severity of illness) when comparing mortality rates among hospitals [28,29]. Similar approaches are necessary for HAI rate comparisons [30].

Many investigators and organizations, including the Joint Commission have rejected a crude rate as a valid indicator of quality of care [31]. The reasons were stated by Dr. Robert Haley, the task force chair and a principal investigator in the SENIC project: "A hospital's crude overall HAI rate was considered to be too time-consuming to collect …, unlikely to be accurate, and thus misleading to interpret, and unusable for interhospital comparison" [32]. Before HAI rates are used for interhospital or intrahospital comparison or as indicators of quality of care, they require risk adjustment. A crude overall HAI rate of a hospital provides no means of adjustment for inpatients' intrinsic or extrinsic risks and is therefore meaningless. The CDC has stated categorically that such a rate should not be used for interhospital comparison or measure of quality [33].

Are the monitored populations adjusted for their level of risk?

The importance of risk adjustment of device-associated infection rates in ICUs has been described previously [34]. In these ICUs, there is one dominant risk factor for HAI—exposure to medical devices and invasive procedures. Unlike ICU infections where one risk factor

predominates, the risk of SSI for patients who have undergone surgical procedures is related to a number of factors, including the operative procedure performed, the degree of microbiologic contamination of the operative field, the duration of operation, the existing infection at other anatomic sites, and the intrinsic risk of the patient [13,15,16,35,36]. Because infection control practices cannot ordinarily alter or eliminate these risks, SSI rates must be adjusted for these risks before the rates can be used for comparative purposes. SSI rates traditionally have been categorized by operative procedure, surgeon, and wound class, in an attempt to account for some of these factors. It remains difficult to account for variations in a patient's intrinsic susceptibility to infection.

An SSI risk index that effectively adjusts SSI rates for most operations has been developed by CDC [37]. This risk index uses a scoring system ranging from 0 to 3 and consists of scoring each operation by counting the number of risk factors present from among the following: (1) a patient with an American Society of Anesthesiologists (ASA) preoperative assessment score of 3, 4, or 5; (2) an operation classified as contaminated or dirty-infected (as opposed to "clean"); and (3) an operation lasting over T hours where T is the approximate 75th percentile of the duration of surgery for the various operative procedures reported to the CDC database. The CDC risk index is a better predictor of SSI risk than is the traditional wound classification system and performs well across a broad range of operative procedures. The risk index also predicts varying SSI risks within a wound class, suggesting, for example, that all clean operations do not carry the same risk of wound infection. SSI rates should generally be stratified by risk categories before comparisons are made among institutions and surgeons or across time.

Do analysis and dissemination of aggregated data occur in a simple and timely fashion?

The analysis, interpretation, and dissemination of data are essential characteristics of a surveillance system. The feedback also must be in a form that personnel in an individual hospital can easily understand. To include an individual hospital in the aggregated data, the sample size (e.g., number of patients undergoing an operative procedure or number of device days in an ICU) must be sufficient so that the calculated rate for the hospital (surgeon, unit) adequately estimates the true rate. This is based on the size of the rate denominator. The number of hospitals (surgeons, units) that provide data must also be sufficient to adequately estimate the distribution of the rate.

If patient care personnel perceive the value of surveillance information, they will alter behavior. This requires dissemination of rates, in a simple and routine manner, to those who need to know. The NNIS/NHSN aggregating system achieves this goal by publishing regular reports [38,39]. Moreover, surveillance data can demonstrate whether or not infection rates are changing (i.e., falling, rising, remaining steady) within a hospital. The use of risk-adjusted infection rates and feedback of the distributions of these rates by the aggregating institution back to participating hospitals have helped refine outcome measures that provide more meaningful rates for interhospital comparison [33].

What approach exists to examine the data for inaccuracies or inconsistencies?

The hospital and the aggregating institution share the responsibility for ensuring that data are as accurate as possible. The aggregating institution must have an organized, systematic approach to examine data for inaccuracies. These should include estimates of sensitivity and specificity of the system, edit checks in software to prevent inaccuracy of data entry, and training of data collectors. For example, in one participating NHSN facility, of 150 coronary artery bypass graft (CABG) operations, 97% were ASA score = 1 (normal, healthy patient). Of all other CABG procedures reported to NHSN, only 4% were ASA = 1. Following an investigation, the hospital corrected the inaccuracies in their ASA scores and sent more consistent CABG data. The assessment of the sensitivity and specificity of HAI case finding by an independent, trained observer will add to the credibility of the surveillance system, will help determine ways to adjust rates for hospitals that vary in size and case mix, and will offer ways to improve surveillance activities.

Sensitivity is the ratio of the number of events (e.g., patients with HAI) reported divided by the number of events that actually occurred. Specificity is the reported number of patients without HAI divided by the actual number without HAI. Predictive value positive is the proportion of reported infections that are indeed true infections. Low sensitivity (i.e., missed infections) in a surveillance system is usually more common than low

specificity (i.e., patients reported to have infections who did not actually have infections).

An evaluation of the sensitivity, specificity, and predictive value positive of CDC HAI definitions has been carried out previously [40]. During 1994–1995, CDC completed a pilot study to determine if a chart review methodology could be used to evaluate the accuracy of HAI data reported to CDC. In this study, patient records from NNIS hospitals that had infection control practitioners trained in the application of NNIS criteria were independently reviewed. The numbers of infections reported to CDC were compared to the numbers detected independently. Discrepancies and CDC confirmation were also analyzed. Reviewers detected 77% of reported infections and detected twice as many infections at the four major sites combined—bloodstream, respiratory, urinary tract, and surgical site—as did the hospitals. The sensitivity for reported bloodstream infections, pneumonia, and SSIs were 86%, 69%, and 68% respectively. The specificity for these three infections ranged from 97.9% to 98.7% suggesting that participating hospitals were not overreporting these infections. In conclusion, CDC ICU data were found to be sufficiently accurate and reliable to be used for interhospital comparison.

Data with hospital identifiers that can be made available to the media or the courts may encourage inaccurate reporting of HAI and the misuse of such information. Sensitivity and specificity of infection case finding in the surveillance system could, therefore, be adversely affected. This makes implementation of an ongoing method to obtain regular estimates of the sensitivity, specificity, and predictive value positive of a surveillance system even more critical. External comparisons may be linked to marketing of a particular hospital's services but this endeavor may compromise the confidentiality status of the participating hospital. If rates are used for marketing, there will be an incentive to obtain lower rates. This use of external comparison should be strongly discouraged, because too many uncertainties exist in the data collection, often by hundreds of different data collectors.

Are the data risk-adjusted by anatomic site, service, and device?

HAI rates differ by service and medical specialty areas. Reports from the SENIC project show that surgery patients are not only at highest risk for surgical wound infection but are also at higher risk of pneumonia (four times higher), and for urinary tract infection and bloodstream infection (one and one-half times higher) than medical service patients. These results, however, reflected combined data from the ICU and hospital-wide components, and were not risk-adjusted. By the early 1990s, CDC had begun to report HAI rates that had been adjusted for service. For example, NNIS data collected during 1990–1994 showed a stepwise decrease in HAI rates (calculated as the number of infections per 1,000 patient days) by service as follows: burn or trauma service (15.0), cardiac surgery service (12.5), neurosurgery service (12.0), high-risk nursery (9.8), general surgery service (9.2), and oncology service (7.0). Lowest rates were found on the pediatric service (3.3), the well-baby nursery (1.7), and the ophthalmology service (0.6). In subsequent CDC report summaries from January 1992 through June 2004, HAI rates are risk-adjusted for device use and type of ICU [38]. CDC data has also shown that medical service inpatients appear to be at greater risk of contracting *Clostridium difficile*–associated disease compared with inpatients on the surgical, pediatric, or obstetrics and gynecology services [41]. Because of this variability of HAI occurrence with service, risk adjustment according to service is mandatory when conducting interhospital and intrahospital comparison of HAI rates.

Are rates adjusted by hospital type and geographic region?

It has long been apparent that overall HAI rates differ substantially from one hospital to another. In the mid-nineteenth century, Sir James Y. Simpson found that the rate of death from infection of amputated extremities varied directly with the size of the hospital in which the operation was performed (with larger hospitals having higher rates), a phenomenon he called "hospitalism" [42].

Among the numerous analyses of CDC hospital data carried out over the years, characteristics consistently found to be associated with higher HAI rates include affiliation with a medical school (i.e., teaching vs. nonteaching), size of the hospital and ICU categorized by the number of beds (large hospitals and larger ICUs generally had higher infection rates), type of control or ownership of the hospital (municipal, nonprofit, inves-

tor owned), and region of the country [43,44]. These relationships were consistent for each of the four major anatomic sites of infection. In addition, within these four HAI sites, rates of urinary tract infection, surgical wound infection, and bloodstream infection were generally higher in the Northeast and North-central regions, whereas rates of pneumonia were higher in the West. Subsequent CDC NNIS data show increased rates of *Clostridium difficile* and *Acinetobacter* spp. infections in the Northeast [41,45]. For *C. difficile*, the lowest rates were in nonteaching hospitals, intermediate rates were found in teaching hospitals with <500 beds, and highest rates were observed in teaching hospitals with ≥500 beds.

Various analyses of SENIC and NNIS/NHSN data have shown that differences in patient risk factors are largely responsible for interhospital differences in HAI rates. After controlling for patients' risk factors, average lengths of stay, and measures of the completeness of diagnostic workups for infection (e.g., culturing rates), the differences in the average HAI rates of the various hospital groups virtually disappeared. These findings suggest that much of the differences in observable infection rates of various types of hospitals are because of differences in the degree of illness of their patients, intrinsic factors (e.g., age, co-morbid conditions), and whether or not hospitals have functioning HAI surveillance systems. For all of these reasons, an overall HAI rate, per se, gives little insight into whether the facility's infection control efforts are effective.

Does collection and dissemination of HAI data actually lead to a reduction in rates?

CDC data consistently show or indicate changes in the entire distribution of HAI rates following dissemination of comparative rates. Since 1987, when the CDC aggregating system for HAI began reporting device-associated, device day rates to member hospitals, there has been a 7–10% annual reduction in mean rates for device-associated infections among ICUs in participating hospitals [46]. More recent data show that HAI surveillance and participation in a surveillance network do indeed reduce the risk of SSI in surgical patients [47]. During the decade from 1990 to 1999, CDC documented significant decreases in risk-adjusted HAI rates for respiratory, urinary tract, and bloodstream infections [48]. Other reports show statistically significant decreases in the pooled ventilator-associated pneumonia rates among hospitals following dissemination of a CDC report on comparative infection rates in 1991 [48]. Gaynes and colleagues concluded that disseminating risk-adjusted, reliable infection rates within NNIS/NHSN hospitals contributed to these falls in HAI rates when infection control practitioners, patient caregivers, administrators, and other patient-care personnel perceived that there was value in the data, began to rely on them for decision making, and altered their behavior resulting in reduced HAI occurrence and improved quality of patient care [6].

Limitations of rates for interhospital comparison

Although a hospital's surveillance system might aggregate accurate data and generate appropriate risk-adjusted HAI rates for both internal and external comparison, comparison may be misleading for several reasons. First, the rates may not adjust for patients' unmeasured intrinsic risks for infection, which vary from hospital to hospital. For example, a hospital with a large proportion of immunocompromised patients would be expected to have a population at higher intrinsic risk for infection than one without such a population of patients. Second, if surveillance techniques are not uniform among hospitals or are used inconsistently over time, variations will occur in sensitivity and specificity for HAI case finding. Third, the sample size (e.g,. number of patients, admissions/discharges, patient days, or operations) must be sufficient. This issue is of concern for hospitals with fewer than 200 beds, which represent about 10% of hospital admissions in the United States. In most CDC analyses, rates from hospitals with very small denominators tend to be excluded [37,46,49]. On the other hand, a hospital with fewer than 100 beds and with large enough denominators may validly compare its HAI rates with larger hospitals if the data were collected and analyzed in a similar manner to hospitals within the aggregating system.

Lack of severity of illness adjustment
The validity of HAI rates from ICUs, adjusted for extrinsic risk factors, would be enhanced if they were better adjusted with a direct measurement of patients' severity of illness. Properties of a severity of illness score should include both the details regarding the specificity for a particular HAI as well as the anatomic site of infection. CDC researchers developed Severity of Illness Scoring Systems (SISS) that would be useful for adjustment of ICU HAI rates [50], and eleven studies reported use of some type of a SISS. Four studies correlated SISS with all sites of HAI but did not meet with success; six showed some predictive value between SISS and healthcare-associated nosocomial pneumonia. The Acute Physiology and Chronic Health Evaluation (APACHE II) score is the most commonly used SISS but performs inconsistently and may not be available in many ICUs. Thus, although existing scores predict mortality and resource use, none is presently considered a reliable predictor of HAI rates. Until such measures are available, comparative HAI rates will be limited in their use as definitive indicators of quality of care.

Difficulties of HAI surveillance in the outpatient and home healthcare settings
Increasing numbers of patients are being treated at home for malignant neoplasms that require intravenous chemotherapy, autoimmune conditions that require immunosuppressive therapy, surgical wound care following hospital discharge, chronic infections (e.g., osteomyelitis or endocarditis) that require long-term antimicrobial therapy, chronic urinary problems or renal failure with in-dwelling urinary catheters, or ambulatory peritoneal dialysis. In addition, increasing numbers of long-term care facilities have established high dependency units to manage critically ill residents, who may acquire infections once they become exposed to medical devices and undergo invasive surgical procedures.

Although numbers of infections acquired during home health care or in long-term care are increasing, formal documentation of infections in these settings remains limited largely because few facilities have designated surveillance personnel or, if they do, the designated personnel are unsure about what numerator or denominator data to collect. One of the few successes has been in the area of ambulatory hemodialysis services. In 1999, CDC established the Dialysis Surveillance Network, a voluntary national system to monitor and prevent infections in patients undergoing hemodialysis

[51,52]. With over 100 participating hemodialysis centers, the Dialysis Surveillance Network collects and reports outcome events, including vascular access site infections, to CDC.

The role of microbiologic surveillance in the control and prevention of HAI

Three decades of CDC data have shown that although overall HAI rates at the main anatomic sites (i.e., bloodstream, respiratory tract, urinary tract, and surgical wounds) in healthcare facilities across the United States have been falling, the rate of HAI caused by resistant pathogens have actually been increasing. Thus, control of antimicrobial resistance remains inextricably linked to the control of transmission of healthcare-associated antimicrobial-resistant pathogens and the infections they cause. The seriousness of the problem was underscored in an editorial in *Infection Control and Hospital Epidemiology* by CA Muto, who made the point that "for as long as CDC has measured the prevalence of hospital-acquired infections caused by multidrug-resistant organisms, it has been increasing" [53]. Measures for the prevention and control of communicable infections include measures to eliminate or contain the reservoirs of infectious agents, curtail the persistence of an organism in a specific setting, interrupt the transmission of infection, or protect the host against infection and disease. This approach requires a detailed knowledge of the epidemiology of the infection. For example, inherent in the measures for the prevention and control of HAI are the education of healthcare workers in infection control practices and procedures through published guidelines, and the implementation of surveillance measures to detect changes in the incidence or prevalence rates of HAI.

The ongoing study of the basic epidemiologic features of infections in various healthcare environments has led to evidence-based recommendations for HAI surveillance, prevention and control programs, which have proved highly successful. For example, the Society for Healthcare Epidemiology of America (SHEA) has established evidence-based guidelines to control the spread of methicillin-resistant *Staphylococcus aureus* (MRSA) and vancomycin-resistant enterococcus (VRE) in acute care settings [54,55]. The tenets of the SHEA guidelines are identification and containment of spread

through (1) active surveillance cultures to identify the reservoir for spread; (2) routine hand hygiene; (3) barrier precautions for patients known or suspected to be colonized or infected with epidemiologically important antimicrobial-resistant pathogens, such as MRSA or VRE; (4) implementation of an antimicrobial stewardship program; and (5) decolonization or suppression of colonized patients [55]. There is now growing evidence that active surveillance cultures do indeed reduce the incidence of MRSA and VRE infections and that programs described in the SHEA guideline are effective and cost-beneficial [56–58]. Identification of MRSA-colonized patients on admission to hospital through the conduct of screening surveillance cultures appears to decrease overall infection rates [59].

There are several issues to consider when interpreting environmental culture data: (1) surfaces do not transmit disease, rather transmission is usually because of healthcare workers not washing their hands or cross-contaminating patient care items; (2) for environmental sampling, there are no benchmarks or standards to compare data generated from different culture methods; and (3) epidemiology and clinical relevance are essential for the interpretation of environmental cultures (just because you isolate a pathogen does not necessarily suggest that an infection has occurred).

Conclusion

Although many healthcare facilities around the country aggregate HAI surveillance data for baseline establishment and interhospital comparison, the comparison of HAI rates is complex, and the value of the aggregated data must be balanced against the burden of their collection. The decision to participate should be discussed at all levels within the hospital–from the hospital administrator to the persons who will be involved in collecting the data. If a hospital does not devote sufficient resources to data collection, the data will be of limited value, because they will be replete with inaccuracies. No national database has successfully dealt with all the problems in collecting HAI data and each varies in its ability to address these problems. Healthcare facilities must be aware of these potential biases when assessing their participation. While comparative data can be useful as a tool for the prevention of HAI, in some instances no data might be better than bad data.

Surveillance methods, effectiveness, and initial results. *J Infect Dis* 1969;**120**(3):305–317.

STUDY QUESTIONS

1. The financial costs and mortality related to healthcare-associated infections (HAI) have increased in recent years. Discuss some of the factors contributing to, or responsible for this trend.

2. Explain how antimicrobial resistance can impact the problem of HAI.

3. Describe the concept of a *comparable rate* and explain how it might be used for different risk factors or comparison of rates.

4. The National Healthcare Safety Network (NHSN) comprises four surveillance components associated with HAI control and prevalence. Explain how each of these components is involved with prevention and control of HAIs.

5. List factors that epidemiologists and healthcare facilities should consider before making decisions to participate in a national database of HAI surveillance. Do you agree? Are they all equally important?

6. What are some limitations of using hospital surveillance rates to make interhospital comparisons?

References

1. Centers for Disease Control and Prevention. Public Health Focus: Surveillance, prevention, and control of nosocomial infections. *MMWR Morb Mortal Wkly Rep* 1992;**41**(42): 783–787.

2. Buie VC, Owings MF, DeFrances CJ, Golosinskiy A. National Hospital Discharge Survey: 2006 summary, National Center for Health Statistics. *Vital Health Stat* 2010;**13**(168).

3. Archibald L, Phillips L, Monnet D, McGowan JE Jr, Tenover F, Gaynes R. Antimicrobial resistance in isolates from inpatients and outpatients in the United States: Increasing importance of the intensive care unit. *Clin Infect Dis* 1997;**24**(2):211–215.

4. Haley RW, Culver DH, White JW, et al. The efficacy of infection surveillance and control programs in preventing nosocomial infections in US hospitals. *Am J Epidemiol* 1985;**121**(2):182–205.

5. Deming WE. Out of the Crisis, Center for Advanced Engineering Study: Cambridge, MA; 1986.

6. Gaynes R, Richards C, Edwards J, et al. Feeding back surveillance data to prevent hospital-acquired infections. *Emerg Infect Dis* 2001;**7**(2):295–298.

7. Eickhoff TC, Brachman PW, Bennett JV, Brown JF. Surveillance of nosocomial infections in community hospitals. I.

8. Thoburn R, Fekety FR Jr, Cluff LE, Melvin VB. Infections acquired by hospitalized patients. An analysis of the overall problem. *Arch Intern Med* 1968;**121**(1):1–10.

9. Kislak JW, Eickhoff TC, Finland M. Hospital-acquired infections and antibiotic usage in the Boston City Hospital—January 1964. *N Engl J Med* 1964;**271**:834–835.

10. Allen-Bridson K, Morrell GC, Horan T. Surveillance of healthcare-associated infections. In: Mayhall CG, ed. *Hospital Epidemiology and Infection Control*, 4th ed. Philadelphia: Lippincott Williams & Wilkins; 2012:1329–1343.

11. Haley RW, Quade D, Freeman HE, Bennett JV. The SENIC Project. Study on the efficacy of nosocomial infection control (SENIC Project). Summary of study design. *Am J Epidemiol* 1980;**111**(5):472–485.

12. Haley RW, Culver DH, White JW, Morgan WM, Emori TG. The nationwide nosocomial infection rate. A new need for vital statistics. *Am J Epidemiol* 1985;**121**(2):159–167.

13. Ehrenkranz NJ. Surgical wound infection occurrence in clean operations; risk stratification for interhospital comparisons. *Am J Med* 1981;**70**(4):909–914.

14. Condon RE, Schulte WJ, Malangoni MA, Anderson-Teschendorf MJ. Effectiveness of a surgical wound surveillance program. *Arch Surg* 1983;**118**(3):303–307.

15. Cruse PJ, Foord R. The epidemiology of wound infection. A 10-year prospective study of 62,939 wounds. *Surg Clin North Am* 1980;**60**(1):27–40.

16. Haley RW, Culver DH, Morgan WM, White JW, Emori TG, Hooton TM. Identifying patients at high risk of surgical wound infection: A simple multivariate index of patient susceptibility and wound contamination. *Am J Epidemiol* 1985;**121**:206.

17. Olson MM, Lee JT Jr. Continuous, 10-year wound infection surveillance. Results, advantages, and unanswered questions. *Arch Surg* 1990;**125**(6):794–803.

18. Stamm WE, Weinstein RA, Dixon RE. Comparison of endemic and epidemic nosocomial infections. *Am J Med* 1981;**70**(2):393–397.

19. Gaynes RP. Surveillance of nosocomial infections: A fundamental ingredient for quality. *Infect Control Hosp Epidemiol* 1997;**18**(7):475–478.

20. Archibald LK, Gaynes RP. Hospital-acquired infections in the United States. The importance of interhospital comparisons. *Infect Dis Clin North Am* 1997;**11**(2):245–255.

21. Emori TG, Culver DH, Horan TC, et al. National nosocomial infections surveillance system (NNIS): Description of surveillance methods. *Am J Infect Control* 1991;**19**(1):19–35.

22. Tokars JI, Richards C, Andrus M, et al. The changing face of surveillance for health care-associated infections. *Clin Infect Dis* 2004;**39**(9):1347–1352.

23. Edwards JR, Peterson KD, Andrus ML, et al. National Healthcare Safety Network (NHSN) Report, data summary for 2006, issued June 2007. *Am J Infect Control* 2007;**35**(5): 290–301.

Most illegal wildlife seizures originate in Southeast Asia, a hotspot for emerging zoonotic diseases because of rapid population growth, high population density, and high biodiversity [38,40]. Herpesvirus and Simian foamy virus, both of which infect humans, have been found in samples of bushmeat illegally imported into the United States [36], suggesting that zoonotic disease transmission through illegal movement of wildlife or wildlife products is likely to occur.

Zoonotic disease outbreaks place a tremendous economic burden on affected countries because of trade restrictions, travel warnings or restrictions, public health efforts to contain the disease outbreak, culling of exposed or diseased animals to prevent spread, and loss of confidence in animal products [34]. Over the past 2 decades, economic losses resulting from emerging zoonotic diseases have totaled more than $200 billion [34]. In 2009, the H1N1 influenza pandemic (referred to as "swine flu" in early media reports) resulted in $1.3 billion in lost revenue to the pork industry. Within 1 month after initial detection of the outbreak, 27 countries had placed official or unofficial bans on pork from the United States because of unjustified claims that the virus could be transmitted through consumption of pork [41]. Similarly, annual costs to government and industry for control measures during the bovine spongiform encephalopathy (BSE) outbreak in the United Kingdom were estimated at $858 million [42].

Zoonotic disease surveillance

Surveillance is essential for controlling infectious diseases and provides critical information on the spread of disease to new areas or hosts. Surveillance can also be used to inform decisions regarding control measures [43]. Surveillance for zoonotic diseases should utilize a multidisciplinary "One Health" approach which incorporates the complex interactions between human and animal health and the environment, as well as the impact of policy, agriculture, and trade on zoonotic diseases [44].

Under a "One Health" approach, human and animal disease surveillance [43–45] are integrated, because disease surveillance in animals offers opportunities to recognize outbreaks or emergence of new diseases before transmission to or detection in human populations [43,44,46]. Effective surveillance hinges on collaboration and communication between public health,

medical, and veterinary partners [44,47]. To increase this collaboration, the American Veterinary Medical Association (AVMA), the American Medical Association (AMA), and Centers for Disease Control and Prevention (CDC) have joined together to promote movement toward an effective, integrated response to public health and animal health emergencies [28].

Approaches to surveillance

To establish and maintain effective systems, zoonotic disease surveillance relies on multiple surveillance methods in human and animal populations—active, passive, laboratory, syndromic, and sentinel surveillance, as well as biosurveillance.

Active surveillance involves outreach to specific groups to collect data on zoonotic diseases in populations and can detect less common diseases or those targeted for eradication. During the worldwide campaign to eradicate rinderpest, as cases became more infrequent, the Global Rinderpest Eradication Program moved to active surveillance using report registries, questionnaire surveys, participatory epidemiology and investigations, and clinical surveillance for new infections [48]. Active surveillance is also used by CDC's Active Bacterial Core Surveillance program to detect methicillin-resistant *Staphylococcus aureus* (MRSA) and by the USDA's bovine spongiform encephalopathy testing program [49,50]. Unfortunately, active surveillance is often labor- and resource-intensive, so it may not be practical for some zoonotic diseases or settings [51].

Passive surveillance is a less-costly option that relies on voluntary reporting by groups such as physicians, veterinarians, or public health workers. Passive surveillance systems are important components of zoonotic disease surveillance worldwide since they are often easier to implement than active surveillance systems, at least in part because there is less reliance on technology [51] Although requirements vary across public health jurisdictions, high-consequence human infections of animal origin (e.g., brucellosis, hantavirus pulmonary syndrome) are reportable in all jurisdictions and they are nationally notifiable. Data on these and all other nationally notifiable diseases are submitted to a national level surveillance system coordinated by the CDC [52].

Laboratory surveillance, a critical element of a robust zoonotic disease surveillance system, is particularly useful for the detection of rare zoonotic infections in human or animal populations [34,53]. Laboratory-based surveillance is often more timely and better than that of clinical surveillance because of automation of electronic laboratory reporting [54]. Laboratory capacity, however, is often in areas most at risk of zoonotic disease outbreaks [34]. Moreover, in some cases it is hard to detect some pathogens through laboratory methods (e.g., *Franciscella tularensis*) [55].

Syndromic surveillance identifies unexpected changes in prediagnostic information from a variety of sources to detect potential outbreaks [56]. Sources include work- or school-absenteeism records, pharmacy sales for over-the-counter pharmaceuticals, or emergency room admission data [51]. During the 2009 H1N1 pandemic, syndromic surveillance of emergency room visits for influenza-like illness correlated well with laboratory diagnosed cases of influenza [57]. Since syndromic surveillance relies on prediagnostic information, a case definition that accurately captures early clinical signs and symptoms of a disease is essential to minimize the reporting of unrelated diseases and to increase specificity of the system [51].

Sentinel surveillance focuses on disease detection activities among specific subpopulations. Sentinel populations are often chosen based on attributes that make the disease easier to detect or the subjects more convenient to sample. Likewise, a clear relationship between the sentinel and target population is necessary to extrapolate findings from one population to the other [58]. Sentinel surveillance systems can detect pathogen spread into new areas, changes in prevalence or incidence of a pathogen over time, the rate and direction of pathogen spread, and the efficacy of control interventions [59]. Sentinel populations may serve as early warnings of increased risk to the target population. Examples are the use of coyotes as a sentinel for plague in humans in the western United States [60] and the use of avian, mosquito, and climatic data to model the risk of human West Nile cases [61]. Monitoring of sentinel populations may be more cost-effective than monitoring of the target population because fewer samples may be needed or subjects may reside in a smaller geographic area [58]. Although not currently well utilized, surveillance systems using companion animals as sentinels have the potential to detect a wide array of zoonotic diseases [3] in a sensitive and timely manner.

Biosurveillance is relatively new approach that involves analysis of health-related data for early threat and hazard warnings, early detection of events, and rapid characterization and response to minimize adverse health effects [62]. Although biosurveillance incorpo-

rates all hazards (e.g., biological, chemical, radiological), biological agents most likely to be used in a terrorist attack are predominantly zoonotic [63]. Biosurveillance may involve syndromic surveillance of hospital admissions, laboratory surveillance from sources such as the Laboratory Response Network, or monitoring of the ambient air or environment [51]. Regardless of the surveillance strategy used, collection of timely and accurate data to provide situational awareness of population health is a primary goal [62].

Integrated approach to surveillance in humans and animals

Barriers to integrated animal and human surveillance in the United States include technology issues and concerns with data sharing and trust among stakeholders [43]. Only 19% of surveillance systems collect both human and animal data for emerging zoonotic diseases [44] and, only half of zoonotic disease data collected from animals or humans was electronically analyzed [64]. This causes a communication barrier between animal and human health officials and slows the response to human disease outbreaks [34]. However, there are some U.S. programs that have successfully integrated animal and human surveillance. The National Antimicrobial Resistance Monitoring System (NARMS), for example, is a surveillance system that involves collaboration between the U.S. Food and Drug Administration (FDA), USDA, and CDC to monitor for antimicrobial resistant pathogens in retail meats, animals, and humans, respectively. Laboratory surveillance for emerging pathogens may suffer from lack of available testing procedures. In some locations, collection of samples for testing may be unpleasant, arduous or hazardous [43]. Also, clinical signs and symptoms as well as severity of illness often vary among different species infected with the same pathogen [34]. Advances in laboratory techniques for screening and detection of pathogens offer opportunities for enhanced detection of emerging zoonotic diseases and should lead to improvements in surveillance for novel organisms in both human and animal populations [43].

Novel zoonotic disease surveillance systems

There are free or low-cost sources of data that may provide reasonable alternatives to formal zoonotic disease surveillance systems [65].

Several Internet-based reporting systems have been described. ProMED, which has more than 60,000 subscribers in 185 countries, uses in-country infectious disease experts to validate reports of emerging disease outbreaks and provides a model for an affordable, Web-based surveillance system for resource-poor countries [43,45]. HealthMap, another news media–based surveillance system, allows users to search for specific diseases and create maps to display similar disease outbreaks and patterns of movement [54]. Data from these Internet-based systems are not as verified as the data from traditional reporting structures; however, these new systems offer advantages in terms of scalability, coverage, and timeliness [66] and provide powerful new tools for real-time reporting and communication of surveillance data.

Another potential tool for zoonotic disease surveillance is the use of mobile phone technology. Participatory surveillance, which collects data contributed by individuals or communities to better understand disease transmission, was developed to meet the needs of the Global Rinderpest Eradication Program [67]. The use of mobile phone–based surveillance is particularly appealing since increases in network coverage, portability, and ease of access have made this technology readily available in many remote areas [43,66]. Community-based reporting systems can augment traditional disease reporting and surveillance in remote areas currently underserved by public health infrastructure.

Lastly, an innovative surveillance model of wildlife populations has been developed to detect novel zoonotic pathogens at high risk of spillover to human populations in resource-poor countries. PREDICT (http://avianflu.aed.org/eptprogram/pdf/Predict_pager_June2010.pdf), an active surveillance model developed by the Emerging Pandemic Threats Program of the U.S. Agency for International Development (USAID), uses risk modelling and sample collection from wildlife in 20 different countries to locate high-risk areas for zoonotic infection where considerable contact between animals and humans occurs [68].

Bioterrorism

The intentional use of zoonotic pathogens as bioterrorism agents became a national concern in the United States in 2001 following the intentional exposure of several individuals to letters contaminated with anthrax delivered through the U.S. Postal System. Most potential bioterrorist agents are zoonotic, can be intentionally introduced into a country to harm human and/or animal health, and may have devastating economic implications [69]. Significant concerns about the threat of agroterrorism (i.e., a bioterrorist attack on agriculture), namely the economic impact on livestock, poultry, and plant production also exist [70].

CDC and the USDA are responsible for monitoring reports of biological agents and toxins and have developed a select agents and toxins list based on the ability of pathogens to cause severe harm to human and animal health. Laboratories are required under federal law to report the identification of a select agent or toxin to CDC or USDA [71,72]. For zoonotic agents, animals can often be used as early warning sentinels of a bioterrorist attack. For example, Q fever may first be detected by a large increase of abortions in animal herds. In some cases, bioterrorism events are first detected by veterinarians who report unusual animal outbreaks to their local health department [69].

Stakeholders

Zoonotic disease surveillance is dependent on collaboration and communication between animal-health and human-health partners, and many national and international organizations are involved. Globally, the World Health Organization (WHO) and the World Organization for Animal Health (Office International des Epizooties, OIE) are involved in zoonotic disease surveillance. The Food and Agricultural Organization of the United Nations (FAO) also participates in zoonotic disease surveillance by monitoring the food supply for livestock diseases that can affect human health [34]. FAO has a joint initiative with WHO and OIE to provide a tripartite global disease tracking system for major animal and zoonotic diseases, called the Global Early Warning and Response System (GLEWS) [73]. In the United States, the USDA has responsibility for animal health surveillance, and CDC is the human health surveillance equivalent at the national level. These two agencies typically collaborate around zoonotic disease issues and outbreaks. During *Salmonella* outbreaks linked to live-poultry contact, the CDC and the USDA's National Poultry Improvement Program work together to investigate source poultry flocks and inform and educate hatcheries, agriculture feed stores, and the public on ways to reduce infections in poultry and humans. In addition, the CDC and the FDA's Center for Veterinary Medicine collaborate on surveillance for zoonotic diseases related to animal feed, feeder rodents, and small turtles. At the state and local levels, health departments collaborate with physicians and healthcare providers, veterinarians, and laboratories to detect unusual health events and investigate outbreaks.

National surveillance and reporting

In the United States, states mandate which human and animal diseases are reportable within their borders; and local jurisdictions within states can make additional reporting requirements. The five zoonotic diseases most commonly listed as reportable are brucellosis (50 states), anthrax (50 states), rabies (49 states), exotic Newcastle disease (48 states), and highly pathogenic avian influenza (47 states) [74]. Nationally, the USDA in collaboration with the U.S. Animal Health Association (USAHA) and the American Association of Veterinary Laboratory Diagnosticians (AAVLD), collect data monthly on confirmed OIE-reportable diseases from state veterinarians through the National Animal Health Reporting System (NAHRS) [75]. The CDC and the Council of State and Territorial Epidemiologists (CSTE) collaborate in updating a list of nationally notifiable diseases that includes several zoonotic diseases (Table 10.1).

Global surveillance and reporting

Internationally, there are separate reporting requirements and mechanism for human and animal diseases [43]. In 2005, the International Health Regulations (IHR) were adopted to prevent and control the spread of four diseases (smallpox, polio, human influenza caused by a new subtype, and SARS); the IHR require reporting of any case to WHO [76]. Two of the four diseases (novel subtype human influenza and SARS) are zoonotic; influenza virus in particular is of zoonotic importance as multiple human infections have resulted from animal exposure [77–79]. SARS, which rapidly emerged in 2003, is thought to have originated from the exotic live-market animal trade (masked palm civet cats, Chinese ferret-badgers, and raccoon dogs) with bats as a possible reservoir host [80,81]. Under the IHR, other zoonotic diseases are also notifiable to WHO in the event of serious public health impact, an unusual or unexpected disease event, or a significant risk of international spread. Examples include pneumonic plague, viral hemorrhagic fevers (Ebola, Lassa, and Marburg), West Nile fever, and Rift Valley fever [76].

The veterinary equivalent of the IHR, the OIE Terrestrial Animal Health Code, requires participating countries to conduct animal surveillance and notify OIE of outbreaks of animal disease that are on the OIE notifiable diseases list [43]. OIE also maintains an extensive databank called the World Animal Health Information Database (WAHID) Interface that includes notices of disease outbreaks reported by country members, maps of global disease distribution and outbreaks, control measures implemented, and biannual reports of OIE-notifiable disease status in each member country [82].

Initiatives have been undertaken to better integrate animal and human disease reporting worldwide. In 2006, GLEWS was adopted by FAO, OIE, and WHO to provide a united response to human and animal disease emergencies and facilitate data sharing and communication among these three organizations [73]. ProMED provides global surveillance for emerging diseases [83] and is a useful communication tool for electronic reporting of emerging zoonotic diseases globally [84]. In addition, CDC houses the Global Disease Detection program, which responds to or detects zoonotic diseases impacting both humans and animals.

Examples of surveillance for zoonotic diseases

Rabies
Public health importance
Rabies, one of the most important zoonotic diseases globally, is almost uniformly fatal in both animals and people [85]. A member of the lyssavirus family, rabies attacks neurologic tissue and causes serious neurologic symptoms including dysphagia, cranial nerve deficits, abnormal behavior, ataxia, paralysis, altered vocalization, seizures, and death. Rabies can infect all mammals and is most often transmitted through bites from an infected host. The incubation period for rabies typically

Table 10.1 Zoonotic diseases reportable to in humans and animals.[5]

Human cases	Human and animal cases	USDA (animal cases):
Arboviral diseases[2]: • California serogroup virus neuroinvasive disease (La Crosse encephalitis)[1,5] • Eastern equine encephalitis virus disease[1,3] • Powassan virus disease[1] • St. Louis encephalitis virus[1] • West Nile virus disease[1] • Western equine encephalitis virus disease[1]	Anthrax[1,3,4]	Bovine spongiform encephalopathy[2]
Babesiosis[1]	Brucellosis[1,3,4]	Chlamydiosis (avian)[2]
Botulism[1,3]	Glanders[3,4]	Camelpox[2]
Cryptosporidiosis[1]	Hendra virus[3,4]	Cysticercosis (porcine)[2]
Ehrlichiosis[1]	Melioidosis[3,4]	Echinococcosis/hydatidosis[2]
Giardiasis[1]	Nipah virus[3,4]	Highly pathogenic avian influenza (HPAI)[2,4]
Hantavirus pulmonary syndrome[1]	Rift Valley fever virus[3,4]	Japanese encephalitis[2]
Listeriosis[1]	Venezuelan equine encephalitis virus[3,4]	Leishmaniosis[2]
Lyme disease[1]		Newcastle disease virus[2,4]
Monkeypox virus[3]		Screwworm[2] • New World (*Cochliomyia hominivorax*) • Old World (*Chrysomya bezziana*)
Novel influenza A virus infections[1]		Trypanosomosis (tsetse-transmitted)[2]
Plague[1,3]		Vesicular stomatitis[2]
Psittacosis[1]		
Q fever[1,3]		
Rabies[1]		
Rocky Mountain Spotted Fever (Spotted Fever Rickettsiosis)[1]		
Salmonellosis[1]		
SARS-CoV[1,3]		
Shiga toxin-producing *Escherichia coli* (STEC)[1]		
Shigellosis[1]		
Trichinellosis[1]		
Tuberculosis[1]		
Tularemia[1,3]		
Vibriosis[1]		
Viral hemorrhagic fever[1]: • Ebola virus[1,3] • Marburg virus[1,3] • Crimean-Congo hemorrhagic fever virus[1,3] • Lassa virus[1,3] • Lujo virus[1,3] • New World arenaviruses[1,3] (Gunarito, Junin, Machupo, and Sabia viruses)		

Note: Reporting requirements are mandated at the state level, but the CDC and USDA coordinate national surveillance for human and animal diseases respectively.

[1]CDC. Extracted zoonotic diseases from CDC's Nationally Notifiable Diseases [110].

[2]USDA. OIE–confirmed zoonotic diseases reportable to USDA [111].

[3]CDC. Extracted zoonotic diseases from HHS Select Agents and Toxins List [112]. These are select agents reportable by federal law to CDC.

[4]USDA. Extracted zoonotic diseases from HHS Select Agents and Toxins List [112]. These are select agents reportable by federal law to USDA.

[5]In most reported cases, California serogroup virus neuroinvasive disease is caused by La Crosse encephalitis [90].

lasts 3–12 weeks, although longer incubation periods have been reported [24]. In humans, prevention of rabies following a potential exposure consists of post-exposure prophylaxis (PEP). This involves washing the wound with soap and water, followed by infiltration of rabies immunoglobulin around the wound and a series of rabies vaccinations, if indicated [85].

Reservoir hosts for rabies in the continental United States include bats, raccoons, skunks, and foxes. Transmission of rabies virus variants typically occurs in distinct geographic areas and among members of the same species [85]. Surveillance is an essential tool for monitoring spread of rabies variants into new geographic areas and detecting spillover into new host species. In 2007, CDC declared the canine rabies variant eliminated from the United States [86]. Since then, oral rabies vaccination programs in wildlife have become key management tools for preventing the reemergence of the canine rabies variant [85].

Rabies surveillance

Surveillance for rabies in both humans and animals in the United States is laboratory based. Throughout the country, 126 laboratories are able to perform direct fluorescent antibody testing on postmortem brain tissue samples [87]. Results and supplemental information, including species, point location, vaccination history if available, rabies variant if positive, and human or domestic animal exposures are sent to CDC for monitoring of disease trends [88]. Each year, rabies is ruled out in more than 99,000 animals tested; 90% of these are wild animals [85]. The costs saved by avoiding administration of unnecessary PEP through testing of suspect animals are enough to more than cover the expenses involved in maintaining the laboratory surveillance system [85].

Rabies in other countries

Although only 33 human cases of rabies have been reported in the United States since 2002, rabies is an important cause of death in many countries, particularly in Africa and Asia [85]. Rabies is still underreported throughout the developing world, and 100-fold underreporting of human rabies is estimated for most of Africa [44]. Reasons for underreporting include lack of public health personnel, difficulties in identifying suspect animals, and limited laboratory capacity for rabies testing. Studies indicate that proxy measures (e.g., reporting incidence of bite injuries from suspect animals) can provide a valuable source of surveillance data [44]. New initiatives involving mobile telephone technologies are being evaluated to address some of these deficits in reporting [3].

Brucellosis
Public health importance

Brucellosis is a bacterial zoonotic disease caused by the *Brucella* organism and is transmissible to humans primarily through consumption of unpasteurized milk or dairy products (e.g., soft cheeses), direct exposure to birthing tissues or vaginal fluids of infected animals, or laboratory-associated inhalational exposure [6]. Symptoms of *Brucella* infection include malaise, night sweats, and recurrent fever in people; symptoms can persist and progress to arthritis and systemic involvement [89]; and endocarditis and death can also occur [6]. Laboratorians, veterinarians, veterinary personnel, and hunters are at risk through occupational or recreational exposure [6,90]. *Brucella* is classified as a category B bioterrorism agent [90] because of its potential for aerosolization [70]. Brucellosis is a nationally notifiable disease in the United States and other countries [90,91].

Animal brucellosis surveillance

The key to preventing brucellosis in humans is to control or eliminate infections in animals [91–93]; therefore, veterinarians are crucial to the identification, prevention, and control of brucellosis [89]. Brucellosis primarily affects livestock and wild animals including cattle, pigs, sheep, goats, and horses, as well as wild animals such as bison, deer, and elk [94]. Brucellosis remains a high-priority zoonotic disease for USDA because of the economic impact from animal production losses and because of the risk to public health. Since 1954, an ongoing eradication program involving surveillance testing of cattle at slaughter, testing at livestock markets, and whole-herd testing on the farm, has decreased the percentage of infected cattle herds from 11.5000% to 0.0001%. Except for endemic brucellosis in wildlife in the Greater Yellowstone Area, all 50 states and territories in the United States are free of bovine brucellosis [94].

USDA continues to conduct brucellosis surveillance in domestic cattle and bison primarily on samples collected at slaughter. Additional surveillance is conducted in endemic areas such as Greater Yellowstone. Veterinary diagnostic laboratories also routinely perform laboratory-based surveillance on samples submitted from cows with abortion or infertility problems. Lastly, because of U.S. import requirements, USDA–accredited veterinarians test animals imported from non–brucellosis-free countries [94]. According to FAO guidelines, once countries are brucellosis-free, additional surveillance involves targeted testing in border areas where reintroduction can occur from illegal activities, testing any animals that are moved or quarantined, and testing imported breeding age animals and imported semen and embryo products [92].

Human brucellosis surveillance

In 2010, 115 human cases of brucellosis were reported to National Notifiable Diseases Surveillance System (NNDSS), with more than half of cases reported from Arizona, California, Florida, and Texas. Studies have shown a high prevalence of brucellosis in Hispanic populations, predominantly associated with consumption of unpasteurized dairy products and travel to endemic countries [95–97]. Up to 14% of elk hunters, veterinarians, hunting guides, ranchers, park employees, and state veterinary laboratory employees in the Greater Yellowstone Area have been exposed to brucellosis [98]. Additional seroprevalence studies are needed to track prevalence of disease in humans and wildlife in other states like Alaska where human cases of brucellosis have been associated with consumption or handling of game meat [99,100].

Plague
Public health importance

Plague is a rapidly progressive zoonotic disease in humans caused by the bacteria *Yersinia pestis*. Because of its high mortality rate in humans in the absence of early treatment, *Y. pestis* is viewed as one of the most pathogenic human bacteria [101]. In the United States, plague is most often found in the Southwest where it is transmitted by fleas and maintained in rodent populations [102]. Deer mice and voles typically serve as main-

tenance hosts (i.e., enzootic hosts) for *Y. pestis* in the United States, and these animals are often resistant to plague [102]. In contrast, in amplifying host species such as prairie dogs, ground squirrels, chipmunks, and wood rats, plague spreads rapidly and results in high mortality [103].

Human infections with *Y. pestis* can result in bubonic, pneumonic, or septicemic plague, depending on the route of exposure. Bubonic plague is most common; however, pneumonic plague poses a more serious public health risk since it can be easily transmitted person-to-person through inhalation of aerosolized bacteria (e.g., when a person coughs) or from close contact with infected animals (Figure 10.2) [6]. Septicemic plague is characterized by bloodstream infection with *Y. pestis* and can occur secondary to pneumonic or bubonic forms of infection or as a primary infection [6,60].

Plague outbreaks are often correlated with animal die-offs in the area [104], and rodent control near human residences is important to prevent disease [103]. In 2010, two cases of plague were reported from the same household in Oregon. The probable source of infection was a dog in the household that tested seropositive for *Y. pestis*. The do t was most likely infected with infected by fleas. As illustrated in Figure 10.2, in endemic areas, household pets can be an important route of plague transmission and flea control in dogs and cats is an important prevention measure [105].

Plague surveillance

An effective surveillance system for plague is necessary to monitor incidence and distribution of disease. Surveillance is also needed to obtain information on animal sources of human infection and other risk factors for humans, to identify flea and rodent species causing disease, and to detect epidemiologic trends [106]. When plague is detected through surveillance, healthcare providers and the public can be notified, and public health messaging and control measures can be implemented to prevent further infections [107]. Plague surveillance involves monitoring three populations for infection: vectors (e.g., fleas), humans, and rodents [106]. In the United States, fleas are monitored for the presence of plague [103], and data obtained on *Y. pestis* infection rates in fleas helps determine which species are the best vectors of plague and the animal hosts that fleas most prefer [106].

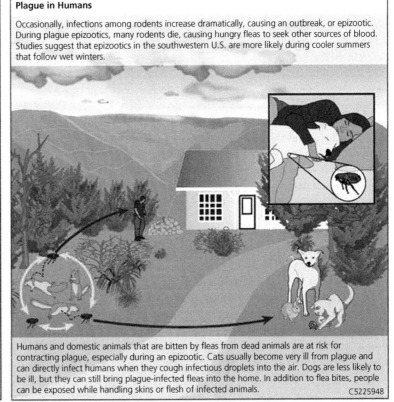

Plague in Nature

Plague occurs naturally in the western U.S., especially in the semi-arid grasslands and scrub woodlands of the southwestern states of Arizona, Colorado, New Mexico and Utah.

The plague bacterium (*Yersinia pestis*) is transmitted by fleas and cycles naturally among wild rodents, including rock squirrels, ground squirrels, prairie dogs and wood rats.

Plague in Humans

Occasionally, infections among rodents increase dramatically, causing an outbreak, or epizootic. During plague epizootics, many rodents die, causing hungry fleas to seek other sources of blood. Studies suggest that epizootics in the southwestern U.S. are more likely during cooler summers that follow wet winters.

Humans and domestic animals that are bitten by fleas from dead animals are at risk for contracting plague, especially during an epizootic. Cats usually become very ill from plague and can directly infect humans when they cough infectious droplets into the air. Dogs are less likely to be ill, but they can still bring plague-infected fleas into the home. In addition to flea bites, people can be exposed while handling skins or flesh of infected animals.

C5225948

Figure 10.2 Plague maintenance cycle in the United States. Plague is caused by infection with *Yersinia pestis*, which can result in various forms of disease depending on route of exposure (e.g., bubonic plague through person-to-person contact.) As shown in this figure, human and domestic animals bitten by fleas are at risk of plague infection. Source: Centers for Disease Control and Prevention.

In the past 20 years, the numbers of human cases of plague reported in the United States have varied from 1 to 17 cases per year [90]. When a new human case is suspected, active surveillance to identify additional cases should be implemented [106], and suspect plague cases should be reported to the local or state health department immediately [107]. A full patient history, including travel during the incubation period, should be obtained; and patient contacts should be identified and tested for infection. Collection of clinical specimens for evidence of *Y. pestis* infection [106] and environmental investigations should be conducted to locate potential plague-infected rodents, infected pets, or infected fleas in the home or workplace [104,106]. The use of syn-

dromic surveillance to detect pneumonic plague has also been proposed [56]. Data taken from sources such as emergency departments or electronic medical records can be cross-referenced with animal data queries. For example, human counts of gastrointestinal symptoms with rapidly progressive respiratory symptoms coinciding with reports of an atypical number of cat or rodent die-offs may point to active plague infections in an area [56].

In the United States, plague surveillance in animals is conducted by state health departments, universities, CDC, and USDA. USDA's National Wildlife Disease Program (NWDP) collects samples from multiple animal species during routine wildlife blood sample collection and submits these samples to CDC for *Y. pestis* testing [60]. Since rodent species are the main reservoirs of the bacteria, these animals can be used for sentinel surveillance to provide an early warning of the public health risk to humans [106]. Rodent surveillance involves tissue and serum sample collection from dead or live rodents, observation of rodent activity, and collection of fleas from rodents to test for *Y. pestis* [106]. Rodent die-offs can often be an early indicator of a plague outbreak [103], so dead rodents should be tested if large numbers are reported in an area [106]. Seroprevalence surveys on live rodents may be performed routinely in plague endemic areas to detect antibodies to *Y. pestis* and identify infected animal hosts and the species of flea found on these animals [106].

In addition, several carnivore species in North America depend on rodents for a large part of their diet and can be infected with plague [102,106]. Thus, a rise in *Y. pestis* seroprevalence in carnivores can suggest an increase of plague activity in rodents. Because of the wide home range of carnivores, carnivore serosurveys are reportedly a more sensitive indicator of plague activity than rodent surveillance [60,106] and may more closely correspond to an increase in human cases of plague [108].

Conclusions

Zoonotic disease surveillance is crucial for protection of human and animal health. An integrated, sustainable system that collects data on incidence of disease in both animals and humans is necessary to ensure prompt detection of zoonotic disease outbreaks and a timely and focused response [34]. Currently, surveillance systems for animals and humans operated largely independently [34]. This results in an inability to rapidly detect zoonotic diseases, particularly novel emerging diseases, that are detected in the human population only after an outbreak occurs [109]. While most industrialized countries have robust disease surveillance systems, many developing countries currently lack the resources to conduct both ongoing and real-time surveillance [34,43]. To decrease the global burden of zoonotic disease, local, national and international stakeholders must work together to improve existing systems, increase the speed and transparency of communication, and enhance the integration of human and animal surveillance data.

STUDY QUESTIONS

1. Define the "One Health" approach. What are its implications for zoonotic disease surveillance?
2. Briefly discuss the level of support for integration of data from humans and animal surveillance systems
3. Provide a brief response to a funding agency that needs to know the reasons for the recent increase in detection of zoonotic diseases.
4. What are some of the reasons that animal and human disease monitoring systems have typically operated separately?
5. Suggest some approaches or ideas that could streamline surveillance for zoonoses.
6. Identify some of the human populations that are at higher risk of acquiring zoonotic diseases.
7. Describe some of the ecologic and environmental factors that lead to emerging zoonotic diseases.

References

1. Krauss H, Weber A, Appel M, et al. *Zoonoses: Infectious Diseases Transmissable from Animals to Humans.* Washington, DC: ASM Press; 2003.
2. Woolhouse ME, Gowtage-Sequeria S. Host range and emerging and reemerging pathogens. *Emerg Infect Dis* 2005;**11**(12):1842–1847.
3. Day MJ, Breitschwerdt E, Cleaveland S, et al. Surveillance of zoonotic infectious disease transmitted by small companion animals. *Emerg Infect Dis* 2012;**18**(12):e1.
4. Goode B, O'Reilly C, Dunn J, et al. Outbreak of *Escherichia coli* O157: H7 infections after Petting Zoo visits, North Carolina State Fair, October–November 2004. *Arch Pediatr Adolesc Med* 2009;**163**(1):42–48.
5. Keen JE, Wittum TE, Dunn JR, Bono JL, Durso LM. Shiga-toxigenic *Escherichia coli* O157 in agricultural fair livestock, United States. *Emerg Infect Dis* 2006;**12**(5):780–786.
6. Colville JL, Berryhill DL. *Handbook of Zoonoses: Identification and Prevention.* St. Louis, MO: Mosby Elsevier; 2007.
7. Howden KJ, Brockhoff EJ, Caya FD, et al. An investigation into human pandemic influenza virus (H1N1) 2009 on an Alberta swine farm. *Can Vet J* 2009;**50**(11):1153.
8. Löhr C, DeBess E, Baker R, et al. Pathology and viral antigen distribution of lethal pneumonia in domestic cats due to pandemic (H1N1) 2009 influenza A virus. *Vet Pathol* 2010;**47**(3):378–386.
9. McMillian M, Dunn JR, Keen JE, Brady KL, Jones TF. Risk behaviors for disease transmission among petting zoo attendees. *J Am Vet Med Assoc* 2007;**231**(7):1036–1038.

10. National Association of State Public Health Veterinarians. Compendium of measures to prevent disease associated with animals in public settings, 2011. *MMWR Morb Mortal Wkly Rep* 2011;**60**(RR–04):1–24.

11. Manini MP, Marchioro AA, Colli CM, Nishi L, Falavigna-Guilherme AL. Association between contamination of public squares and seropositivity for *Toxocara* spp. in children. *Vet Parasitol* 2012;**188**(1–2):48–52.

12. Won KY, Kruszon-Moran D, Schantz PM, Jones JL. National seroprevalence and risk factors for *Zoonotic Toxocara* spp. infection. *Am J Trop Med Hyg* 2008;**79**(4):552–557.

13. Schantz PM, Glickman LT. Toxocaral visceral larva migrans. *N Engl J Med* 1978;**298**(8):436.

14. Uga S, Minami T, Nagata K. Defecation habits of cats and dogs and contamination by *Toxocara* eggs in public park sandpits. *Am J Trop Med Hyg* 1996;**54**:122–126.

15. Baker WS, Gray GC. A review of published reports regarding zoonotic pathogen infection in veterinarians. *J Am Vet Med Assoc* 2009;**234**(10):1271–1278.

16. Myers KP, Olsen CW, Setterquist SF, et al. Are swine workers in the United States at increased risk of infection with zoonotic influenza virus? *Clin Infect Dis* 2006;**42**(1):14–20.

17. Gray G, Baker W. The importance of including swine and poultry workers in influenza vaccination programs. *Clin Pharmacol Ther* 2007;**82**(6):638–641.

18. Croft DR, Sotir MJ, Williams CJ, et al. Occupational risks during a monkeypox outbreak, Wisconsin, 2003. *Emerg Infect Dis* 2007;**13**(8):1150.

19. Centers for Disease Control and Prevention. Multistate outbreak of human *Salmonella* typhimurium infections associated with aquatic frogs—United States, 2009. *MMWR Morb Mortal Wkly Rep* 2010;**58**(51):1433–1436.

20. Centers for Disease Control and Prevention. Update: Potential exposures to attenuated vaccine strain *Brucella abortus* RB51 during a laboratory proficiency test—United States and Canada, 2007. *MMWR Morb Mortal Wkly Rep* 2008;**57**(2):36–39.

21. Miller C, Songer J, Sullivan J. A twenty-five year review of laboratory-acquired human infections at the National Animal Disease Center. *Am Ind Hyg Assoc J* 1987;**48**(3):271–275.

22. Weinstein RA, Singh K. Laboratory-acquired infections. *Clin Infect Dis* 2009;**49**(1):142–147.

23. Trevejo RT, Barr MC, Robinson RA. Important emerging bacterial zoonotic infections affecting the immunocompromised. *Vet Res* 2005;**36**(3):493–506.

24. Psarros G, Riddell IVJ, Gandhi T, Kauffman CA, Cinti SK. Bartonella henselae infections in solid organ transplant recipients: Report of 5 cases and review of the literature. *Medicine* 2012;**91**(2):111.

25. Wallon M, Peyron F, Cornu C, et al. Congenital Toxoplasma infection: Monthly prenatal screening decreases transmission rate and improves clinical outcome at 3 years. *Clin Infect Dis* 2013;**56**(9):1223–1231.

26. Elshamy M, Ahmed AI. The effects of maternal brucellosis on pregnancy outcome. *J Infect Dev Ctries* 2008;**2**(3):230–234.

27. Centers for Disease Control and Prevention. Vital signs: Listeria illnesses, deaths, and outbreaks—United States, 2009–2011. *MMWR Morb Mortal Wkly Rep* 2013;**62**(22):448–452.

28. American Veterinary Medical Association. One health: A new professional imperative. One Health Initiative Task Force Final Report. 2008.

29. Chomel BB, Belotto A, Meslin FX. Wildlife, exotic pets, and emerging zoonoses. *Emerg Infect Dis* 2007;**13**(1):6–11.

30. Woodford MH. Veterinary aspects of ecological monitoring: The natural history of emerging infectious diseases of humans, domestic animals and wildlife. *Trop Anim Health Prod* 2009;**41**(7):1023–1033.

31. Kilpatrick AM, Randolph SE. Drivers, dynamics, and control of emerging vector-borne zoonotic diseases. *Lancet* 2012;**380**(9857):1946–1955.

32. Ogden NH, Lindsay LR, Morshed M, Sockett PN, Artsob H. The emergence of Lyme disease in Canada. *CMAJ* 2009;**180**(12):1221–1224.

33. Rogers DJ, Randolph SE. Climate change and vector-borne diseases. *Adv Parasitol* 2006;**62**:345–381.

34. Keusch G. *Sustaining Global Surveillance and Response to Emerging Zoonotic Diseases*. Washington, DC: National Academy Press; 2009.

35. Karesh WB, Cook RA, Bennett EL, Newcomb J. Wildlife trade and global disease emergence. *Emerg Infect Dis* 2005;**11**(7):1000–1002.

36. Smith KM, Anthony SJ, Switzer WM, et al. Zoonotic viruses associated with illegally imported wildlife products. *PLoS ONE* 2012;**7**(1):e29505.

37. Larkin M. Monkeypox spreads as US public-health system plays catch-up. *Lancet Infect Dis* 2003;**3**(8):461.

38. Rosen GE, Smith KF. Summarizing the evidence on the international trade in illegal wildlife. *Ecohealth* 2010;**7**(1):24–32.

39. Sonricker Hansen AL, Li A, Joly D, Mekaru S, Brownstein JS. Digital surveillance: A novel approach to monitoring the illegal wildlife trade. *PLoS ONE* 2012;**7**(12):e51156.

40. Jones KE, Patel NG, Levy MA, et al. Global trends in emerging infectious diseases. *Nature* 2008;**451**(7181):990–993.

41. Butler D, President, National Pork Producers Council. Testimony of the National Pork Producers Council on the U.S. pork industry economic crisis: Hearing before the US House Committee on Agriculture, Subcommittee on Livestock, Dairy, and Poultry (Oct 22, 2009).

42. Rocourt J, Moy G, Vierk KA, et al. *Foodborne Disease in OECD Countries: Present State and Economic Costs*. Paris: OECD Publications; 2003.

43. Halliday J, Daborn C, Auty H, et al. Bringing together emerging and endemic zoonoses surveillance: Shared

challenges and a common solution. *Philos Trans R Soc Lond B Biol Sci* 2012;**367**(1604):2872–2880.

44. Vrbova L, Stephen C, Kasman N, et al. Systematic review of surveillance systems for emerging zoonoses. *Transbound Emerg Dis* 2010;**57**(3):154–161.

45. Morens DM, Fauci AS. Emerging infectious diseases in 2012: 20 years after the institute of medicine report. *MBio* 2012;**3**(6):e00494-12.

46. Kahn LH. Confronting zoonoses, linking human and veterinary medicine. *Emerg Infect Dis* 2006;**12**(4):556–561.

47. Kruse H, Kirkemo AM, Handeland K. Wildlife as source of zoonotic infections. *Emerg Infect Dis* 2004;**10**(12): 2067–2072.

48. Mariner JC, Jeggo MH, van't Klooster GG, Geiger R, Roeder PL. Rinderpest surveillance performance monitoring using quantifiable indicators. *Rev Sci Tech* 2003;**22**(3): 837–847.

49. Schuchat A, Hilger T, Zell E, et al. Active bacterial core surveillance of the emerging infections program network. *Emerg Infect Dis* 2001;**7**(1):92–99.

50. U.S. Department of Agriculture. Bovine spongiform encephalopathy. 2002. Available at http://www.ces.uga.edu/Agriculture/agecon/outlook/cattle/factsheet.pdf (accessed April 8, 2014).

51. Kman NE, Bachmann DJ. Biosurveillance: a review and update. *Adv Prev Med* 2012;**2012**:1–9.

52. Centers for Disease Control and Prevention. National Notifiable Diseases Surveillance System (NDSS): CDC; 2012. Available at http://wwwn.cdc.gov/nndss/ (accessed March 21, 2013).

53. Merianos A. Surveillance and response to disease emergence. *Curr Top Microbiol Immunol* 2007;**315**:477–509.

54. Sintchenko V, Gallego B. Laboratory-guided detection of disease outbreaks: Three generations of surveillance systems. *Arch Pathol Lab Med* 2009;**133**(6):916–925.

55. Gunnell MK, Lovelace CD, Satterfield BA, Moore EA, O'Neill KL, Robison RA. A multiplex real-time PCR assay for the detection and differentiation of *Francisella tularensis* subspecies. *J Med Microbiol* 2012;**61**(Pt 11):1525–1531.

56. Babin S. Using syndromic surveillance systems to detect pneumonic plague. *Epidemiol Infect* 2010;**138**(01): 1–8.

57. Westheimer E, Paladini M, Balter S, Weiss D, Fine A, Nguyen TQ. Evaluating the New York City emergency department syndromic surveillance for monitoring influenza activity during the 2009–10 influenza season. *PLoS Curr* 2012;**4**:e500563f3ea181.

58. Halliday JE, Meredith AL, Knobel DL, Shaw DJ, Bronsvoort BM, Cleaveland S. A framework for evaluating animals as sentinels for infectious disease surveillance. *J R Soc Interface* 2007;**4**(16):973–984.

59. McCluskey BJ. *Use of Sentinel Herds in Monitoring and Surveillance Systems. Animal Disease Surveillance and Survey Systems.* Ames, IA: Iowa State Press; 2008:119–133.

60. Bevins SN, Baroch JA, Nolte DL, Zhang M, He H. Yersinia pestis: Examining wildlife plague surveillance in China and the USA. *Integr Zool* 2012;**7**(1):99–109.

61. Kwan JL, Park BK, Carpenter TE, Ngo V, Civen R, Reisen WK. Comparison of enzootic risk measures for predicting West Nile disease, Los Angeles, California, USA, 2004–2010. *Emerg Infect Dis* 2012;**18**(8):1298–1306.

62. Centers for Disease Control and Prevention. Concept plan for the implementation of the national biosurveillance strategy for human health [Internet]. U.S. Department of Health and Human Services. 2010. Available at http://www.cdc.gov/osels/phsipo/pdf/Concept_Plan_V1+5+final+for+print+KMD.PDF (accessed April 8, 2014).

63. Ryan CP. Zoonoses likely to be used in bioterrorism. *Public Health Rep* 2008;**123**(3):276–281.

64. Scotch M, Rabinowitz P, Brandt C. State-level zoonotic disease surveillance in the United States. *Zoonoses Public Health* 2011;**58**(8):523–528.

65. Keller M, Blench M, Tolentino H, et al. Use of unstructured event-based reports for global infectious disease surveillance. *Emerg Infect Dis* 2009;**15**(5):689–695.

66. Freifeld CC, Chunara R, Mekaru SR, et al. Participatory epidemiology: Use of mobile phones for community-based health reporting. *PLoS Med* 2010;**7**(12):e1000376.

67. Jost CC, Mariner JC, Roeder PL, Sawitri E, Macgregor-Skinner GJ. Participatory epidemiology in disease surveillance and research. *Rev Sci Tech* 2007;**26**(3):537–549.

68. Morse SS, Mazet JA, Woolhouse M, et al. Prediction and prevention of the next pandemic zoonosis. *Lancet* 2012; **380**(9857):1956–1965.

69. Gubernot DM, Boyer BL, Moses MS. Animals as early detectors of bioevents: Veterinary tools and a framework for animal-human integrated zoonotic disease surveillance. *Public Health Rep* 2008;**123**(3):300.

70. Spickler AR, Roth JA, Lofstedt J. *Emerging and Exotic Diseases of Animals.* Ames, IA: CFSPH Iowa State University; 2010.

71. USDA APHIS. Part II. 7 CFR Part 331 and 9 CFR Part 121 Agricultural Bioterrorism Protection Act of 2002; possession, use, and transfer of biological agents and toxins; final rule. *Fed Register* 2005;**70**:13241–13292.

72. CDC and Office of Inspector General. Possession, use, and transfer of select agents and toxins. Final rule. *Fed Regist* 2005;**70**:13293–13325.

73. World Health Organization. *Global Early Warning System for Major Animal Diseases, Including Zoonoses (GLEWS).* Geneva: WHO; 2007.

74. Allen H. Reportable animal diseases in the United States. *Zoonoses Public Health* 2011;**59**(1):44–51.

75. U.S. Department of Agriculture. National Animal Health Reporting System. 2012. Available at http://www.aphis.usda.gov/wps/portal/aphis/ourfocus/animalhealth?1dmy&urile=wcm%3Apath%3A/aphis_content_library/sa_our_focus/sa_animal_health/sa_monitoring_and

_surveillance/sa_disease_reporting/ct_usda_aphis _animal_health (accessed April 8, 2014).

76. World Health Organization. *International Health Regulations (2005)*, 2nd ed. Geneva: World Health Organization; 2008.

77. Centers for Disease Control and Prevention. Notes from the field: Highly pathogenic avian influenza A (H7N3) virus infection in two poultry workers—Jalisco, Mexico, July 2012. *MMWR Morb Mortal Wkly Rep* 2012;**61**(36): 726–727.

78. Centers for Disease Control and Prevention. Update: Isolation of avian influenza A(H5N1) viruses from humans—Hong Kong, 1997–1998. *MMWR Morb Mortal Wkly Rep* 1998;**46**(52–53):1245–1247.

79. Nalluswami K, Nambiar A, Lurie P, et al. Swine-origin influenza A (H3N2) virus infection in two children–Indiana and Pennsylvania, July–August 2011. *MMWR Morb Mortal Wkly Rep* 2011;**9**:60.

80. Wang L, Eaton B. Bats, civets and the emergence of SARS. In: Childs JE, Mackenzie JS, Richt JA, eds. *Wildlife and Emerging Zoonotic Diseases: The Biology, Circumstances and Consequences of Cross-Species Transmission*. Springer: Berlin, Heidelberg, New York; 2007; 315:325–344.

81. Shi Z, Hu Z. A review of studies on animal reservoirs of the SARS coronavirus. *Virus Res* 2008;**133**(1):74–87.

82. Office International des Epizooties. World Animal Health Information Database (WAHID) Interface. 2012. Available at http://www.oie.int/wahis_2/public/wahid .php/Wahidhome/Home (accessed June 26, 2013).

83. Morse SS, Rosenberg BH, Woodall J. ProMED global monitoring of emerging diseases: Design for a demonstration program. *Health Policy (New York)* 1996;**38**(3):135–153.

84. Cowen P, Garland T, Hugh-Jones ME, et al. Evaluation of ProMED-mail as an electronic early warning system for emerging animal diseases: 1996 to 2004. *J Am Vet Med Assoc* 2006;**229**(7):1090–1099.

85. Blanton JD, Dyer J, McBrayer J, Rupprecht CE. Rabies surveillance in the United States during 2011. *J Am Vet Med Assoc* 2012;**241**(6):712–722.

86. Centers for Disease Control and Prevention. US declared canine-rabies free [Internet]. CDC. 2007. Available at http://www.cdc.gov/news/2007/09/canine_rabies.html (accessed March 19, 2013).

87. Centers for Disease Control and Prevention. Protocol for postmortem diagnosis of rabies in animals by direct fluorescent antibody testing [Internet]. CDC. 2003. Available at http://www.cdc.gov/rabies/pdf/rabiesdfaspv2.pdf (accessed March 21, 2013).

88. Centers for Disease Control and Prevention. Compendium of animal rabies prevention and control, 2011. *MMWR Morb Mortal Wkly Rep* 2011;**60**(RR–6):1–17.

89. Glynn MK, Lynn TV. Zoonosis update. *J Am Vet Med Assoc* 2008;**233**:900–908.

90. Centers for Disease Control and Prevention. Summary of notifiable diseases—United States, 2010. *MMWR Morb Mortal Wkly Rep* 2012;**59**(53):1–111.

91. Seleem MN, Boyle SM, Sriranganathan N. Brucellosis: A re-emerging zoonosis. *Vet Microbiol* 2010;**140**(3): 392–398.

92. Robinson A. *Guidelines for Coordinated Human and Animal Brucellosis Surveillance*. Rome: FAO; 2003.

93. Lee HS, Her M, Levine M, Moore GE. Time series analysis of human and bovine brucellosis in South Korea from 2005 to 2010. *Prev Vet Med* 2012;**110**(2): 190–197.

94. The National Surveillance Unit, APHIS, USDA. National Bovine Brucellosis Surveilance Plan [Internet]. 2012. Available at http://www.aphis.usda.gov/animal_health/ animal_diseases/brucellosis/downloads/nat_bruc_surv _plan.pdf (accessed March 19, 2013).

95. Logan LK, Jacobs NM, McAuley JB, Weinstein RA, Anderson EJ. A multicenter retrospective study of childhood brucellosis in Chicago, Illinois from 1986 to 2008. *Int J Infect Dis* 2011;**15**(12):e812–e817.

96. Troy SB, Rickman LS, Davis CE. Brucellosis in San Diego: Epidemiology and species-related differences in acute clinical presentations. *Medicine* 2005;**84**(3):174–187.

97. Shen MW. Diagnostic and therapeutic challenges of childhood brucellosis in a nonendemic country. *Pediatrics* 2008;**121**(5):e1178–e1183.

98. Luce R, Snow J, Gross D, et al. Brucellosis seroprevalence among workers in at-risk professions: Northwestern Wyoming, 2005 to 2006. *J Occup Environ Med* 2012;**54**(12): 1557–1560.

99. Hueffer K, Parkinson AJ, Gerlach R, Berner J. Zoonotic infections in Alaska: Disease prevalence, potential impact of climate change and recommended actions for earlier disease detection, research, prevention and control. *Int J Circumpolar Health* 2013;**72**:19562.

100. Brody JA, Huntley B, Overfield TM, Maynard J. Studies of human brucellosis in Alaska. *J Infect Dis* 1966;**116**(3): 263–269.

101. Stenseth NC, Atshabar BB, Begon M, et al. Plague: Past, present, and future. *PLoS Med* 2008;**5**(1):e3.

102. Abbott RC, Rocke TE. Plague: U.S. Geological Survey Circular 1372, 79 p., plus appendix. 2012. Available at http:// pubs.usgs.gov/circ/1372 (accessed April 8, 2014).

103. Witmer GW. *Rodent Ecology and Plague in North America*. University of Nebraska-Lincoln, Lincoln, Nebraska: USDA National Wildlife Research Center-Staff Publications; 2004:400. Available at http://digitalcommons.unl.edu/ cgi/viewcontent.cgi?article=1395&context=icwdm _usdanwrc (accessed April 8, 2014).

104. Centers for Disease Control and Prevention. Human plague—four states, 2006. *MMWR Morb Mortal Wkly Rep* 2006;**55**(34):940–943.

105. Centers for Disease Control and Prevention. Notes from the field: Two cases of human plague—Oregon, 2010. *MMWR Morb Mortal Wkly Rep* 2011;**60**(7):214.

106. Dennis D, Gage K, Gratz N, Poland J, Tikhonov I. *Plague Manual: Epidemiology, Distribution, Surveillance and Control.*

Geneva: World Health Organization; 1999. WHO/CDS/CSR/EDC/99.2.

107. Centers for Disease Control and Prevention. Fatal human plague—Arizona and Colorado, 1996. *MMWR Morb Mortal Wkly Rep* 1997;**46**(27):617–620.

108. Brown HE, Levy CE, Enscore RE, et al. Annual seroprevalence of *Yersinia pestis* in coyotes as predictors of interannual variation in reports of human plague cases in Arizona, United States. *Vector Borne Zoonotic Dis* 2011; **11**(11):1439–1446.

109. Heymann DL, Dixon M. Infections at the animal/human interface: shifting the paradigm from emergency response to prevention at source. *Curr Top Microbiol Immunol* 2013;**366**:207–215. [Epub 14 Dec 2012].

110. Centers for Disease Control and Prevention. 2012 case definitions: Nationally notifiable conditions infectious and non-infectious cases. 2012. Available at http://www .ct.gov/dph/lib/dph/infectious_diseases/pdf_forms_/2012 _nationally_notifiable_diseases_case_definitions.pdf (accessed June 27, 2013).

111. World Organisation for Animal Health. OIE-listed diseases, infections and infestations in force in 2014. OIE. 2014. Available at http://www.oie.int/animal-health-in -the-world/oie-listed-diseases-2014/ (accessed April 9, 2014).

112. Centers for Disease Control and Prevention and U.S. Department of Agriculture. HHS and USDA Select Agents and Toxins [Internet]. 2012. Available at http://www .selectagents.gov/resources/List_of_Select_Agents_and _Toxins_2012-12-4.pdf (accessed June 27, 2013).

CHAPTER 11

Surveillance of viral hepatitis infections

Daniel R. Church,[1] Gillian A. Haney,[1] Monina Klevens,[2] and Alfred DeMaria, Jr.[1]

[1] *Massachusetts Department of Public Health, Jamaica Plain, MA, USA*
[2] *Centers for Disease Control and Prevention, Atlanta, GA, USA*

Introduction

In the United States, public health surveillance activities for viral hepatitis vary among jurisdictions. At the national level, the Centers for Disease Control and Prevention (CDC) provide recommendations, guidance, and analysis. In addition to participating in the national surveillance network (National Notifiable Diseases Surveillance System [NNDSS]), state and local health departments are responsible for the development and implementation of their own surveillance systems and adoption of national guidelines. Local policies and resources determine the extent to which surveillance and epidemiological strategies can be implemented and achieved. State and local health departments rely on the active participation of clinical providers and laboratories for key laboratory, clinical, and epidemiological information. Other data sources may also be utilized to further the understanding of the infections, diseases, and disease patterns.

Use of these data supports a range of public health activities. These may include disease prevention and control, program and policy development, evaluation, and resource allocation. However, because surveillance methodologies across the diseases have not been uniformly funded, established, or assessed, viral hepatitis surveillance systems are still evolving.

Clinical background of viral hepatitis

Hepatitis—inflammation of the liver—can have many causes, both infectious and noninfectious. The hepatitis viruses (A through E) are unrelated viruses that primarily cause communicable hepatitis. Prior to the elucidation of specific viral etiologies for hepatitis in the 1960s and 1970s, hepatitis was classified as short-incubation "infectious" hepatitis and long-incubation "serum" hepatitis. Infectious hepatitis was characterized by acute infection, often foodborne with a fecal–oral route of transmission and occurrences in outbreaks or clusters. Serum hepatitis was most commonly recognized as a consequence of blood transfusion and injection drug use, as well as a complication of contaminated medical injections. Hepatitis A and E are etiologic agents causing hepatitis most consistent with what was called infectious hepatitis; and hepatitis B and C are long-incubation, bloodborne, and (particularly hepatitis B) sexually transmitted. Hepatitis D virus is a "defective" virus that depends completely on hepatitis B coinfection to replicate and generally causes more severe disease as a consequence of coinfection.

Blumberg reported Australia antigen in the serum of leukemia patients in 1965 [1] and recognized it as a marker for hepatitis B in 1968 [2]—first designated "hepatitis-associated antigen" (HAA) and then "hepatitis

Concepts and Methods in Infectious Disease Surveillance, First Edition. Edited by Nkuchia M. M'ikanatha and John K. Iskander.
Published 2014 by John Wiley & Sons, Ltd.

B surface antigen" (HBsAg). Hepatitis A virus (HAV) was identified in stool in 1973 [3], and a serologic test for IgM antibody became available after 1977 [4]. Once hepatitis A and B were defined etiologically, there remained hepatitis cases that were "non-A, non-B," in particular long-incubation hepatitis, primarily related to transfusion of blood products, as well as some epidemic infectious hepatitis that was not hepatitis A. After years of seeking the etiologic agent, hepatitis C virus (HCV) was identified, and a serologic test for anti-hepatitis C antibody was reported in 1989 [5,6]. Hepatitis D virus (HDV) was originally thought to be a "delta antigen" of HBV [7]; but, subsequently, it was demonstrated to be a distinct agent that was completely dependent on hepatitis B virus (HBV) infection [8]. Hepatitis E virus (HEV), as a cause of epidemic hepatitis with a fecal–oral transmission route, was first identified in 1983 [9] and was associated retrospectively with earlier outbreaks.

Acute hepatitis of any cause has similar, usually indistinguishable, signs and symptoms. Acute illness is associated with fever, fatigue, nausea, abdominal pain, followed by signs of liver dysfunction, including jaundice, light to clay-colored stool, dark urine, and easy bruising. The jaundice, dark urine, and abnormal stool are because of the diminished capacity of the inflamed liver to handle the metabolism of bilirubin, which is a breakdown product of hemoglobin released as red blood cells are normally replaced. In severe hepatitis that is associated with fulminant liver disease, the liver's capacity to produce clotting factors and to clear potential toxic metabolic products is severely impaired, with resultant bleeding and hepatic encephalopathy. Characteristic laboratory findings of liver damage of any cause are elevations of bilirubin and liver enzymes, such as alanine transaminase (ALT) and aspartate transaminase (AST) [10]. Acute hepatitis may be associated with ALT (or AST) levels from 5 to greater than 100 times the upper limit of normal. Other tests used to evaluate liver function are tests for alkaline phosphatase (a measure of damage and dysfunction), gamma glutamyl transpeptidase (GGT, a measure of liver cell dysfunction), albumin (a protein product of reduced liver function), and measures of clotting. None of these tests is entirely specific to liver disease.

Chronic hepatitis—persistent and ongoing inflammation that can result from chronic infection—usually has minimal to no signs or symptoms; but it might result in fatigue and other nonspecific symptoms. There are a number of methods of assessing the extent of liver damage, including liver biopsy and other less-invasive procedures and tests. Ongoing chronic hepatitis can result in scarring (fibrosis) of the liver that can lead to progressive liver disease and severe damage characterized by cirrhosis (scarring with nodular distortion of the liver architecture) [11]. Cirrhosis leads to severe dysfunction in the metabolic clearing and synthetic functions of the liver, as well as restriction of the blood flow from the gastrointestinal tract through the portal vein to the liver. This portal hypertension leads to risk for gastrointestinal bleeding and shunting of blood to the systemic circulation, further reducing the clearance of potentially toxic substances by the liver tissue that remains. Portal hypertension and low serum albumin contribute to the collection of fluid in the abdominal cavity constituting ascites. A possible complication of chronic inflammation and fibrosis of the liver from any cause is liver cancer.

HAV and HEV infections cause acute disease worldwide, which is self-limited and associated with a low case fatality rate (<1% for A and ~2–4% for E); but hepatitis E has approximately a 10-fold higher mortality rate in pregnant women. Many cases of both infections are subclinical (without recognized illness). The presentation of symptoms is age related. That is, among children <6 years of age, illness is mostly asymptomatic; whereas, among adults, illness is mostly symptomatic (Table 11.1). An effective vaccine to prevent hepatitis A has been available for more than 15 years, and incidence rates of hepatitis A are dropping wherever it is used in routine childhood immunization programs. Hepatitis E has 4 genotypes with different epidemiologic characteristics, but similar disease [12]. While primarily transmitted by the fecal–oral route, infection has also been described as resulting from exposure to products from infected animals.

Hepatitis B and C viruses cause acute hepatitis as well as chronic hepatitis. The acute component is often not recognized as an episode of acute hepatitis, and the chronic infection may have little or no symptoms for many years. With hepatitis B, clearance of infection is age related, as is presentation with symptoms. Over 90% of infants exposed to HBV develop chronic infection, while <1% have symptoms; 5–10% of adults develop chronic infection, but 50% or more have symptoms associated with acute infection. Among those who

Table 11.1 Summary of viral hepatitis A–E, inclusive of serologic tests in clinical use.

Hepatitis	Virus abbreviation	Older nomenclature	Transmission	Chronic	Vaccine	Incubation period, days (range)	Serologic marker	Time to being detectable after infection, range in days	Interpretation
A	HAV	Infectious, epidemic, short incubation	Fecal-oral or foodborne	No	Yes	28 (15–50)	Total antibody	18–21	Past or present infection, immunity
							Anti-HAV IgM	18–21	Recent or current infection
B	HBV	Serum, long incubation	Bloodborne or sexual transmission	Yes (5–90% depending on age)	Yes	90 (45–160)	HBsAg	10–28	Acute or chronic infection
							HBeAg	10–28	Acute or chronic infection with high viral replication
							Anti-HBs Ab	160–240	Past infection, vaccine immunity
							Anti-HBc IgG	45–60	Past or current infection
							Anti-HBc IgM	45–60	Acute or recent infection
							Anti-HBe Ab	90–120	Clearance of HBeAg
							HBV DNA	7–28	Active infection
C	HCV	Non-A, non-B	Bloodborne or sexual transmission	Yes (55–85%)	No	45 (14–180)	Anti-HCV Ab	60–90	Past or current infection
							Anti-HCV	60–90	HCV antibody true positive, past or current infection
							RIBA+		
							HCV RNA	7–14	Current infection
D	HDV	Delta	Only with HBV	Yes, with HBV	HBV vaccine	15–56	Anti-HDV Ab*	Unknown	HDV coinfection or superinfection, HDV viremia
							RT-PCR*		
E	HEV	Epidemic or acute, short incubation	Fecal-oral or zoonotic	No	No	40 (15–60)	Anti-HEV IgG*	21–28	Past or present infection
							Anti-HEV IgM*	21–28	Current or recent infection

*No FDA–approved test available in the United States.

acquire hepatitis C, 15–45% clear the infection; the remainder have lifelong infection unless treated specifically for hepatitis C. (Currently available treatment can result in sustained viral response in 70–90% of those infected). HDV infection can occur as a coinfection with HBV, in which case the course is similar to HBV infection alone; HDV can also superinfect someone with chronic HBV infection, leading to a tendency for more progressive liver disease [13].

A number of laboratory tests (antibody, antigen, and nucleic acid) have provided markers of viral hepatitis that can be used to diagnose infection, monitor patients, and categorize cases for surveillance purposes. These laboratory tests and the basic characteristics and epidemiology of the forms of viral hepatitis are summarized in Table 11.1. Currently, acute hepatitis A, acute hepatitis B, chronic hepatitis B, HBV perinatal infection, acute hepatitis C, and past or present hepatitis C are nationally notifiable for public health surveillance purposes in the United States.

Epidemiology of viral hepatitis

Much of what is known about the epidemiology of viral hepatitis was derived from observations of outbreaks prior to the identification of specific etiologic agents. The development of diagnostic laboratory tests enabled the investigation of cases that could be identified clinically or through serologic surveillance. Public health and military investigations helped define "infectious," "epidemic," and "serum" hepatitides as clinical and epidemiologic entities [14,15]. Specific diagnosis of hepatitis A, hepatitis B (and D), and later hepatitis C allowed for inquiry into risk factors and behaviors associated with infection. Current studies are further defining the epidemiology of hepatitis E.

Investigation of the incidence of viral hepatitis in the United States has been pursued in the past via sentinel surveillance studies of acute hepatitis that CDC funded in six counties around the United States [16]. The Sentinel Counties Study of Viral Hepatitis was a population-based study conducted in seven U.S. counties: Contra Costa, California; San Francisco, California; Multnomah, Oregon; Jefferson (Birmingham), Alabama; Denver (Denver), Colorado; Pinellas (St. Petersburg), Florida; and Pierce (Tacoma), Washington from 1996 to 2006 [17]. All patients in those regions who

were identified with acute viral hepatitis were reported to the respective county health department. Case definitions used for this study required both clinical and serologic criteria. Serum specimens from patients with acute disease were collected within 6 weeks of onset of illness and tested for serologic markers of acute infection with known hepatitis viruses. To obtain epidemiologic information, each patient was interviewed by a trained study nurse, who used a standard questionnaire. The questionnaire collected select demographic, clinical, and risk-factor information for the 2–6 weeks preceding onset of illness. The data collected from this study have been instrumental in understanding the epidemiology of viral hepatitis infections in the United States. However, the understanding of the extent of the epidemics determined by this study and other ongoing disease surveillance is limited because data are only received on individuals accessing care. Asymptomatic acute infection and poor or unavailable measurements for high risk populations, including injection drug users and immigrants from endemic countries, have resulted in questionable estimates of the prevalence and incidence of hepatitis B and C. Further, a lack of understanding of the different types of viral hepatitis by many medical providers [18] has led to many undiagnosed individuals living with chronic infection, who are not captured in disease surveillance systems.

Serologic surveys of various population groups have helped to define demographic and risk correlates of infection. Clinical and population research and observation has produced a risk profile for all of the types of viral hepatitis. A summary of the major risk factors, correlates, and screening recommendations are presented in Table 11.2. These data inform understanding of transmission parameters and what is needed for prevention of transmission. A particularly valuable source of information on the correlates of infection with hepatitis viruses is the National Health and Nutrition Examination Survey (NHANES) [19]. This periodic survey that is performed by the CDC samples the general population. Medical and behavioral histories are collected, as well as clinical specimens that may be tested for markers of infection. However, institutionalized populations, including those that are incarcerated or live in college and university housing are not included in the sampling; and this likely contributes to underestimates of HCV infection [20].

Table 11.2 Summary of viral hepatitis A–E risk history and screening recommendations

Hepatitis type	Relevant risk behaviors/history	Screening recommendation
A	• Travelers to regions with intermediate or high rates of HAV infection • Sex partners of infected persons • Household members or caregivers of infected persons • Men who have sex with men • Users of certain illegal drugs (injection and non-injection) • Persons with clotting-factor disorders	• No screening for chronic infection; screen only those with evidence of acute liver disease of unknown etiology
B	• Infants born to infected mothers • Sex partners of infected persons • Persons with multiple sex partners • Persons with a sexually transmitted disease • Men who have sex with men • Injection drug users • Household contacts of infected persons • Healthcare and public safety workers exposed to blood on the job • Hemodialysis patients • Residents and staff of facilities for developmentally disabled persons • Travelers to regions with intermediate or high rates of Hepatitis B (HBsAg prevalence of 2%)	• All pregnant women • Persons born in regions with intermediate or high rates of hepatitis B (HBsAg prevalence of 2%) • U.S.-born persons not vaccinated as infants and whose parents were born in regions with high rates of hepatitis B (HBsAg prevalence of ≥ 8%) • Infants born to HBsAg-positive mothers • Household, needle sharing, or sex contacts of HBsAg-positive persons • Men who have sex with men • Injection drug users • Patients with elevated liver enzymes (ALT/AST) of unknown etiology • Hemodialysis patients • Persons needing immunosuppressive or cytotoxic therapy • HIV-infected persons • Donors of blood, plasma, organs, tissues, or semen
C	• Current or former injection drug users • Recipients of clotting-factor concentrates before 1987 • Recipients of blood transfusions or donated organs before July 1992 • Long-term hemodialysis patients • Persons with known exposures to HCV (e.g., healthcare workers after needle sticks, recipients of blood or organs from a donor who later tested positive for HCV) • HIV-infected persons • Infants born to infected mothers	• All people born between 1945 to 1965 [55] • Persons who currently inject drugs or who have injected drugs in the past, even if once or many years ago • Recipients of clotting factor concentrates before 1987 • Recipients of blood transfusions or donated organs before July 1992 • Long-term hemodialysis patients • Persons with known exposures to HCV • HIV-infected persons • Children born to infected mothers. (Do not test before age 18 months.) • Patients with signs or symptoms of liver disease (e.g., abnormal liver enzyme tests) • Donors of blood, plasma, organs, tissues, or semen
D	• Those infected with or at risk for HBV virus; perinatal transmission rare	• All HBsAg+ persons [1]
E	• Persons living in or traveling to endemic countries with exposure to contaminated water • Zoonotic transmission possible; significance undetermined	• No screening for chronic infection. Only screen those with evidence of acute liver disease of unknown etiology

Source: Except where noted, adapted from CDC, *Morbidity and Mortality Weekly Report*, September 19, 2008; 57 (RR-8): 8–10 and October 16, 1998; 47 (RR-19): 20–26.

Purpose of viral hepatitis surveillance

The purpose of conducting surveillance is to inform public health action. Acute hepatitis infections are routinely investigated to determine a source of infection (e.g., food, healthcare facility, household contact), to identify contacts, and to limit further transmission [21,22]. Surveillance data can serve as infrastructure to conduct special studies that clarify the role of a specific mode of transmission. For example, concerns about outbreaks of hepatitis B and C among residents of assisted living facilities prompted a surveillance-based case control study among persons >55 years of age to assess risk factors for viral hepatitis [23].

Primarily because of resource constraints, the potential utility of chronic hepatitis surveillance registries for case management has not been established [24]. However, there are a number of reasons to perform surveillance of these infections. First, the routine screening, reporting, and subsequent case management of pregnant women for HBV infection can help insure prevention of chronic infection in the newborn [25]. Second, because acute HBV and HCV infections are frequently not clinically apparent and are underreported, reports of past or present infection may be the only way to identify likely acute infections. Third, surveillance of chronic infection is an important component in the determination of resource allocation and evaluation. Identification of populations at highest risk can guide development of appropriate services. These may include prevention services (e.g., provision of sterile needles and syringes), testing programs, and linkage to care. Finally, linkage to clinical care may be useful in ensuring that individuals with chronic viral hepatitis receive appropriate medical care, including antiviral treatment. It has also been suggested that identification and follow-up of all individuals with chronic HBV or HCV infection can be used to detect other at-risk or infected individuals (e.g., family and household contacts, drug sharing partners) and to ensure appropriate preventive screening or care [18]. Box 11.1 summarizes key reasons to conduct acute and chronic viral hepatitis surveillance.

There have also been discrete studies that have identified other potential uses of chronic viral hepatitis surveillance data. Characterization of a sample of cases reported with chronic hepatitis C was used in New York City to identify where services were needed and found

Box 11.1 Summary of purposes of viral hepatitis surveillance.

Acute viral hepatitis surveillance:
- Detect recent transmission of viral hepatitis, including outbreaks, and inform control measures.
- Define epidemiology and emerging issues.
Chronic viral hepatitis surveillance:
- Prevent perinatal HBV transmission.
- Support the identification of acute viral hepatitis infections.
- Inform service delivery needs, resource allocation, and policy development.
- Link newly diagnosed patients to health care.
- Identify contacts and link to screening and other services.

that while most chronically infected individuals had health insurance, many were not vaccinated and were still susceptible to hepatitis A and/or B [26]. An increase in reported HCV infection among persons between the ages of 15 and 25 in Massachusetts led to the identification of heroin injection as a primary mechanism for exposure. This resulted in prioritization of prevention programs and provider education [27]. San Francisco has routinely used information about cases of chronic hepatitis B to target educational materials in appropriate languages [28].

Analyses using matching with other data sources, such as HIV/AIDS surveillance or refugee health programs, can broaden understanding of risk and disease burden. Matching of case registries may also lead to opportunities for efficient integration of services. For jurisdictions with services in place, surveillance data can support programmatic evaluation, in terms of impact of prevention programs and screening initiatives. For example, surveillance of disease incidence is critical to effective vaccination program implementation and evaluation [29]. Data on incidence of disease supplement data on seroprevalence, vaccination coverage, and adverse events associated with vaccination. In the U.S. vaccination program for hepatitis A, surveillance data described high rates of hepatitis A disease in select racial/ethnic and geographic populations. This information was the basis for the first hepatitis A vaccination recommendations immediately following the availability of the vaccine in the United States [30]. Since then, the vaccination recommendations have expanded in coverage. Currently, hepatitis A vaccine is part of the U.S. childhood immunization schedule recommended by the Advisory Committee on Immunization Practices (ACIP) [31]. Hepatitis surveillance data also served to evaluate the impact of vaccination and provided guidance for the U.S. policy [32]. Surveillance continues to be essential for the elimination of indigenous transmission of hepatitis A; clusters are quickly detected and vaccination offered as postexposure prophylaxis [22].

Surveillance methods

Infection caused by each hepatitis virus presents its own unique set of surveillance requirements and challenges. Acute and chronic viral hepatitis virus infections are nationally notifiable in the United States; however, reporting of viral hepatitis and other diseases is mandated at the state level. Reporting of chronic hepatitis B and C is not required in all jurisdictions. The CDC, on the advice of the Council of State and Territorial Epidemiologists (CSTE), establishes standard case definitions and minimal case reporting requirements that may be updated from time to time. Recent case definitions are presented in Table 11.3. Local and state health departments are charged with gathering and triaging reports for surveillance case classification determination and follow-up.

In general, surveillance begins with a report of at least one positive result of a laboratory marker for viral hepatitis. Reports typically contain minimal information (perhaps just patient name and date of birth) requiring surveillance staff to collect additional data that will allow elimination of duplicate records and follow-up. Most health departments start the investigation by contacting the healthcare provider associated with the most recent positive laboratory result. CDC recommendations for case follow-up include the collection of specific data elements [33]. Health departments attempt to collect this information from providers, thereby realistically limiting data to information that may be found in a medical record. For example, the New York City Department of Health and Mental Hygiene collected country of birth on a sample of persons reported with chronic hepatitis B infection [21]. When providers were unable to report country of birth, surveillance staff contacted patients directly by telephone.

Standardizing case report forms across disease categories allows for improved opportunities to analyze data across notifiable diseases. This is particularly relevant for viral hepatitis where coinfection has clinical implications in the case of HBV and HCV coinfection, as well as for coinfection with HIV [34].

Acute viral hepatitis

Timely identification of acute viral hepatitis is critical for implementing effective control measures. This requires access to both clinical and laboratory information, including in some instances, laboratory test results generally not reported to health departments, such as negative serology results for other hepatitis viral infections and liver function test results.

In the case of HAV, which is transmitted by fecal–oral routes, it is particularly relevant to determine whether a case is a food handler (broadly defined to include anyone who handles something that others ingest, including nurses administering oral medications and dental professionals, as well as cooks, waiters, and other food handlers.) to reduce the risk for widespread transmission. Isolation measures may be implemented. HAV infection in children is often asymptomatic, which may lead to transmission within households, and daycare and school settings. The problem may become apparent with identification of secondary and tertiary cases. Identification of contacts at risk for exposure to HAV whenever cases are identified can permit the use of vaccine and immune globulin to prevent further transmission. For situations where a source case has not been identified, examination of the geographic distribution and risk history of cases may establish potential linkages between cases, as well as identification of a common exposure or risk behavior.

Timely identification and linkage to care for individuals with acute HCV can result in prompt therapy that is more effective in attaining a sustained virologic response than treatment later in the course of infection [35]. However, most people with acute hepatitis C infection are asymptomatic and there are no specific serologic markers for acute infection. It is also challenging to classify acute HCV infection as the CDC recommended case definition [33] relies on ruling out of other causes of acute hepatitis (e.g., negative results of tests for HAV and HBV infection) and supportive clinical data.

in determining surveillance classification and relevant follow-up. Tests and results should automatically be associated with a relevant disease(s) in order to create and/or append to a disease event within a surveillance system. New evidence suggests that certain viral hepatitis laboratory tests, specifically anti-HAV IgM, may have a lower positive predictive value than previously thought [45]. Acute hepatitis B may be less likely to be identified through laboratory testing alone [45].

Laboratory test result information may often be limited in scope and insufficient for viral hepatitis case classification and follow-up. Laboratory information systems do not always contain complete information on case address, race, ethnicity or country of origin, all of which can be useful for viral hepatitis evaluation and response. It is therefore desirable to employ a system that can synthesize information from disparate clinical and laboratory systems to allow health departments to obtain the full range of required demographic, clinical, and epidemiological data.

Increased adoption of electronic health records (EHR) may support case finding activities and assist health departments with automatically obtaining initial supporting data [46]. Disease detection algorithms mining EHR have also been found to assist in case-finding activities for acute viral hepatitis infection with a high degree of sensitivity and specificity [45,47]. However, EHR may not provide all the relevant clinical and epidemiologic information to complete a full case investigation. Therefore, additional follow-up with clinicians may still be required.

Surveillance systems can be highly automated and support electronic inputs from laboratory information systems, electronic medical records and administrative data. Technologies that allow for the rapid entry of data can be incorporated. Optical character recognition (OCR) software can scan information into an electronic format, prompt user review of potential errors, store images for quality assurance and finally transmit data to a surveillance system.

Given the highly confidential nature of viral hepatitis and other public health surveillance data, strict security measures are necessary. Role-based access ensures individuals only have access to cases under their jurisdiction and purview. Security and confidentiality policies and procedures are critical elements for implementation of any surveillance system, but are especially important in automated systems with Web-based access.

Follow-up efforts can benefit from automation. For diseases that require an immediate response, such as hepatitis A, a pager message or other electronic notification can automatically be sent to appropriate public health professionals. For high-volume diseases, such as hepatitis B and C, automated triage of cases to prompt a specific review and response can improve efficiency. Predetermined criteria to sort data as they enter a system can be established. Work flows, defined as electronic in-boxes or queues, hold cases until a specific response is completed and allow for prioritization, communication, and response prompts. In 2007, CSTE discussed and approved the requirement that case definitions should comply with American Health Information Community standards for "automated case reporting from electronic health records or other clinical care information systems." Since 2010, all five notifiable types of viral hepatitis have case definitions that are in compliance with this standard.

Case study

Surveillance of viral hepatitis in Massachusetts

In Massachusetts, viral hepatitis public health response is enhanced through the use of numerous automated systems and workflows. These include sending out case report forms to ordering providers based on a laboratory report, with available information already completed. Upon return, the form is electronically imaged and sent using an HL7 message to the surveillance system. If specific clinical and laboratory criteria are met, the case is sent to an epidemiologist's workflow to assess whether or not it is acute viral hepatitis infection and determine appropriate follow-up measures.

The state was able to identify and expedite enhanced surveillance of an emerging epidemic of HCV infection in young injection drug users [27]. Cases of HCV among people 15–25 years of age are automatically classified as "suspect acute HCV infection" and sent to an epidemiologist for enhanced follow-up. A separate workflow prompts the sending of an acute case report form to ordering providers to obtain additional risk and clinical information. Once the information is returned, the case flows into a final workflow for the epidemiologist to review new information and assign a surveillance case classification status.

To prevent HBV transmission to newborns, the state established several workflows to identify and follow pregnant women with chronic hepatitis B infection. Relevant positive hepatitis B laboratory reports are automatically assessed for gender and age and triaged to ascertain pregnancy status. If determined to be pregnant, the case is prioritized to receive case management services following delivery to ensure the infant receives appropriate immune globulin and vaccination. This has led to an increase in identification of the HBV-infected pregnant women and improved timeliness of follow-up of newborns and other household contacts [48]. The surveillance system allows for documentation of all case management activities and enables state and local officials to share information in real time.

Conclusions

Given the environment of limited resources for viral hepatitis surveillance, more efficient methods are warranted. The most obvious option in the short term is to maximize the use of electronic laboratory reporting and electronic health records, since there is evidence that they provide timely and complete data [49]. CDC could fund jurisdictions to support the implementation of electronic disease notification from electronic health records. A protocol for sampling within special populations of cases might improve efficiency and yield actionable data by decreasing the number of cases requiring follow-up investigations. For example, the New York State Department of Health (NYDOH) conducts investigations of persons under 30 years of age who have been reported with HCV infection. From one cluster of cases investigated by NYDOH, it was determined that ongoing transmission was occurring in an educational facility in one New York county [50]. Other populations that might be efficiently sampled for investigation include persons over 50 and under 19 years of age, in whom acute or recent infections might be related to healthcare and drug use related exposures, respectively. Investigation of potential risk factors for infection in the older cohort may be useful for identifying potential healthcare transmissions given the increased likelihood that people in older age groups will have contact with the healthcare system. Persons with hepatitis B and who are under 19 years

of age may be investigated as potential childhood vaccination failures given that all people under 18 years should have been part of a universal HBV vaccination program (in some states, the threshold age may be higher).

A second option to improve hepatitis surveillance might be to integrate with other infectious disease data management systems leading to economies of scale. A third would be to integrate programmatic surveillance follow-up with other infectious disease surveillance activities such as having STD disease investigation specialists follow up with cases of acute HBV or HCV to identify contacts. Since prevention and services are moving toward integrated approaches [51], it may make particular sense to target both STD and HIV programs. Where populations at risk overlap, integration might yield efficiencies, but no evaluations have yet been conducted.

In addition, partner notification services linked with surveillance activities have been successful at identifying new undiagnosed cases of sexually transmitted infections, including HIV infection [52]. These methodologies have been found to have utility in identifying drug injection partners among people diagnosed with HCV infection [53]. Further exploration and expansion of this type of program may be helpful at addressing incident cases among drug users. While use of surveillance systems to link people to HCV treatment has not been found to be successful, additional support and the availability of new and more effective treatments may improve outcomes [54]. Serosurveillance activities may also be useful supplements to standard surveillance practices to develop better estimates of hepatitis B and C incidence and prevalence in targeted, medically underserved communities.

In summary, surveillance for viral hepatitis is a critical function of public health departments. It poses many challenges and may require significant investment. A well-designed surveillance system will provide the information necessary to assess disease burden and emerging trends and to inform program and policy development. Leveraging surveillance mechanisms for other diseases with common risk factors (e.g., tuberculosis, sexually transmitted infections, HIV), as well as use of emerging technologies, offer opportunities to implement a robust, flexible, sustainable and efficient system that addresses the complex needs posed by viral hepatitis.

Table 12.1 Examples of strategies for STD surveillance.

Characteristic	Case reporting	Sentinel surveillance	Opportunistic surveillance: Positivity in screened populations	Opportunistic surveillance: Administrative data	Population-based studies
Population	Entire population	Representative sample of population	Persons tested or screened for STDs	Persons receiving care in health system	Representative sample of population
Methods	Case reports submitted by health-care provider or laboratory	Data collected from a sample of sites, following common protocols	Review of positivity (number of positive tests divided by number of tests completed)	Review of routinely collected data such as billing, pharmacy, and laboratory records	Probability survey of defined population
Strengths	Routinely collected; national coverage	Allows for detailed information to be collected; flexible	Accounts for changes in screening coverage	Large volume of data; often has unique identifiers to create cohorts	Can estimate population prevalence
Weaknesses	Does not account for changes in population screened or diagnostic tests used; limited variables collected	May not be representative of population of interest	Not generalizable to the unscreened population; trends affected by changes in screening criteria	Limited information available; not generalizable to persons not in care	Expensive and labor intensive; not timely
Example	Nationally notifiable: chlamydia, gonorrhea, syphilis, and chancroid	STD Surveillance Network (SSuN); Gonococcal Isolate Surveillance Project (GISP)	National Job Training Program	Medicaid data	National Health and Nutrition Examination Survey (NHANES)

health care (e.g., they may not be screened for rectal infections) or may result in their being inaccurately categorized as heterosexual on case reports. Sex workers may also fear that disclosure would result in criminal prosecution. Transgender persons may not identify as such, or the surveillance system may only accept gender values of male, female, or missing. Effectively using surveillance data in decision making is contingent on understanding what information may be missing because of systemic bias in the available data.

Strategies for STD surveillance

Strategies for STD surveillance include case reporting; sentinel surveillance; opportunistic surveillance, includ-

ing use of administrative data and positivity in screened populations; and population-based studies (Table 12.1). Given the multiple challenges in effectively conducting surveillance for STDs, the choice of strategy depends on the type of STD and the population of interest. Inference involving multiple data sources and strategies is often necessary to monitor prevalence and incidence of STDs.

Case reporting

State and local laws require that healthcare providers or laboratories report communicable diseases to public health authorities by submitting case reports. Four STDs are reportable conditions in all 50 states: chlamydia, gonorrhea, syphilis, and chancroid [3]. Other STDs, such as neonatal herpes, nongonococcal urethritis, and

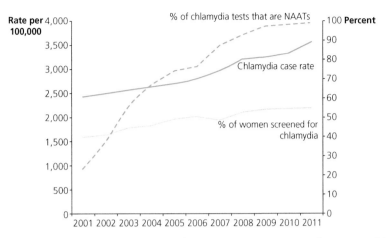

Figure 12.1 Trends in chlamydia case rates among women aged 15–24 years [3], percentage of women aged 16–24 years tested for chlamydia through Medicaid [29], and use of NAAT for screening for chlamydia in women aged 15–24 tested in family planning clinics [54].

Lymphogranuloma venereum, are reportable in some states [25]. Although case reporting has relied historically on individual providers to complete case reports, the use of laboratory reporting for reportable STDs has increased in the last 2 decades. Increasing use of electronic lab reports has likely improved the timeliness and completeness of case reporting [26]. Additionally expanded use of electronic medical records to aid in reporting should further improve the completeness of case reports, particularly for common STDs such as chlamydia [27].

Case reports are the foundation of STD surveillance as they are collected annually, national in scope, available in every locality, and provide important (albeit limited) demographic information such as age, race/ethnicity, and gender to monitor epidemiologic trends and describe health inequities. Additionally, case-report data can aid in prevention and control programs. For example, when a syphilis infection is reported, public health staff contacts the patient to ensure treatment is completed (secondary prevention) and to provide risk reduction counselling and partner notification services (primary and secondary prevention).

Case reports can also provide a sampling frame for probability samples for sentinel surveillance. For example, in the STD Surveillance Network (SSuN) a sample of all reported cases of gonorrhea in participating areas are selected for enhanced interviews to collect additional information not reported on the case-report

form, such as sexual behaviors and clinical signs and symptoms [28].

Trends in case-report data must be carefully interpreted. Case-report data are heavily influenced by advances in diagnostic test technology and, for STDs that are usually asymptomatic, by changes in screening coverage. A prominent example of this is found in chlamydia reporting. From 2001 to 2011 reported case rates of chlamydial infection have steadily increased, and rates are considerably higher among females than males [3]. However, this does not necessarily mean that chlamydia incidence is increasing or that incidence is higher in females, however, as these trends must be considered in the context of the U.S. chlamydia control program (Figure 12.1). As untreated chlamydia can lead to infertility, the CDC recommends that all sexually active young females be screened annually for chlamydia [20]. In the United States, screening coverage has increased steadily since 2001 [29]. During the same time period, an increasing number of tests were completed using nucleic acid amplification tests (NAATs), which are more sensitive than previously used chlamydia tests [3]. Consequently increasing rates in females likely reflect an expanding control program. More infections were identified because more women were screened and they were screened using more sensitive tests. Thus, chlamydia case-report data must be interpreted in the context of trends in testing and diagnostic technology.

Sentinel surveillance

When it is not feasible to conduct surveillance on the entire population, sentinel surveillance strategies may be used. For STDs, sentinel surveillance is often used for monitoring trends in infections that are not nationally reportable or for obtaining information that is not routinely collected on case reports (e.g., individual sexual behavior information or antimicrobial resistance of isolates). The sentinel system may be based on a representative sample of geographic locations, clinics, providers, or patients. For example, the SSuN, in addition to collecting enhanced interview data on a sample of patients diagnosed with gonorrhea, also monitors STDs, STD-related sequelae, and STD-service utilization in a national sample of STD clinics. Findings from SSuN have furthered the understanding of the epidemiology of genital warts by monitoring prevalence by sex and by the sex of the sex partner [3] and by adhering to HIV testing recommendations among patients infected with gonorrhea [30].

Because a limited number of sites are involved, sentinel surveillance allows collection of detailed information. Additionally, sentinel surveillance systems are often flexible and can allow additional data to be collected as epidemics emerge or change. For example, little was known about antimicrobial resistance to *Trichomonas vaginalis*. For a defined period of time, six clinics in SSuN systematically collected specimens from women undergoing physical examinations. Specimens were assayed for susceptibility to antibiotics and provided the first estimates of prevalence of antimicrobial resistance of this protozoan [31]. A key factor in success of sentinel surveillance is that participating sites must follow common protocols to ensure comparability across sites. However, even with common protocols, the sample selected may not be generalizable to the population of interest. Caution must be used in extrapolating estimates from sentinel surveillance to the full population of interest.

Opportunistic surveillance

Some surveillance strategies take advantage of data collected for other purposes to opportunistically monitor trends in STDs. Two examples are monitoring positivity among persons screened or tested for STDs and use of administrative data, such as billing, pharmacy, and laboratory records.

Positivity in populations tested or screened for STDs is calculated as the number of positive tests divided by the total number of tests. Positivity is useful for STD surveillance because estimates take into account any changes in screening coverage (e.g., the denominator increases if more screening occurs). Additionally, as positivity estimates are generally collected in smaller, defined populations, detailed information on persons tested can be collected and compared to the basic demographic data available from case reports. One example of this type of surveillance is the routine monitoring of chlamydia and gonorrhea positivity among females screened in family planning and prenatal care clinics [3].

Positivity can estimate prevalence in the population screened [32], particularly if screening coverage is high. For example, all entrants to the National Job Training Program, a vocational program for socioeconomically disadvantaged youths aged 16–24 years, are routinely screened for chlamydia and gonorrhea. As such, trends in positivity can be interpreted as trends in prevalence in that population [33]. It is important to note that positivity among screened populations is not generalizable to the nonscreened population. First, populations screened may not be representative of the general population or may be a population at higher risk that seeks care for reasons related to STDs. Consequently, positivity in screened populations is likely to be an overestimate of prevalence in the general population. Temporal trends in positivity may be influenced by changes in populations tested and changes in screening criteria [34]. If a clinic begins to target screening to a high-risk population, clinic positivity will increase independent of changes in the underlying population prevalence.

Administrative data, including billing, pharmacy, and laboratory records, provide a rich data source for STD surveillance, particularly for monitoring STDs in patients covered by private health insurance. Administrative data are routinely collected as part of healthcare service delivery and are captured electronically. While not intended for public health surveillance, these data can be used to track trends in STD incidence and prevalence, as well as adverse sequelae, in defined populations. Administrative data are particularly useful for monitoring trends in conditions that are not based solely on a laboratory diagnosis, such as pelvic inflammatory disease [35], as they use multiple sources of clinical care information.

Administrative data may also be used to monitor adherence to STD-related clinical care guidelines. Since 1999, chlamydia screening of sexually active young women has been included as a performance measure for commercial and Medicaid health insurance plans [36]. Federal clinics within the Indian Health Service monitor indicators of STD-related services, such as the proportion of all patients diagnosed with an STD who are tested for HIV [37]. Using routine review of administrative data, facilities can individually track their progress on indicators and apply continuous quality-improvement strategies. Data can also be aggregated nationally in order to better understand patterns of STD-related healthcare services.

Similar to other STD surveillance strategies, there are strengths and limitations to using administrative-based data sources. A primary strength is the large volume of data (i.e., many records on many patients over many time periods). However, administrative data often are missing key demographic variables (e.g., race/ethnicity) [38] and few contain behavioral risk-factor data, limiting their utility. It is often possible to triangulate among multiple data types (e.g., billing data and laboratory results), having the benefit of combining health services data with morbidity data. However, using electronic records for surveillance often relies on diagnosis codes, such as International Classification of Diseases, 9th Revisions (ICD-9) codes, to indicate infection or morbidity. Unfortunately administrative codes may not always align with surveillance case definitions [39] and may be used inconsistently or incorrectly [40], so validation (e.g., verification of codes in comparison with a case definition) is often necessary prior to use. Finally, although electronic records can increase the accessibility and usefulness of databases, datasets are often large and unwieldy. Thus analysis of these datasets requires both extensive computing (e.g., file space) and personnel resources (e.g., trained data managers).

Population-based studies

Using population-based studies as a surveillance strategy can overcome the inherent limitation of other surveillance strategies: that is, that they are biased by healthcare-seeking behavior. By design, case-based and test-based surveillance monitor infections diagnosed by providers. As many STDs are asymptomatic, it is likely that many infections are never diagnosed. To capture true population prevalence, monitoring disease in a nationally representative sample is ideal. The National Health and Nutrition Examination Survey (NHANES) interviews a representative sample of the general population and tests of participants for a variety of STDs, including tests for many infections that are not reportable such as HSV and HPV. Prevalence estimates from NHANES are the bases for national STD prevalence estimates [5,7]. Population-based studies have been used to monitor STD-related sequelae [3,41], risk behaviors associated with STDs [42], and the implementation of prevention and control programs [23,43].

Although many population-based studies are designed to be nationally representative, population-based studies may also be conducted locally. In Baltimore, the Monitoring Sexually Transmitted Infections Survey Program (MSSP), conducted during 2006–2009, sampled residents aged 15–35 years and asked participants to complete a telephone audio–computer assisted self-interview and mail a urine sample for STD testing [44]. In New York City, a local NHANES includes testing for STDs [45]. Both the MSSP and New York City NHANES generate local prevalence estimates that can assist local STD programs in creating targeted prevention messages.

Population-based studies are useful for surveillance, particularly for estimating population prevalence, but they are not widely utilized. Designing and implementing a sampling framework that is representative of a large population requires extensive financial and personnel resources. Few localities have the resources necessary for such studies. Additionally, it may take years for national survey data to become available for analysis and interpretation. As timeliness is an important criterion for the usefulness of a surveillance system [46], population-based survey data may not be suitable for timely public health action.

Case studies

Monitoring antibiotic-resistance gonorrhea

The Gonococcal Isolate Surveillance Project (GISP) was established in 1986 as a sentinel surveillance program designed to monitor trends in antimicrobial resistant *Neisseria gonorrhoeae* infections [17]. GISP includes a network of approximately 30 municipal STD clinics and

5 regional laboratories. Urethral culture specimens are collected monthly from the first 25 male patients who present at each clinic with urogenital symptoms (such as discharge or dysuria). These culture specimens are then tested to determine the minimum inhibitory concentration for seven antibiotics currently or historically used to treat uncomplicated urogenital gonococcal infections. Although GISP is limited to male patients with urogenital symptoms who present at STD clinics, the data collected through the surveillance system has greatly augmented the limited data collected through case-based reports of gonorrhea infections. GISP has facilitated the prospective monitoring of *Neisseria gonorrhoeae* infections that have reduced susceptibility to different classes of antibiotics, and GISP has helped inform changes to the CDC STD Treatment guidelines. Following increases in the proportion of GISP specimens with reduced susceptibility to fluoroquinolones, such as ciprofloxacin, the CDC discontinued recommending this class of antibiotic as a treatment for *Neisseria gonorrhoeae* infections among MSM in 2004 [48] and among all persons in 2007 (Figure 12.2) [49]. More recently, CDC revised treatment guidelines to respond to decreased susceptibility of GISP specimens to oral cephalosporins [50]. GISP is an excellent example of a sentinel surveillance system that helps augment case-based reporting in order to provide a broad and varied geographic perspective on an epidemic.

Should neonatal herpes be a reportable condition?

Determining which diseases and conditions should be included in mandatory case reporting requires balancing the benefits to the public health system (e.g., utility of the data) with the costs and burdens of case reporting. While many epidemiologists and public health practitioners follow the mantra "the more data, the better," the costs (in both dollars and human resources) of developing and maintaining a robust case-based reporting system can be large. Case-based surveillance has been mandated for chlamydia, gonorrhea, syphilis, and chancroid nationally; but expansion of state-initiated mandatory reporting for other STDs is controversial.

One particular STD that has been under consideration for mandatory reporting is neonatal herpes, a relatively rare but severe herpes infection of a newborn [51]. As of 2010, only 15 states had mandated provider reporting of neonatal herpes [25]. Advocates suggest that the severity of the infection and the opportunity for prevention support mandated case reporting for neonatal herpes [51,52]. However, others argue that the significant resources needed to establish robust surveillance for this rare outcome, the challenge of translating neonatal herpes surveillance data to actionable public health intervention, and the availability of other data sources, such as administrative clinical or billing data, lessen the need for mandated neonatal herpes reporting

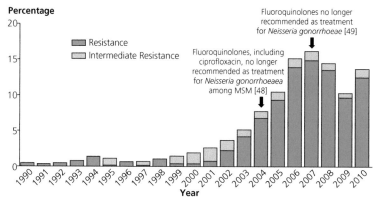

Figure 12.2 Percentage of *Neisseria gonorrhoeae* isolates with resistance or intermediate resistance to ciprofloxacin, 1990–2010, obtained from the Gonococcal Isolate Surveillance Project (GISP) [55]. Note: Resistant isolates have ciprofloxacin minimum inhibitory concentrations (MICs) $\geq 1\,\mu g/mL$. Isolates with intermediate resistance have ciprofloxacin MICs of 0.125–0.500 $\mu g/mL$. Susceptibility to ciprofloxacin was first measured in GISP in 1990. Source: CDC, *Sexually Transmitted Disease Surveillance*, 2010. 2011, Department of Health and Human Services: Atlanta, GA.

[53]. Future evaluations are necessary to assess the relative utility and potential for impact of both case-based and administrative data-based surveillance.

Conclusion

STDs are important sources of morbidity in the United States, and STD surveillance plays an important role in effectively preventing and controlling infections. Surveillance data can help describe the overall burden of disease in populations and are the foundation of prevention efforts. From identifying most at-risk populations to monitoring health services utilization to developing screening and treatment recommendations, surveillance data help ensure that limited resources are most effectively used. Although there are numerous challenges to STD surveillance, data from multiple sources can provide useful surveillance information to describe specific STD epidemics and inform control efforts.

STUDY QUESTIONS

1. Give two examples of how STD surveillance can be used to inform prevention and control activities for STDs.
2. STDs are often considered a "hidden epidemic." What is meant by this, and how does this impact surveillance of STDs?
3. A local health department notices that the number of reported chlamydial infections in their county has increased steadily over the past decade. Give two possible reasons that reported cases have increased.
4. What is meant by "opportunistic" surveillance?
5. Discuss two ways that increased use of electronic medical records could impact STD surveillance.
6. Name one strength and one weakness of using population-based surveys for STD surveillance.
7. Discuss two ways that changes in healthcare access in the United States could impact STD surveillance.
8. Should neonatal HSV disease be reportable to public health authorities? Research the issue briefly and argue for or against it.

References

1. Bean W. *Sir William Osler: Aphorisms from His Bedside Teachings and Writings*. Bean WB, ed. New York: Henry Schuman; 1950.
2. Centers for Disease Control and Prevention. Summary of notifiable diseases—United States, 2010. *MMWR Morb Mortal Wkly Rep* 2012;**59**(53):1–111.
3. Centers for Disease Control and Prevention. *Sexually Transmitted Disease Surveillance, 2011*. Atlanta, GA: Department of Health and Human Services; 2012. November 2011.
4. Farley TA, Cohen DA, Elkins W. Asymptomatic sexually transmitted diseases: The case for screening. *Prev Med* 2003;**36**(4):502–509.
5. Satterwhite CL, Torrone E, Meites E, et al. Sexually transmitted infections among US women and men: Prevalence and incidence estimates, 2008. *Sex Transm Dis* 2013;**40**(3):187–193.
6. Centers for Disease Control and Prevention. Racial disparities in nationally notifiable diseases—United States, 2002. *MMWR Morb Mortal Wkly Rep* 2005;**54**(1):9–11.
7. Forhan SE, Gottlieb SL, Sternberg MR, et al. Prevalence of sexually transmitted infections among female adolescents aged 14 to 19 in the United States. *Pediatrics* 2009;**124**(6):1505–1512.
8. Purcell DW, Johnson CH, Lansky A, et al. Estimating the population size of men who have sex with men in the United States to obtain HIV and syphilis rates. *Open AIDS J* 2012;**6**:98–107.
9. Pathela P, Braunstein SL, Schillinger JA, Shepard C, Sweeney M, Blank S. Men who have sex with men have a 140-fold higher risk for newly diagnosed HIV and syphilis compared with heterosexual men in New York City. *J Acquir Immune Defic Syndr* 2011;**58**(4):408–416.
10. San Francisco Department of Public Health. MSM Surveillance Supplement. STD Control Section, 2012.
11. Holmes K. *Sexually Transmitted Disease*, 4th ed. New York: McGraw-Hill; 2008.
12. World Health Organization. Investment case for eliminating mother-to-child transmission of syphilis: Promoting better maternal and child health and stronger health systems. 2012.
13. Kohlhoff SA, Hammerschlad MR. Gonococcal and chlamydial infections in infants and children. In: Cohen MS, ed. *Sexually Transmitted Diseases*. New York: McGraw Hill; 2008:1613–1628.
14. Jerman P, Constantine NA, Nevarez CR. Sexually transmitted infections among California youth: Estimated incidence and direct medical costs, 2005. *Calif J Health Promot* 2007;**5**(3):80–91.
15. Owusu-Edusei K Jr, Chesson HW, Gift TL, et al. The estimated direct medical cost of selected sexually transmitted infections in the United States, 2008. *Sex Transm Dis* 2013;**40**(3):197–201.
16. Galvin SR, Cohen MS. The role of sexually transmitted diseases in HIV transmission. *Nat Rev Microbiol* 2004;**2**(1):33–42.
17. Cohen MS. Sexually transmitted diseases enhance HIV transmission: No longer a hypothesis. *Lancet* 1998;**351**(Suppl 3):5–7.

18. Bernstein KT, Marcus JL, Nieri G, Philip SS, Klausner JD. Rectal gonorrhea and chlamydia reinfection is associated with increased risk of HIV seroconversion. *J Acquir Immune Defic Syndr* 2010;**53**(4):537–543.

19. Stein CR, Kaufman JS, Ford CA, Leone PA, Feldblum PJ, Miller WC. Screening young adults for prevalent chlamydial infection in community settings. *Ann Epidemiol* 2008; **18**(7):560–571.

20. Workowski KA, Berman S, CDC. Sexually transmitted diseases treatment guidelines, 2010. *MMWR Recomm Rep* 2010;**59**(RR-12):1–110.

21. Chow JM, de Bocanegra HT, Hulett D, Park HY, Darney P. Comparison of adherence to chlamydia screening guidelines among Title X providers and non-Title X providers in the California Family Planning, Access, Care, and Treatment Program. *J Womens Health (Larchmt)* 2012;**21**(8): 837–842.

22. Hoover KW, Butler M, Workowski K, et al. STD screening of HIV-infected MSM in HIV clinics. *Sex Transm Dis* 2010;**37**(12):771–776.

23. Tao G, Hoover KW, Leichliter JS, Peterman TA, Kent CK. Self-reported Chlamydia testing rates of sexually active women aged 15-\–25 years in the United States, 2006–2008. *Sex Transm Dis* 2012;**39**(8):605–607.

24. Molano M, Van den Brule A, Plummer M, et al. Determinants of clearance of human papillomavirus infections in Colombian women with normal cytology: A population-based, 5-year follow-up study. *Am J Epidemiol* 2003;**158**(5): 486–494.

25. Council of State and Territorial Epidemiologists. State Reportable Conditions. 2007. Available at http://www.cste.org/?StateReportable (accessed March 31, 2014).

26. Overhage JM, Grannis S, McDonald CJ. A comparison of the completeness and timeliness of automated electronic laboratory reporting and spontaneous reporting of notifiable conditions. *Am J Public Health* 2008;**98**(2): 344–350.

27. Centers for Disease Control and Prevention. Automated detection and reporting of notifiable diseases using electronic medical records versus passive surveillance—Massachusetts, June 2006–July 2007. *MMWR Morb Mortal Wkly Rep* 2008;**57**(14):373–376.

28. Newman LM, Dowell D, Bernstein K, et al. A tale of two gonorrhea epidemics: Results from the STD surveillance network. *Public Health Rep* 2012;**127**(3):282–292.

29. National Committee for Quality Assurance. The state of healthcare quality 2012. Washington DC: 2012.

30. Bradley H, Asbel L, Bernstein K, et al. HIV testing among patients infected with *Neisseria gonorrhoeae*: STD surveillance network, United States, 2009–2010. *AIDS Behav* 2013;**17**(3):1205–1210.

31. Kirkcaldy RD, Augostini P, Asbel LE, et al. *Trichomonas vaginalis* antimicrobial drug resistance in 6 US cities, STD Surveillance Network, 2009–2010. *Emerg Infect Dis* 2012;**18**(6): 939–943.

32. Dicker LW, Mosure DJ, Levine WC. Chlamydia positivity versus prevalence. What's the difference? *Sex Transm Dis* 1998;**25**(5):251–253.

33. Bradley H, Satterwhite CL. Prevalence of *Neisseria gonorrhoeae* infections among men and women entering the National Job Training Program—United States, 2004–2009. *Sex Transm Dis* 2012;**39**(1):49–54.

34. Miller WC. Epidemiology of chlamydial infection: Are we losing ground? *Sex Transm Infect* 2008;**84**(2):82–86.

35. Scholes D, Satterwhite CL, Yu O, Fine D, Weinstock H, Berman S. Long-term trends in *Chlamydia trachomatis* infections and related outcomes in a U.S. managed care population. *Sex Transm Dis* 2012;**39**(2):81–88.

36. Centers for Disease Control and Prevention. Chlamydia screening among sexually active young female enrollees of health plans—United States, 2000–2007. *MMWR Morb Mortal Wkly Rep* 2009;**58**(14):362–365.

37. Reilley B. HIV/STI screening: Four key indicators tracked at the service unit and national level. How is your facility performing? *IHS Prim Care Provid* 2012;**37**(4):80–81.

38. Mark DH. Race and the limits of administrative data. *JAMA* 2001;**285**(3):337–338.

39. Ratelle S, Yokoe D, Blejan C, et al. Predictive value of clinical diagnostic codes for the CDC case definition of pelvic inflammatory disease (PID): Implications for surveillance. *Sex Transm Dis* 2003;**30**(11):866–870.

40. O'Malley KJ, Cook KF, Price MD, Wildes KR, Hurdle JF, Ashton CM. Measuring diagnoses: ICD code accuracy. *Health Serv Res* 2005;**40**(5 Pt 2):1620–1639.

41. Chandra A, Stephen EH. Infertility service use among U.S. women: 1995 and 2002. *Fertil Steril* 2010;**93**(3): 725–736.

42. Eaton DK, Kann L, Kinchen S, et al. Youth risk behavior surveillance—United States, 2011. *MMWR Surveill Summ* 2012;**61**(4):1–162.

43. Liddon NC, Hood JE, Leichliter JS. Intent to receive HPV vaccine and reasons for not vaccinating among unvaccinated adolescent and young women: Findings from the 2006–2008 National Survey of Family Growth. *Vaccine* 2012;**30**(16):2676–2682.

44. Eggleston E, Rogers SM, Turner CF, et al. *Chlamydia trachomatis* infection among 15- to 35-year-olds in Baltimore, MD. *Sex Transm Dis* 2011;**38**(8):743–749.

45. Schillinger JA, McKinney CM, Garg R, et al. Seroprevalence of herpes simplex virus type 2 and characteristics associated with undiagnosed infection: New York City, 2004. *Sex Transm Dis* 2008;**35**(6):599–606.

46. German RR, Lee LM, Horan JM, et al. Updated guidelines for evaluating public health surveillance systems: Recommendations from the Guidelines Working Group. *MMWR Recomm Rep* 2001;**50**(RR-13):1–35, quiz CE1-7.

47. Schwarcz SK, Zenilman JM, Schnell D, et al. National surveillance of antimicrobial resistance in *Neisseria gonorrhoeae*. The Gonococcal Isolate Surveillance Project. *JAMA* 1990;**264**(11):1413–1417.

48. Centers for Disease Control and Prevention. Increases in fluoroquinolone-resistant *Neisseria gonorrhoeae* among men who have sex with men–United States, 2003, and revised recommendations for gonorrhea treatment, 2004. *MMWR Morb Mortal Wkly Rep* 2004;**53**(16):335–338.

49. Centers for Disease Control and Prevention. Update to CDC's sexually transmitted diseases treatment guidelines, 2006: Fluoroquinolones no longer recommended for treatment of gonococcal infections. *MMWR Morb Mortal Wkly Rep* 2007;**56**(14):332–336.

50. Centers for Disease Control and Prevention. Update to CDC's sexually transmitted diseases treatment guidelines, 2010: Oral cephalosporins no longer a recommended treatment for gonococcal infections. *MMWR Morb Mortal Wkly Rep* 2012;**61**(31):590–594.

51. Handsfield HH, Waldo AB, Brown ZA, et al. Neonatal herpes should be a reportable disease. *Sex Transm Dis* 2005;**32**(9):521–525.

52. Handsfield HH, Stone KM, Wasserheit JN. Prevention agenda for genital herpes. *Sex Transm Dis* 1999;**26**(4): 228–231.

53. Bauer HM. Monitoring trends and epidemiologic correlates of neonatal herpes: Is mandated case reporting the answer? *Sex Transm Dis* 2011;**38**(8):712–714.

54. Torrone EA, Weinstock HS. *Chlamydia Surveillance: Need for New Approaches* in *National STD Prevention Conference*. 2012. Minneapoli, MN.

55. Centers for Disease Control and Prevention. *Sexually Transmitted Disease Surveillance, 2010.* 2011, Department of Health and Human Services: Atlanta, GA.

CHAPTER 13

Surveillance for HIV in the United States

Eve D. Mokotoff[1] and James J. Gibson[2]

[1] *HIV Counts, Ann Arbor, MI, USA*
[2] *South Carolina Department of Health and Environmental Control (Retired), Columbia, SC, USA*

Introduction: biology and natural history of HIV

The human immunodeficiency virus (HIV) is a single-stranded RNA virus that contains a reverse transcriptase enzyme. When HIV enters the human cell, it transcribes the viral RNA into host-recognizable DNA that directs the cell to manufacture more copies of the virus. When persons first become infected with HIV via sex or exposure to blood, they usually undergo a brief illness resembling infectious mononucleosis but then have no remarkable symptoms for approximately 8–10 years until they develop stage 3 HIV infection (AIDS). As the immune system is progressively damaged by HIV infection, the patient becomes more susceptible to certain infections and cancers, many of which were extremely uncommon before the HIV epidemic; these are referred to as "opportunistic illnesses" (OIs). Presence of these OIs or a very low level of CD4 cells define stage 3 (Table 13.1) [1]. Common HIV-related OIs include *Pneumocystis* pneumonia, candida esophagitis, and Kaposi's sarcoma. It was the increase in incidence of such OIs in the early 1980s that allowed the initial detection of the HIV epidemic and that was the initial hallmark of AIDS.

When a person is first infected with HIV, the amount of virus in his blood peaks within 3 weeks and then drops (Figure 13.1). The probability of transmitting HIV to another person is roughly proportional to the concentration of virus in a person's blood, known as "viral load," which is an indicator of both the patient's health status and his potential to infect others. Although it is not yet routinely possible to cure HIV infection (i.e., eliminate the virus from the person's body), the development of effective and safe antiretroviral drugs has radically changed the natural course of disease. Highly active antiretroviral therapy (HAART) can slow or stop production of new virus, rendering the person's viral load undetectable. This can bring the HIV-infected person back to health; but even with an undetectable viral load, the infected individual still has HIV-infected cells and must take antiretroviral treatments (ART) for life. This is very difficult to do consistently; yet it is critical, because the virus is capable of very rapid mutation; and intermittent medication adherence will cause resistance of the patient's virus to the drugs he is receiving, necessitating a change to other antiretroviral drugs that may be more toxic and expensive.

During the time after initial infection when a person displays minimal symptoms (usually years) a person's HIV status is only detectable by testing. Thus the number of newly identified HIV infections in a population in a year is not a measure of the true incidence of infection, but rather reflects new diagnoses and is related to the intensity and effectiveness of testing in that community. True incidence is currently measured using a special testing algorithm that integrates information on the testing history of all persons diagnosed with HIV in the population [2].

The initial indicator of the course of the epidemic, the AIDS death rate, is no longer useful for that purpose because of prolonged survival of persons in care. Today at least four key characteristics of the epidemic should be monitored: (1) rate of occurrence of new infections and the demographic and behavioral characteristics of those persons, (2) proportion of diagnosed HIV-infected persons in care and taking treatment consistently, (3)

Concepts and Methods in Infectious Disease Surveillance, First Edition. Edited by Nkuchia M. M'ikanatha and John K. Iskander.

Table 13.1 HIV infection stage* based on age-specific CD4+ T-lymphocyte count or CD4+ T-lymphocyte percentage of total lymphocytes.

Stage	Age on date of CD4+ T-lymphocyte test					
	<1 yr		1–5 yrs		≥6 yrs	
	Cells/μL	%	Cells/μL	%	Cells/μL	%
1	≥1,500	≥34	≥1,000	≥30	≥500	≥26
2	750–1,499	26–33	500–999	22–29	200–499	14–25
3	<750	<26	<500	<22	<200	<14

*The stage is based primarily on the CD4+ T-lymphocyte count. The CD4+ T-lymphocyte count takes precedence over the CD4 T-lymphocyte percentage, and the percentage is considered only if the count is missing. There are three situations in which the stage is not based on this table: (1) if the criteria for stage 0 are met, the stage is 0 regardless of criteria for other stages (CD4 T-lymphocyte test results and opportunistic illness diagnoses); (2) if the criteria for stage 0 are not met and a stage-3–defining opportunistic illness has been diagnosed, then the stage is 3 regardless of CD4 T-lymphocyte test results; and (3) if the criteria for stage 0 are not met and information on the above criteria for other stages is missing, then the stage is classified as unknown.

Source: Selik RM, Mokotoff ED, Branson B, Owen SM, Whitmore S, Hall HI. *MMWR* Recomm Rep. 2014 Apr 11;63(RR-03):1–10.

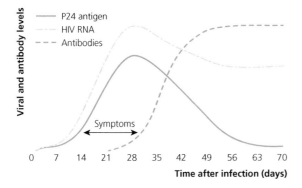

Figure 13.1 Viral load and antibody levels following initial HIV infection
Source: Das G, Baglioni P, Okosieme O. Easily Missed? Primary HIV Infection. BMJ 2010; 341:c4583. Reproduced with permission of BMJ Publishing Group Ltd.

proportion with an undetectable viral load, and (4) rate of antiviral drug resistance. Measurement of all these parameters is the responsibility of the HIV surveillance program.

Surveillance implications of the unique epidemiology of HIV

The surveillance systems for all stages of HIV infection, including stage 3 (AIDS), are the most highly developed, complex, labor-intensive, and expensive of all routine infectious disease surveillance systems. This additional complexity and cost is justified by the enormous cost of HIV disease to society and by the numerous opportunities for prevention of the disease and its complications [3].

The epidemiology of HIV impacts surveillance and data use in ways that are nearly unique among human diseases. Its natural course with a long period of asymptomatic infectivity, usually ending in stage 3 and death when untreated, and its modes of transmission often determined by specific behaviors that carry social stigma (e.g., men having sex with men, sharing of intravenous drug equipment) contribute to HIV's distinctiveness. These special characteristics of the natural course and distribution of HIV disease determine the design and methods of HIV surveillance (Table 13.2).

Although some behaviorally based prevention interventions (e.g., individual counseling and testing) are relatively inexpensive and simple to implement, others are expensive and difficult to maintain. Consequently, HIV control programs have added more treatment-based methods in recent years. These consist primarily of routine and, in some populations, repeated and frequent testing for HIV with an emphasis on diagnosing every infected person as quickly as possible, linking them to clinical care, prescribing ART, monitoring for retention in care, and maintaining an undetectable viral load. This approach is referred to as "treatment as prevention." Another treatment-based strategy is

Table 13.2 How HIV's epidemiology and its natural course, as well as the use of data, differ from most infectious diseases.

Disease characteristic/Data Use	Implications for Surveillance
Asymptomatic infectious latent period 8–10 years. Much transmission occurs during early acute phase.	• Surveillance counts newly diagnosed cases. Special surveillance is required to measure true incidence (new infections).
Long, natural course without Rx. There is no cure, but expensive Rx prolongs life.	• Surveillance is ongoing until death. • Data are acquired from multiple sources. • Case registry contains hundreds of variables (eHARS) and ongoing deduplication is conducted. Source of each data element must be captured.
Clinical disease presentations are diverse and vary by age group.	• Adherence to complex age-specific case definitions is required.

Surveillance data are used to allocate substantial prevention and care dollars.	• HIV requires:
	  ○ active surveillance so that case identification can be complete and accurate,
	  ○ adherence to complex case definitions, and
	  ○ scrupulous data editing and deduplication.

Transmission is determined by specific personal behaviors (risk factors).	• Demographic and transmission risk data must be accurate and complete.
There is serious stigma in many communities throughout the United States and overseas.	• Mandatory reporting and notification of partners must be continually justified. • HIV surveillance requires strict adherence to confidentiality and security guidelines.

pre-exposure prophylaxis (PrEP) which consists of giving ART to uninfected people before they are exposed to HIV [4]. Surveillance data are used to evaluate the success of these strategies, increasing the need to collect ongoing detailed patient care data and broadening the scope of HIV surveillance.

HIV surveillance data are used for many purposes: delivering direct patient services (prevention counseling, linkage to and retention in care, adherence to ART, and assisting patients with notifying their sexual partners), monitoring the scope, geographic distribution and secular trends of HIV infection, monitoring risk behavior to target prevention and planning, evaluating prevention and care programs, and contributing to applied research.

The impact of stigma on the development of HIV surveillance systems

In the United States, initial cases of AIDS were described in 1981 among young, white, gay men with very high

numbers of sexual partners [5]. The need for public health to conduct surveillance for a disease that was spreading rapidly with high mortality rates and engendering fear among the first-infected populations was urgent. Surveillance was viewed with suspicion among the affected groups, who had already experienced discrimination on the basis of their sexual orientation. However, because of the urgency to understand this frightening syndrome, name-based AIDS surveillance was not opposed by AIDS advocacy groups. Public health officials at the state or local health-department level established a traditional surveillance system based on collection of name, address, date of birth, and presumed mode of transmission. Names are collected by state and local health departments for several reasons: (1) they enable state and local public health officials to determine if subsequent case reports are the same or a different person; (2) they facilitate contact with the patient to assist in notifying sex- or needle-sharing partners about their potential exposure to HIV; (3) they allow updating of the case reports with vital status (i.e., death) and, in the current era of ART, with laboratory data that measure immune system status and viral load;

and (4) they allow the health department to contact the patient to assist with linkage to and reengagement in care. Contacting partners of persons diagnosed with HIV has increased in importance as we have gained evidence that getting HIV infected persons into care early can decrease their viral load improving their long-term health and decreasing their risk of transmitting HIV [6]. Contacts who are found to be HIV-negative can be provided with risk-reduction counseling. Confidentiality concerns were lessened by removing names of cases from data forwarded to the Centers for Disease Control and Prevention (CDC). Instead, in national data, cases were identified only by Soundex code [7] and date of birth.

Surveillance data could describe how and to whom HIV was spreading; but, during the early course of the HIV epidemic, the political context of discrimination against gay men produced opposition to surveillance of persons with HIV who had not progressed to AIDS. This opposition was widespread because persons who had not yet progressed to severe HIV disease had more to lose if their infection status was known because of ongoing stigma associated with a positive status [8]. Nonetheless, by 2006, 21 years after the virus was identified and an antibody test was developed to diagnose it, all 50 states had name-based HIV surveillance systems.

The unique epidemiology and political context of HIV have important implications for the public health response. HIV's social stigma underscores the need for surveillance programs to maintain the highest standards of data security and confidentiality, and also emphasizes that public health must justify mandatory reporting.

Surveillance methods for HIV

Case identification

Surveillance for any disease must begin with a case definition so that a single standard is used to decide who to include as a case. The HIV case definition varies by age group, because the human immune and clinical response to HIV infection and the interpretation of the different tests varies with age (Table 13.1). For example, for the first 12–18 months of life a perinatally infected infant will have circulating antibodies from maternal infection, which mask the presence or absence of an infant immune response [9].

Since the beginning of the HIV epidemic, case definitions for HIV infection and AIDS have undergone several revisions to respond to changes in methods of diagnosis of HIV infection and the opportunistic illnesses (OIs) that defined AIDS. By 2008, HIV testing was more integrated into medical care, and laboratory tests for HIV became extraordinarily sensitive and specific. These changes continued and are reflected in the 2014 revised surveillance case definition for HIV infection [1]. Unlike case definitions before 2008, which were separate for non-AIDS HIV infection and AIDS, the 2014 version is an HIV definition and classification system presenting AIDS as stage 3—the most severe stage of a continuum of HIV infection based on either a low CD4 count or percentage or one or more stage 3 defining opportunistic illnesses (Table 13.1) [1]. The 2014 definition also includes a stage for early HIV infection (stage 0) recognized by a negative HIV test within 6 months of HIV diagnosis, because current (2014) testing algorithms are more sensitive during early infection than previous tests. This is important for public health purposes because early infection includes the most highly infectious period when intervention might be most effective in preventing further transmission. The HIV case definitions described here are for public health surveillance only and are too rigid to be a basis for making a clinical diagnosis [1].

Data sources and case-finding

HIV infection may be detected at any point during the progression of the disease, and thus the reportable events range from detection in an asymptomatic person, through occurrence of initial symptoms of disease, low CD4 counts, an OI defining stage 3, or detection only at death (Figure 13.2).

Reporting of HIV by healthcare providers and clinical laboratories is mandated in all jurisdictions in the United States. However, because of underreporting, active surveillance is necessary to ensure complete ascertainment. Active surveillance involves health department staff regularly contacting potential sources of new cases such as hospitals, physicians' offices, and correctional facilities to obtain case reports. Case reports can be completed by health department staff through review of paper or electronic medical records at provider sites and/or through securely accessing their electronic medical record off site. Public health departments may also help sites to complete case report forms using

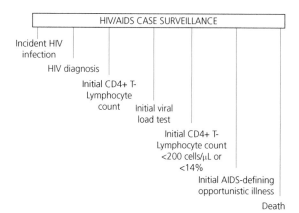

Figure 13.2 Sentinel events in HIV/AIDS case surveillance. Source: Nkuchia M. M'ikanatha, Ruth Lynfield, Chris A. Van Beneden and Henriette de Valk, eds. *Infectious Disease Surveillance*. Blackwell Publishing, 2007. Reprinted with permission of John Wiley & Sons.

health department telephone support, or they may simply require the site to complete the case report form and mail it in or submit it electronically. Some health departments encourage sites to complete the HIV case report form online, using electronic disease reporting systems that are used for all notifiable diseases.

Establishing an active surveillance system for HIV involves the following basic activities:
- Identifying reporting sources
- Establishing reporting routines with the laboratories that perform diagnostic tests
- Establishing communication with clinicians who diagnose and care for persons living with HIV and motivating them to report and/or establishing a procedure for reviewing medical records to complete case report forms including ascertainment of risk factors
- Establishing electronic reporting of laboratory tests
- Analyzing the data and distributing statistical reports—both so the data are used and as feedback to reporting sources

When a case report is first received in the surveillance unit from a reporter outside of the health department it must be reviewed by trained staff to ensure that it is complete, meets the case definition, and is not missing required variables such as name, race, sex, or date of birth. CDC will not accept as a valid case one that is missing a required variable: state ID number, last name Soundex code, sex at birth, date of birth, vital status, date of death (if dead), race/ethnicity, date of first positive HIV test result or physician diagnosis of HIV, and (if applicable) date of first condition qualifying the case as stage 3 using the current case definition. Although not required by CDC, mode of transmission (risk) is critically important for the users of surveillance data. When it is missing, follow-up is done to obtain the information.

Electronic laboratory reporting

Electronic laboratory reporting (ELR) is laboratory data (results) that arrive in an electronic format (e.g., HL-7, ASCII, spreadsheet). However, once they arrive at the health department results must be standardized, validated, entered, and/or uploaded or transferred into an electronic database that can be matched to the HIV registry. Reported laboratory results that do not match previously reported HIV cases must be distributed to staff for follow-up and reporting. The complex process includes monitoring data quality for errors and missing values, parsing, and uploading the data automatically into the database. Figure 13.3 illustrates the flow of ELR for HIV surveillance in Michigan.

Reporting of individual HIV-related laboratory results (e.g., positive confirmatory HIV antibody tests, viral detection results, and CD4 counts) directly by laboratories to surveillance programs can support key surveillance objectives and facilitate timely case ascertainment [10]. Receipt of laboratory results that indicate a new case leads to (1) medical chart abstractions done either electronically at the health department, (2) visiting the site, or (3) triggering a reminder to a healthcare provider to report. Laboratory reporting has become the most frequent mechanism for both learning of new cases and staging a case of HIV, for example, as stage 3 if a CD4 count <200 cells/μL or <14% in a person age 6 or older is reported (Table 13.1). Laboratory results are also used to monitor access to care for persons newly diagnosed, estimate the level of unmet need for medical care, and assess viral load.

Prior to the advent of HAART in the mid-1990s, surveillance consisted primarily of collecting initial HIV diagnosis, followed by monitoring of progression to AIDS and death. The current need to monitor adherence to treatment and care has led to surveillance to collect results of all CD4 count and viral load tests conducted on HIV-infected persons. Treatment guidelines recommend such testing quarterly [11], leading to

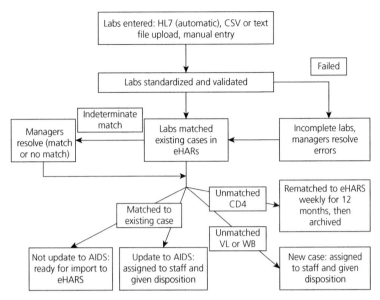

Figure 13.3 Flow of electronic laboratory data in Michigan.

dozens of laboratory tests being reported for each HIV-infected person in care; hence, the need to receive laboratory results electronically and efficiently has increased. While all states require reporting at some level of CD4 count or viral load results (e.g., <200 μL or detectable viral loads), not all states require reporting of all levels and not all send these data to the CDC for inclusion in national reports. As of January 2013, 39 states, Puerto Rico, and the District of Columbia required reporting of all levels of CD4 and viral load test results; 19 of these areas had reported at least 95% of the results to CDC [12].

Surveillance activities specific to HIV

The activities listed in the previous section, including establishing a case definition, conducting active surveillance, and relying upon laboratory reporting, can apply to surveillance for other infectious diseases. There are other approaches used specifically in surveillance for HIV: linkage with other disease registries, evaluation requirements and published performance standards established by the funding agency (CDC) and local jurisdictions, and the requirement to analyze and distribute the data.

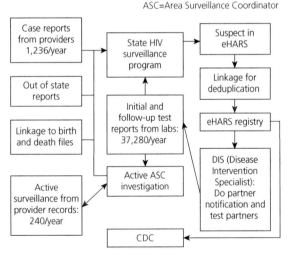

Figure 13.4 Flow of case reports, lab test, risk factor, demographic information in HIV Surveillance: South Carolina, calendar year 2010. Source: Division of Surveillance and Technical Support, South Carolina Department of Health and Environmental Control, Columbia SC.

Data sources and data flow

Although data flow varies somewhat from one jurisdiction to another, the basic reporting sources and processes are the same. Figure 13.4 shows the main data sources and routing for the South Carolina HIV

Surveillance Program in 2010. To maximize case detection, programs seek patient-level data on HIV test results from a variety of sources. Data are received from medical provider case reports, laboratories doing diagnostic or other clinical tests regarding HIV, linkages to files of death and birth certificates, other state health departments, and active surveillance by area surveillance coordinators (ASCs). Prompted by lab reports of positive HIV tests, ASCs obtain completed case report forms from provider medical records and collect other key information such as patient race/ethnicity and risk-factor behavior.

Disease intervention specialists (DIS) are another important source of surveillance information. Their primary role is to obtain names of sexual partners from each new case and test those partners to detect new cases; but, during their interview of each new case, DIS can also obtain reliable information, such as risk-factor behavior, that is otherwise difficult to obtain. Once potential cases are shown to satisfy the case definition, they are entered into the HIV registry—eHARS—and a de-identified extract of this data is sent to the CDC.

Record linkage and registry matches

Because complete detection of HIV infection is important for both prevention and care, surveillance programs go to great lengths to assure complete reporting. This can be accomplished by record linkage, which can be defined as the comparison of two different data sets that both contain at least one key identifying variable in common (usually name and date of birth) in order to bring records of the same person from the two sets together. The purposes are to find cases of HIV that have not been detected by other case-finding methods, as well as to collect missing information on cases already reported. Matching with death registries can find previously unreported cases, as well as update vital status on those already in the registry. Because sexually transmitted disease (STD) investigations include identification of partners, matching with an STD database for cases that have both HIV and another STD can identify behavioral risk factors for reported cases. For example, if a male patient names another male as a partner in an STD investigation, the risk status can be updated to "sex with male" in the HIV case record. Linking the HIV case registry with the state hospital discharge claims database can be used to study HIV comorbidities, the range of hospital charges for HIV-related illnesses, or the propor-

tion of HIV-related hospitalizations for patients without health insurance. Other external databases that have proven particularly valuable include hepatitis B and C registries, tuberculosis registries, and client registries for the AIDS Drug Assistance Program (ADAP).

Matching case registries to state Ryan White HIV care program data can find cases that have gone undetected by the regular surveillance system, if access to their program data can be negotiated. The program was named for Ryan White, a teenager who died in 1990 of AIDS acquired as a result of receiving HIV infected blood treatments for hemophilia. Because of fear and lack of complete information on how HIV was transmitted, he was expelled from middle school; and he subsequently became a spokesperson for HIV infected persons [13,14]. Federally funded Ryan White programs exist in each jurisdiction and provide comprehensive HIV clinical care or simply antiretroviral drugs (through ADAP) to medically indigent patients. They may or may not be managed by the health department and may not be administratively connected to HIV surveillance.

Evaluation of HIV surveillance programs and performance standards

Several essential quality characteristics of HIV surveillance data must be assessed on a regular basis. These include completeness of case identification, timeliness of reporting, thoroughness of removal of duplicate cases from the registry, risk-factor ascertainment, and accuracy of case data (Table 13.3).

Completeness of case ascertainment

The standard set by CDC for completeness is that at least 85% of diagnosed cases are reported to public health within the year of diagnosis. This can be accomplished by including reporting from multiple sources (e.g., healthcare provider, laboratory, and vital statistics) to maximize the likelihood that all persons diagnosed with HIV infection are reported to the health department.

Most jurisdictions measure completeness using a CDC-provided statistical program to conduct capture-recapture analysis on their reported cases [15]. This method compares the multiple independent documents reported for each case, but it can only be used to estimate the completeness of reporting for jurisdictions that had reported at least 30 newly diagnosed cases at 12 months after the close of the year of diagnosis and

Table 13.3 Performance attributes, minimum performance measures, and activities to achieve maximum performance.

Attribute	Minimum performance measure	Examples of activities to achieve acceptable performance
Accuracy: Interstate	≤5% duplicate case reports	• Participate in routine interstate duplication review (RIDR). • Conduct interstate reciprocal case notification.
Accuracy: Intrastate	≤5% duplicate case reports ≤5% incorrect matched surveillance reports	• Verify accuracy of key patient identifiers. • Assess accuracy of matching algorithms. • Complete annual 5% random sample of records for reabstraction.
Completeness of case ascertainment	≥85% of diagnosed cases reported to public health for a given diagnostic year	• Include reporting from multiple sources (e.g., healthcare provider, laboratory, vital statistics).
Timeliness of case reporting	≥66% of cases reported to public health within 6 months of diagnosis	• Electronic reporting • Active surveillance driven by laboratory reporting
Risk-factor ascertainment	≥85% of cases (or representative sample) with identified HIV exposure risk factor	• Healthcare provider education • Patient and provider risk assessment tools • Matching to other public health databases with risk factor information

Source: Centers for Disease Control and Prevention.

where each reporting source had reported at least 20% of the cases. For jurisdictions that do not meet those criteria, CDC recently began using an alternative approach that estimates the total number of diagnoses that occurred in a particular year by modeling reporting delay patterns seen among cases in the previous 5 years (CDC, personal communication).

Timeliness of case reporting

The standard set by CDC for timeliness is that more than 66% of cases are reported to public health within 6 months of diagnosis. Methods for achieving this include electronic laboratory reporting of tests diagnostic of HIV and securely accessing electronic medical records.

Intra- and interstate deduplication and case residency

It is critical that reports that appear to be duplicates be reconciled as the same or different people. In the early years of the epidemic, infected persons died rapidly, minimizing duplicate reports. Consequently, states and CDC used residence at diagnosis as the basis for assigning cases to specific jurisdictions. However, since the mid-1990s when HAART came into use and death rates plummeted, it became increasingly evident that collect-

ing and assigning cases by current known residence was more useful for both prevention and care planning.

The increase in life expectancy among HIV-infected persons allowed them to start living more normal lives; and consequently they moved more, both within and between states, giving them the opportunity to repeatedly enter and leave care. Each city and state system must have methods for checking whether an individual case is already in the system before entering that person's data as a new infection. In order to keep interstate duplication rates low, CDC ascertains potential duplicates between states using Soundex code and date of birth. The list of potential duplicates is sent to each state program twice a year. This list includes the names of other state(s) where this person may have been reported. Because Soundex codes can represent more than one name, states must compare records to ascertain whether the records refer to the same person. If they do, the states determine where the person was first diagnosed; and the case is then assigned to that state. This process is known as Routine Interstate Duplicate Review (RIDR). Within their jurisdiction, health departments can only know about cases that are tested and/or are receiving care. If the person is tested at home or anonymously and does not enter into care, there is no record to send to the health department. Although anonymous reports can be made in some jurisdictions, such reports cannot be deduplicated and are not counted as cases nationally.

Risk-factor ascertainment

Individual risk factors for HIV acquisition are needed for all cases. These include sexual behaviors, injection drug use, transfusion or transplantation of blood or tissues known to be from an HIV-infected donor, or birth to an HIV-infected mother. Unfortunately, ascertainment of risk factors has become increasingly difficult, particularly in the southern United States [16]. However, demand for this information remains high, because it is needed to target prevention programs to the groups where HIV rates are highest or are increasing.

CDC and Council of State and Territorial Epidemiologists (CSTE) have established national guidelines to assist in ascertainment of risk factors. Methods for maximizing acquisition of risk information include (1) ongoing training of surveillance staff and providers on why risk-factor information is important and how the information is used, (2) discussion of cases without identified risk with facility/provider staff to obtain risk factors initially unknown, and (3) rereviewing of medical records, where risk-factor information is most commonly found in the "History and Physical" sections.

In many states HIV surveillance systems work closely with the staff from the STD program or partner services who interview HIV cases to assist them in notifying sexual partners. This process can reveal whether, for example, a man has had sex with other males (MSM). Because of the stigma associated with MSM behavior, this is the most common mode of transmission for male cases initially reported without known risk factors. In order to successfully use STI records to identify risk, the interviewers must include full name and date of birth in their records (to insure it is the same person as in the HIV registry). It is also critical to set up a method to regularly transfer this information between the two electronic information systems that are usually used by these programs. Although face-to-face interviews of persons with unreported risk were commonly conducted in the past as part of surveillance efforts, because of their resource-intensive nature, face-to-face interviews are now often limited to cases that may represent an unusual mode of transmission (e.g., from healthcare provider to patient).

There is a national effort to represent the mode of HIV transmission more comprehensively in surveillance data, using exposure categories that allow data users to see all ways in which persons may have been infected with HIV. The state of Michigan began using these categories in January 2009 [17].

Evaluating data quality received from all data sources

The commonly used methods for evaluating data quality include chart reabstraction studies and comparisons between the case report form and the electronic registry (eHARS). In reabstraction studies, field surveillance staff supervisors repeat data collection from a sample of previously reviewed medical records of presumed HIV cases, or they perform dual abstraction of the same record at the same time. Such studies address accuracy and systematic errors but do not address case completeness or timeliness. Staff may also compare a sample of case records entered from different reporting sources to the information actually entered in eHARS in order to evaluate and correct errors. As more reporting is done electronically and data entry of paper case report forms becomes less common, this activity will become less important; but, in 2014, paper case report forms still represented the majority of reports in most surveillance systems.

Evaluating data received from laboratories and providers

Analyzing data from providers and laboratories for completeness and timeliness is necessary so that training and other interventions can be targeted to underperforming reporters. Some jurisdictions have begun creating Provider and Laboratory Feedback Reports to provide information on performance and to identify where improvements are needed. These reports give the surveillance program a system for continuous quality improvement (CQI).

Data management

A critical part of collecting HIV data is maintaining the database. Regularly scheduled data checking and "cleaning" should be part of ongoing work routines. In Michigan, statistics are produced on a quarterly basis; and, in preparation for producing those reports, standard cleaning programs are run. The database is closed to new entry during the first week of the quarter while errors are investigated and corrected. After cleaning is completed, the database is "frozen" (i.e., saved with no further changes allowed) and is used for analysis.

A standard analytic program can be used to produce lists of cases with suspect state identification numbers or death information, inconsistent or incomplete patient addresses, or other questionable diagnostic and demographic information. To identify potential duplicates, a list of cases that match on Soundex code and date of birth is generated. For both steps, original case report forms may need to be compared and duplicates or errors reconciled. Additional data cleaning projects are developed periodically based on errors that are revealed when responding to data requests.

HIV surveillance systems need methods to manage reports for cases that may be reported with more than one value for the same identifier. This can be done by maintaining fields for multiple names, multiple dates of birth and, if needed, multiple social security numbers. The Michigan program suggests that, if local laws allow, maintaining a "non-case file" should be considered. This file can include electronic or paper case report forms that have been completed on an individual later discovered to be uninfected. Rather than dispose of these reports, they are maintained, using the same security and confidentiality procedures as for cases, in the event that the person presents for care again with questionable HIV status.

Role of information technology staff and data managers

Access to information technology (IT) support staff is essential to the functioning of HIV surveillance. Programs must make data inaccessible to unauthorized persons, while making it accessible to authorized users. Many larger surveillance programs have internal IT staff while others depend on staff from a separate IT unit or assistance from contractors. The staff maintains the databases on secure servers, installs updates, and sets up folder structures to facilitate communication and transmission of electronic documents between central office and the field. IT staff also sets up and maintains complex equipment, guides data encryption systems, and may set up and maintain ELR systems. The staff

member responsible for certifying program compliance with data confidentiality and security requirements needs some understanding of IT principles and procedures to effectively evaluate program policies and to assure that security techniques are up to date.

A staff person trained in IT usually has a background in systems analysis and computer programming or general information technology, but usually lacks training in public health or a significant understanding of the HIV epidemic. Therefore, a well-functioning HIV surveillance unit should have at least one HIV data manager who manages the surveillance registry and coordinates the quarterly cleanings. This person may also be responsible for generating custom analyses and quality assurance reports, preparing reports for funders and the public, linking surveillance files with other databases (e.g., the National Death Index; the TB, STD, or hepatitis databases; state hospital discharge claims data), and communicating regularly with HIV prevention and care programs to assure their data needs are met and that the data are being properly interpreted. This person may also participate in setting up the systems to process ELR data, converting them into a format that is compatible with the surveillance database, importing the converted records, and assuring that the imported data are complete and accurate. The IT staff and data manager must also work together to perform database updates and troubleshoot problems with the HIV registry software as they occur.

Training and technical assistance for HIV surveillance staff

HIV Surveillance programs require personnel with a range of specialized epidemiologic, informatics and managerial skills. Principles of epidemiologic analysis, surveillance methods, and statistical software programming skills can be acquired from formal education; but managing a high-quality HIV surveillance program requires specialized knowledge and skills. These may include information about the local epidemiology of HIV transmission, practical methods of seeking disease reporting from reluctant medical providers, the ability to write programs to transfer data from one database to another, understanding of data analysis methods, searching for the "needle" of the gender of a patient's sexual partners in the "haystack" of a massive patient medical record, applying detailed CDC HIV case definitions, assuring compliance with confidentiality and security practices, sharing key data with the HIV prevention and care and STD programs, and organizing the different members of the surveillance team so that each is assigned to do the work they do best. These skills are acquired through attendance at formal orientation or training courses from the CDC or CSTE, and through provision of peer-to-peer technical assistance. Often it is useful to have a new worker shadow their counterpart for several weeks to learn by observing and doing. Experts in specific topics conduct Webinar-based trainings, sometimes accompanied by a Web-delivered "toolkit" of document templates, for HIV surveillance staff. A great deal of technical assistance is provided through both monthly CSTE HIV subcommittee conference calls and more informal communication within the community of state and city HIV surveillance coordinators at their annual meetings. Such focused training not only serves to teach a worker how to do their job but also standardizes how staff works (e.g., applying case definitions in the same way to make data comparable between South Carolina and Michigan), and assures that data accuracy, completeness, and comparability are optimized.

Security and confidentiality

Security and confidentiality are central to the work of HIV surveillance because (1) identifying information may be maintained for decades, (2) the registry includes personal and sensitive information about sexual practices and potentially illegal behaviors, (3) society stigmatizes some of these behaviors, and (4) maintenance of provider and community trust is essential to system success. In 2011, CDC published updated guidelines that jurisdictions must follow to maintain funding for active HIV surveillance [18]. These data security and confidentiality guidelines apply to HIV surveillance and prevention grantees, as well as to STD, hepatitis, and TB surveillance programs. They were updated to ease data sharing between and within public health agencies. Because data sharing practices vary substantially from jurisdiction to jurisdiction, it is recommended that surveillance programs seek legal advice from their agencies.

The federal Health Insurance Portability and Accountability Act (HIPAA) Privacy Rule [19] can be misinterpreted by some providers as applying to public health and preventing them from cooperating with reporting. However, the Privacy Rule allows a covered entity (e.g., the providers) to disclose protected health information (i.e., the subset of health information that can identify an individual) to a public health authority without the authorization of the individual [20]. It may be helpful to share with providers a letter from the Director of Public Health (or other recognizable senior official) stating this exclusion.

Integrating security and confidentiality into daily work and holding mandatory annual confidentiality trainings should be parts of standard operating procedures. Michigan and South Carolina have found that collecting anecdotes of "real-life" situations and using them as scenarios for discussion makes the trainings more meaningful. Examples could include a field investigator who has had identified patient records stolen from an unlocked car parked at a shopping center or a fax with protected health information sent to the wrong number.

Uses of HIV surveillance data

HIV generates enormous costs to the public and government for medical care and prevention programs (i.e., direct costs), as well as lost wages, human disability, pain, and premature death (i.e., indirect costs). Thus public health must provide valid and understandable information to justify these public expenditures, to increase effectiveness and efficiency of programs, and to focus on prevention and promote use of health services.

As HIV-infected persons live longer as a consequence of ART, the scope of HIV surveillance has expanded to include the lifetime impact of HIV care and treatment activities. For example, surveillance data are relied on to measure progress toward the goals of the National HIV/AIDS Strategy, which include reducing new HIV infections, increasing access to care, improving health outcomes for people living with HIV, and reducing HIV-related disparities [21].

Integrating the surveillance program into the work of the prevention and care programs can increase accurate and productive use of the data. In practice, this means producing, at least annually, statistical reports that display the data requested most often by data users. If staffing levels allow, including surveillance epidemiologists as part of prevention and/or care planning groups places someone who is familiar with the data in a place where decisions are being made about prioritizing populations. Distributing regular statistical reports will also facilitate dissemination of this vital information.

Data from surveillance programs are commonly analyzed to generate several types of reports, including the following:

- Evaluations of the effectiveness of prevention and care programs. For example, "concurrent diagnosis" —defined as initial HIV diagnosis at stage 3—indicates failure of screening or reporting [22].
- Ad hoc analyses to drive program and agency decisions regarding prevention activities focused on risk groups and behaviors, the relative effectiveness of alternative prevention or care activities, and prioritizing legislative budget requests.
- Regular annual reports of the descriptive epidemiology of HIV for use by senior management, funding agencies, community-based planning groups, the press, and interested members of the public. The last page of the National HIV Statistics includes links to all states' websites with their HIV statistical report [23].
- Analyses for program partners who work in related or similar health areas (e.g., STD, tuberculosis, hepatitis, family planning, general acute disease control, and cancer registries.)
- Special ad hoc analyses for interested partner groups such as state departments of correction or education, academic researchers, and the news media.
- Annual and semiannual reports on the organization's progress toward the required objectives of their federal funding agencies: CDC and the Health Resources and Services Administration.
- Essential variables commonly used in such analyses include the basic demographic characteristics of race-ethnicity, sex at birth, current gender, HIV transmission category (the hierarchical summary classification of each case's HIV risk factors), residence at first diagnosis and the most-current known residence, the person's HIV infection stage, whether the person is in adequate HIV care/treatment, and whether the person's viral load is undetectable (low enough to

prevent infectiousness and progression to stage 3). Analyses that show time trends can be particularly useful [22].

The program should have clear policies and procedures for data analysis and dissemination. The data release policy should include rules or policies/procedures (1) to prevent release of information that could identify an individual, including minimum table cell sizes and minimum denominators and numerators for calculating rates; (2) to assess the appropriateness of data requests from outside the program; (3) to determine how analyses will be released and who within the program will do those releases; (4) to monitor adherence to data confidentiality and security rules, including the release of datasets to external researchers with continued protection of confidentiality of that data and return or destruction of data after completion of analysis; and (5) to determine authorship of publications resulting from analysis of surveillance data.

Expanded surveillance

Incidence surveillance

HIV incidence is the measure of new HIV infections in a given period. In recent years, CDC has developed technology and methodology to more directly measure the number of new HIV infections in the United States [2]. These incidence estimates are used to monitor the HIV epidemic in this country and to guide prevention policies and programs created to serve those communities and populations most affected by HIV.

The methodology used to calculate incidence estimates is known as the Serologic Testing Algorithm for Recent HIV Seroconversion (STARHS). STARHS uses results of the BED Assay, along with data on testing history and antiretroviral use collected on newly diagnosed cases, to estimate incidence for the whole population, including those not yet diagnosed. The BED assay [24] is an enzyme immunoassay that estimates recency of infection by detecting the level of anti-HIV IgG after seroconversion. Test results are not accurate on an individual basis, but across a large population this testing provides the foundation to estimate the number and rate of new HIV infections occurring each year in the population.

The BED assay is performed on available serum left over from diagnostic, confirmed-positive specimens. The remaining serum is sent without name to the New York State STARHS laboratory for testing after HIV infection has been confirmed. If the original diagnostic specimen is not available, a subsequent blood specimen obtained within 3 months of HIV diagnosis is obtained for testing. This methodology is expensive and imprecise and is only available in 25 states. Although the purpose of incidence surveillance is to describe the "leading edge" of the epidemic, the data have not been available as rapidly as needed; and the system is still maturing.

CDC plans to introduce other methods for measuring incidence and held a consultation in the fall of 2011 [25] to discuss the future of incidence surveillance. Ideally, incidence would be measured based on a test run by clinicians as a routine part of the care of HIV-infected persons; and data produced on all persons in care could be extrapolated to all HIV-infected persons, including those who have not yet been diagnosed.

Molecular HIV surveillance

The International AIDS Society recommends genotype testing for newly diagnosed HIV positive individuals at entry into care [26]. In Michigan, such testing is increasing; and at present roughly half of all HIV cases that present for care following diagnosis have a genotype performed within 6 months (unpublished data, Michigan Department of Community Health). Genotyping data allow estimation of transmitted HIV drug resistance and determination of HIV subtype; in some cases, this information may affect clinical options such as type of antiretroviral medicines prescribed.

Recently, the concept of using HIV genotype sequence data to determine stage of infection or recency of infection has been proposed, and preliminary results [25] are encouraging. HIV genotype surveillance may add to our understanding of the transmission dynamics present in populations and may help target prevention efforts to more effectively disrupt identified chains of transmission.

Behavioral surveillance

Behavioral surveillance for populations at high risk began in 2003. The National HIV Behavioral Surveillance (NHBS) system conducts surveys in cities with high levels of HIV among MSM, intravenous drug users (IDUs), and heterosexuals at high risk to determine individual risk behaviors, testing behaviors, and use of prevention services. In the first cycle, MSM were interviewed in 17 cities. The second cycle interviewed IDUs in 25 cities. In 2006, CDC expanded the system to include heterosexuals at high risk [27].

Clinical surveillance

The Medical Monitoring Project (MMP) is an expanded surveillance project designed to produce nationally and locally representative data on people who are living with HIV and receiving care in the United States. The CDC funds 23 state and local health departments to conduct MMP. The MMP aims to gain a deeper understanding of health-related experiences and needs of people living with HIV. Information is collected from medical records and patient interviews. The goals of the project are to provide local and national estimates of behaviors and clinical outcomes of persons receiving medical care for HIV, describe their health-related behaviors, determine the accessibility and use of prevention and support services, increase knowledge about the care and treatment provided, and examine how these factors vary by geographic region and patient characteristics. The system is still evolving and under-represents people who have begun receiving clinical care recently [28].

Conclusion

Surveillance for HIV infection uses the same principles and methods as used for other diseases, however, it uses additional methods to optimize case detection and completeness of patient information, to track disease course as well as entry into and retention in care, to monitor effectiveness of prevention and treatment, and to ensure data accuracy and timeliness. The investment in this complex surveillance system is justified by the enormous impact of HIV on health and healthcare costs and the resulting need to make primary and secondary prevention as effective as possible.

Acknowledgments

We are grateful to the staff of the CDC Public Health Library and Information Center for bibliographic assistance.

STUDY QUESTIONS

1. Why are HIV infected persons subject to stigma? How has stigmatization affected how surveillance for HIV has developed and affected the methods that are used?
2. Why has active surveillance been considered necessary for effective monitoring of the HIV epidemic? What are the implications of the need for active surveillance on funding and personnel?
3. Surveillance for HIV today includes far more than the classic initial counting and description of incident cases. Describe what other activities are included and why this expansion of the scope of surveillance has been necessary.
4. Complete HIV case detection and ongoing collection of CD4 and viral load counts is important to allow effective and efficient HIV prevention and treatment programs. However, this goal must be balanced with the need to assure confidentiality and security of surveillance data. List some of the data collection methods that can threaten, or give the appearance of threatening, personal privacy and confidentiality. How would you explain these methods to an HIV infected person or concerned citizen?
5. What are the most important functions of the various types of personnel (e.g., IT, epidemiology, training, administrative support) in conducting HIV surveillance?

References

1. Selik RS, Mokotoff ED, Branson B, Owen SM, Whitmore S, Hall, HI. CDC. 2014 Revised surveillance case definition for HIV infection—United States. MMWR, April 11, 2014 / 63(RR03);1–10. Available at http://www.cdc.gov/mmwr/preview/mmwrhtml/rr6303a1.htm?s_cid=rr6303a1_e (accessed April 10, 2014).

2. Centers for Disease Control and Prevention. Estimated HIV incidence in the United States, 2007–2010. *HIV Surveil Suppl Rep* 2012;**17**(4):1–26. Available at http://www.cdc.gov/hiv/pdf/statistics_hssr_vol_17_no_4.pdf (accessed April 6, 2014).

3. U.S. Department of Health and Human Services, Health Resources and Services Administration, HIV/AIDS Programs. n.d. Grantee allocations & expenditures: 2009 Ryan White HIV/AIDS program spending. Available at http://hab.hrsa.gov/data/reports/granteeallocations.html (accessed April 7, 2014).

4. CDC. US Public Health Service Preexposure Prophylaxis for the Prevention of HIV Infection in the United States – 2014: A Clinical Practice Guideline. Available at http://www.cdc.gov/hiv/pdf/guidelines/PrEPguidelines2014.pdf (accessed May 28, 2014).

5. Shilts R. *And the Band Played on: Politics, People, and the AIDS Epidemic.* New York: St. Martin's Press; 1987.

6. Holtgrave DR, Maulsby C, Wehrmeyer L, Hall HI. Behavioral factors in assessing impact of HIV treatment as prevention. *AIDS Behav* 2012;**16**:1085–1091.

7. U.S. National Archives and Records Administration. 2007, May 30. The soundex indexing system. Available at http://www.archives.gov/research/census/soundex.html (accessed January 25, 2013).

8. Burris S. Surveillance, social risk, and symbolism: Framing the analysis for research and policy. *J Acquir Immune Defic Syndr* 2000;**25**:S120–S127.

9. Caldwell MB, Oxtoby MJ, Simonds RJ, Lindegren ML, Rogers MF. 1994 revised classification system for human immunodeficiency virus infection in children less than 13 years of age. *MMWR Recomm Rep* 1994;**43**(RR-12):1–10. Available at http://www.cdc.gov/mmwr/PDF/rr/rr4312.pdf (accessed April 7, 2014

10. Klevens RM, Fleming PL, Li J, Karon J. Impact of laboratory-initiated reporting of CD4+ T lymphocytes on U.S. AIDS surveillance. *J Acquir Immune Defic Syndr* 1997;**14**:56–60. Available at http://journals.lww.com/jaids/Fulltext/1997/01010/Impact_of_Laboratory_Initiated_Reporting_of_CD4__T.9.aspx (accessed April 7, 2014).

11. U.S. Department of Health and Human Services, Office of Aids Research Advisory Council, Panel on Antiretroviral Guidelines for Adults and Adolescents. 2013. *Guidelines for the use of antiretroviral agents in HIV-1-infected adults and adolescents.* Available at http://aidsinfo.nih.gov/guidelines/html/1/adult-and-adolescent-treatment-guidelines/5/ (accessed January 20, 2013).

12. Centers for Disease Control and Prevention. Monitoring selected national HIV prevention and care objectives by using HIV surveillance data—United States and 6 dependent areas—2011. HIV Surveillance Supplemental Report 2013;18(No. 5). Published October 2013. Available at http://www.cdc.gov/hiv/pdf/2011_Monitoring_HIV_Indicators_HSSR_FINAL.pdf (accessed March 13, 2013).

13. Johnson D 1990, April 9. Ryan White dies of AIDS at 18; His struggle helped pierce myths, *The New York Times.* Available at http://www.webcitation.org/5qUYvFtAc (accessed April 7, 2014).

14. U.S. Department of Health and Human Services, Health Resources and Services Administration, HIV/AIDS Programs. n.d. Who was Ryan White? Available at http://hab.hrsa.gov/abouthab/ryanwhite.html (accessed January 20, 2013).

15. Hall HI, Song R, Gerstle JE, Lee LM. Assessing the completeness of reporting of human immunodeficiency virus diagnoses in 2002–2003: Capture-recapture methods. *Am J Epidemiol* 2006;**164**:391–397.

16. McDavid K, McKenna MT. HIV/AIDS risk factor ascertainment: A critical challenge. *AIDS Patient Care STDS* 2006;**20**:285–292. doi: 10.1089/apc.2006.20.285.

17. Michigan Department of Community Health, Bureau of Disease Control, Prevention and Epidemiology, HIV/STD/VH/TB Epidemiology Section. 2013. *Quarterly HIV surveillance report, Michigan, January 2013.* Available at http://www.michigan.gov/documents/mdch/January_2013_ALL_408513_7.pdf (accessed January 20, 2013).

18. Centers for Disease Control and Prevention. 2011. *Data security and confidentiality guidelines for HIV, viral hepatitis, sexually transmitted disease, and tuberculosis programs: Standards to facilitate sharing and use of surveillance data for public health action.* Atlanta, GA: U.S. Department of Health and Human Services, Centers for Disease Control and Prevention. Available at http://www.cdc.gov/nchhstp/programintegration/docs/PCSIDataSecurityGuidelines.pdf (accessed January 20, 2013).

19. Wilson A. Missing the mark: The public health exception to the HIPAA Privacy Rule and its impact on surveillance activity. *Houst J Health Law Policy* 2009;**9**:131–156. Available at http://www.law.uh.edu/hjhlp/Issues/Vol_91/Wilson.pdf (accessed January 21, 2013).

20. Uses and disclosures for which an authorization or opportunity to agree or object is not required, 45 C.F.R. § 164.512(b) 2002. Available at http://www.ecfr.gov/cgi-bin/text- http://www.whitehouse.gov/sites/default/files/uploads/NHAS.pdf (accessed April 7, 2014).

21. White House Domestic Policy Council, Office of National AIDS Policy. n.d. National HIV/AIDS strategy. Available at http://www.whitehouse.gov/administration/eop/onap/nhas (accessed April 7, 2014).

22. Michigan Department of Community Health, Bureau of Disease Control, Prevention and Epidemiology, HIV/STD/VH/TB Epidemiology Section. 2012. *Annual review of HIV trends in Michigan (2006–2010).* Available at http://www.michigan.gov/documents/mdch/MIReport12_378356_7.pdf (accessed January 20, 2013).

23. Centers for Disease Control and Prevention. 2012. Web addresses for reports of state and local HIV surveillance. *HIV Surveil Rep* 2010, **22**:79. Available at http://www.cdc.gov/hiv/pdf/statistics_2011_HIV_Surveillance_Report_vol_23.pdf#Page=84 (accessed April 7, 2014).

24. Parekh BS, Kennedy MS, Dobbs T, et al. Quantitative detection of increasing HIV type 1 antibodies after seroconversion: A simple assay for detecting recent HIV infection and estimating incidence. *AIDS Res Hum Retroviruses* 2002;**18**:295–307.

25. Centers for Disease Control and Prevention. n.d. *Consultation on advancing HIV incidence surveillance summary.* Available at http://www.cdc.gov/hiv/pdf/statistics_cahivis.pdf (accessed May 7, 2013).

26. National Institutes of Health. Last updated 2/12/2013. Guidelines for the Use of Antiretroviral Agents in HIV-1-Infected Adults and Adolescents. Available at http://aidsinfo.nih.gov/guidelines/html/1/adult-and-adolescent-arv-guidelines/6/drug-resistance-testing/ (accessed April 7, 2014).

27. Centers for Disease Control and Prevention. 2012. National HIV Behavioral Surveillance (NHBS). Available at http://www.cdc.gov/hiv/bcsb/nhbs/index.htm (accessed January 21, 2013).

28. Blair JM, McNaghten AD, Frazier EL, Skarbinski J, Heffelfinger JD, Huang P. Clinical and behavioral characteristics of adults receiving medical care for HIV infection: Medical monitoring project, United States, 2007. *Morb Mortal Wkly Rep Surveill Summ* 2011;**60**(SS-11):1–18. Available at http://www.cdc.gov/mmwr/preview/mmwrhtml/ss6011a1.htm?s_cid=ss6011a1_e (accessed January 23, 2013).

Additional resources

Centers for Disease Control and Prevention, HIV/AIDS Statistics and Surveillance. Available at www.cdc.gov/hiv/topics/surveillance/index.htm.

Council of State and Territorial Epidemiologists (CSTE), HIV Surveillance Training Manual. Available at c.ymcdn.com/sites/www.cste.org/resource/resmgr/InfectiousDisease/HIVSurveillanceTrainingManua.pdf?hhSearchTerms=HIV+and+surveillance

Midwest AIDS Training and Education Center (MATEC), HIV Surveillance and Epidemiology Modules. Available at www.matec.info/?page=online

National Alliance of State and Territorial AIDS Directors (NASTAD), State Health Department HIV/AIDS Reporting Requirements. Available at www.nastad.org/Docs/034156_Federal%20Reporting%20Requirements%20-%20June%202011%20update.pdf

CHAPTER 14

Public health surveillance for tuberculosis

Lori R. Armstrong and Roque Miramontes

Centers for Disease Control and Prevention, Atlanta, GA, USA

Introduction

Tuberculosis (TB) occurred in humans as early as 9000 years ago [1]. Surveillance for TB, although it started earlier than for many other diseases, is a relatively recent public health activity. The World Health Organization (WHO) estimates that 8.7 million new cases of TB and 1.4 million deaths from TB occurred in 2011 worldwide [2]. In the United States the first strategy of TB control is the prompt detection and reporting of TB cases [3]. A core responsibility of public health agencies is to assess the extent and character of TB by collecting and analyzing epidemiologic data. TB surveillance data enable public health officials to describe morbidity and mortality, monitor trends in TB incidence, detect potential outbreaks, and define high-risk populations. Since 1953, Centers for Disease Control and Prevention (CDC) has maintained a standardized national TB surveillance system focused on identifying incident TB cases and reporting TB incidence counts, rates, and case follow-up information on an annual basis.

The goal of this chapter is to introduce the reader to the epidemiology of TB and the national TB surveillance system used in the United States. The history of TB surveillance, the TB case definition, the rationale for collection of specific data, the data evaluation, and reporting will be discussed. Additionally, laws pertaining to TB reporting will be covered briefly.

TB is most commonly caused in humans by *Mycobacterium tuberculosis* (MTB) and is usually spread via airborne particles, most commonly by coughing, sneezing, talking, shouting, laughing, and singing. Other species in the *Mycobacterium tuberculosis* complex (*Mycobacterium bovis* and *Mycobacterium africanum*) can also cause disease [4]. Cough is the most common symptom in patients with TB; other frequent findings include lethargy, weight loss, fever, and night sweats.

TB infection can occur anywhere in the body; however, most disease occurs in the lungs. If the disease affects the lungs, symptoms can include coughing, chest pain, and coughing up blood. Viable mycobacteria bacillus can persist in the body for years as an inactive infection, a condition referred to as latent TB infection (LTBI). Although persons with LTBI have no symptoms, they are at risk for the eventual development of active disease. In general, persons with active TB (or TB disease) are symptomatic and can transmit the infection to others. According to the 1999–2000 National Health and Nutrition Examination Survey [5], more than 11 million persons have latent TB infection; and WHO estimates that one of every three individuals worldwide is infected with TB [6]. An estimated 5–10% of persons with LTBI in the general population will eventually develop active TB disease. Persons with latent infection who are immune suppressed for any reason are more likely to develop active disease. It is estimated that

Concepts and Methods in Infectious Disease Surveillance, First Edition. Edited by Nkuchia M. M'ikanatha and John K. Iskander.
Published 2014 by John Wiley & Sons, Ltd.

people infected with human immunodeficiency virus (HIV) are 21–34 times more likely to progress from latent to active TB disease than those without HIV infection [7], and they are more likely to die without treatment [8]. The advancement of latent TB infection to TB disease is dependent upon the degree of immunodeficiency. Those with a higher CD4 count (>350 cells/ μL) will present with TB symptoms that resemble those of individuals without HIV infection. Those with a lower CD4 count (<200 cells/μL) may not have symptoms of active TB disease and, once diagnosed, are more likely to have disseminated TB [9]. CDC began collecting information on HIV testing for TB cases in 1993 in response to a resurgence of TB from 1985 to 1992 [10,11]. In 1993, the prevalence of reported HIV-infection among TB cases was 15% although only 30% of cases were tested for HIV. By 2010, the percentage of all TB cases tested for HIV was 65% and the prevalence of coinfection was 6% [4].

Persons with TB disease can be treated with a 6- to 12-month course of multidrug therapy; however, some cases are caused by organisms that are resistant to these medications. Multidrug-resistant tuberculosis (MDR-TB), as defined by WHO, is TB that is resistant to at least two of the first-line drugs used to treat the disease (e.g., isoniazid and rifampin) [12]. MDR-TB complicates public health efforts to control disease. Some cases of MDR-TB are caused by organisms that are resistant not only to first-line antibiotics but also to the best second-line drugs—fluoroquinolones—and at least one of three injectable drugs. This subtype of MDR-TB, known as extensively drug-resistant TB (XDR-TB) [13], occurs very rarely in the United States. Fewer than six cases of XDR-TB have been reported annually for the years 2003–2009, whereas approximately 100–130 cases of MDR-TB were reported each year during the same time period [4].

From a global perspective, the United States is considered a low morbidity and mortality country for TB. In 2010, the national annual incidence rate for TB was 3.6 per 100,000 persons with 11,182 reported cases of TB (Figure 14.1) [4]. Only 13 states and the District of Columbia had incidence rates above the national rate. In 2009, 547 persons died of TB disease in the United States, representing a rate of 0.2 deaths per 100,000 persons [4].

Foreign-born cases (those born outside the 50 states, District of Columbia, Guam, Puerto Rico, U.S. Virgin

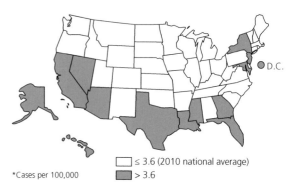

*Cases per 100,000

☐ ≤ 3.6 (2010 national average)
▨ > 3.6

Figure 14.1 Tuberculosis incidence rates, United States, 2010. (Source: Centers for Disease Control and Prevention. Reported Tuberculosis in the United States, 2010. Atlanta, GA: U.S. Department of Health and Human Services, CDC, October 2011. www.cdc.gov/features/dstb2010data/index .html.)

Islands, American Samoa, or those not born in the United States or territories and not of parents who are U.S.-born) were 29% of all reported TB cases in the United States in 1993, when the birth origin of TB cases was first collected for surveillance (Figure 14.2). By 2002, foreign-born cases were over 50% of all reported cases (51%); and in 2010, that proportion reached 60%. The birth country of origin and the number of years that foreign-born patients have resided in the United States are important monitoring indicators for TB control. Since 1991, CDC has required all immigrants and refugees traveling to the United States to be screened for TB [14]. In 2007, the technical instructions accompanying this policy were updated to include sputum culture on suspect cases, drug susceptibility testing, and treatment using directly observed therapy until the patient has completed treatment before allowing them entry into United States [15]. Implementation of the updated instructions is being phased in and may help reduce the number of foreign-born patients with TB disease entering the United States [16].

Other risk factors for TB include residence in correctional and long-term care facilities, homelessness, drug and alcohol abuse, and unemployment. In 2011, the prevalence of homelessness, residing in a correctional facility or residing in a long-term care facility among reported TB cases over age 15 was 5.8%, 4.3%, and 2.3%, respectively. Among reported TB cases over age 15, the prevalence of excess alcohol use was 12.4%;

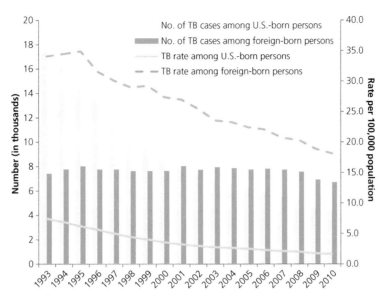

Figure 14.2 Number and rate of tuberculosis (TB) cases among U.S.-born and foreign-born persons, by year reported—United States, 1993–2010. Source: Centers for Disease Control and Prevention, Division of TB Elimination, National TB Surveillance System.

injection drug use, 1.5%; and for non-injection drug use, 7.6% [4].

Laboratory detection of *Mycobacterium tuberculosis*

Laboratory detection of tuberculosis must distinguish between disease and infection. The Mantoux tuberculin skin test (TST) and the interferon-gamma release assay (IGRA) both detect infection but not TB disease. For the TST, purified protein derivative (PPD), an antigen of MTB, measures the delayed hypersensitivity reaction to MTB. It requires at least two patient visits—one to administer the test and another to read the reaction 48–72 hours later. The success of the TST depends on a patient's intact immune function to enable reaction to the antigen and the ability of the health professional to properly read the result. The IGRA identifies the presence of MTB infection by measuring the immune response to the TB proteins in whole blood. A blood sample is required, and the test requires one patient visit to a health-care provider. Both tests have varying sensitivity, and special guidelines should be considered depending on the risk level of the patient being tested [17–19].

For many years, the mainstay of laboratory diagnosis of tuberculosis disease was detection of mycobacteria in a sputum or tissue specimen by acid-fast bacillus (AFB) stain or by culture. Although results for AFB smears can be available within 24 hours, a positive result does not rule out disease caused by nontuberculosis mycobacteria (NTM) or other acid-fast organisms, and many patients are AFB-smear negative but have TB disease. Culture-positive specimens, which can distinguish between NTB and MTB complex, allow for antimicrobial resistance testing (drug susceptibility testing) and genotyping of the MTB organism. In recent years molecular techniques for detecting MTB in a clinical specimen, detecting drug resistance, and defining the origin of the infecting mycobacteria have been developed. Direct detection of genetic material unique to MTB complex can be performed on cultured or fresh specimens using nucleic acid amplification tests (NAATs); these test allow diagnosis of MTB in fresh specimens within 24 to 48 hours [20], enabling the physician to begin treatment with anti-TB medications promptly. In some commercially available or laboratory developed tests, NAAT can also be used to detect genes associated with drug resistance. Traditional culture-based tests for detecting drug resistance involve culturing of the organism in liquid or solid media and can take several weeks to several months to complete. NAAT is still followed up with traditional detection methods in liquid or solid media culture; however, a patient may be started on the anti-TB medications to which their infection is susceptible long before the traditional methods confirm resistance [21].

In addition to diagnosis of TB, molecular characterization of MTB is being used to define the origin of infection. Genotyping techniques are used to determine the genetic makeup of the MTBC DNA. This can aid in identifying the genetic links between two or more infected patients. If the specific genotype matches other infections in the community, health workers can know whether the infection was recently transmitted and can plan appropriate contact tracing to find other infected individuals [22]. Universal genotyping of culture-positive TB specimens started in 2004 in the United States. By 2010, slightly over 88% of reported culture-positive TB cases were being genotyped [23].

TB case verification criteria

The United States employs five separate hierarchical verification criteria for TB cases, which are based on

laboratory confirmation or clinical criteria (Table 14.1). Laboratory criteria are based on confirmation either by isolation of *M. tuberculosis* complex from culture, by identification of microscopic AFB on a specimen smear, or by identification of *M. tuberculosis* complex DNA by NAAT from a clinical sample. AFB culturing of respiratory or tissue samples is the gold standard for confirmation of tuberculosis During 2010-2011, about 75% of TB cases in the United States have been diagnosed by culture, 1% by NAAT, and 1% by AFB positivity. All three methods require well-equipped laboratories with trained and certified laboratory personnel. Most state health departments have full-service certified TB laboratories or contracts with commercial laboratories. Local county public health laboratories and hospitals may have AFB smear capabilities and limited culture or molecular facilities for identifying *M. tuberculosis*. Many state TB programs now require that all reporting entities send clinical samples from suspect TB cases to their respective state public health laboratories.

In the absence of laboratory confirmation of *M. tuberculosis* from a clinical specimen, physicians can confirm a TB case based on clinical criteria (Table 14.1). Patients who have evidence of TB infection based on a positive TB skin test result or positive interferon gamma release

Table 14.1 National TB Surveillance System TB Case Classifications.

Hierarchy	Criteria	Definition
1	Laboratory confirmation • Culture confirmed	Isolation of *M. tuberculosis* complex from a clinical specimen
2	Laboratory confirmation • Nucleic acid amplification test (NAAT)	Demonstration of *M. tuberculosis* complex from a clinical specimen by NAAT
3	Labaoratory confirmation • Positive smear for acid-fast bacilli (AFB)	Demonstration of AFB in a clinical specimen when a culture has not been or cannot be obtained or is falsely negative or contaminated
4	Clinical confirmation	Must meet all the following criteria: • Positive TB skin test result or positive interferon gamma release assay for *M. tuberculosis* • Other signs and symptoms compatible with TB (e.g., abnormal chest radiograph, abnormal chest computerized topography scan, or other chest imaging study, or clinical evidence of current disease) • Treatment with two or more anti-TB drugs • A completed diagnostic evaluation
5	Provider diagnosis	The patient doesn't meet any of the above criteria but the provider believes the patient has a TB diagnosis.

Source: Centers for Disease Control and Prevention. *Reported Tuberculosis in the United States, 2011.* Atlanta, GA: U.S. Department of Health and Human Services, CDC, October 2012

assay (IGRA) for *M. tuberculosis*, who have signs and symptoms compatible with TB (abnormal chest radiograph or abnormal chest computed topography scan or other chest imaging study) or clinical evidence of current disease, who are on treatment with at least two antituberculosis medications, and who have completed a diagnostic evaluation can be clinically confirmed. If all these criteria are absent but the provider still believes the patient has TB, the patient can be confirmed as a clinical TB case by provider diagnosis.

History of tuberculosis surveillance in the United States

The scourge of TB in the United States was well known before there was any attempt to develop a national TB surveillance system. Prior to Robert Koch's 1882 discovery of the bacterium responsible for TB, however, the medical establishment viewed tuberculosis as hereditary and inevitable [24]. In the nineteenth century, the most common index used to measure the effect of tuberculosis on the U.S. population was mortality data. However, reporting of that data was often limited and collected inconsistently across cities and states. During this time, the state of Massachusetts maintained a registry of deaths that was considered to be a reliable source of TB mortality data in that state. In fact, combined mortality data from the cities of New York, Philadelphia, and Boston from 1871 to 1912 was utilized to describe a decrease in mortality from TB at a meeting of the National Association for the Study and Prevention of Tuberculosis in 1912 [25]. Michigan became the first state to mandate the reporting of tuberculosis in 1888 [26]. New York City was another pioneer in the early efforts to prevent TB; registration of cases was among the activities undertaken beginning in 1893 [27,28].

By the early twentieth century, a national death registry maintained by the U.S. Government Office of Vital Statistics was in place and included mortality data from 10 states and the District of Columbia. At that time, those 11 reporting areas represented approximately 40% of the total U.S. population [29]. The campaign against TB was becoming much better organized by 1904 when the National Tuberculosis Association (NTA) was formed. NTA was an early leader in efforts to decrease TB nationwide through education and advocacy. The NTA leadership of the national association was instru-

mental in bringing the 6th International Tuberculosis Conference to Washington, D.C., in 1908 and in the formation of state TB associations in Colorado, Kansas, Michigan, Wisconsin, Texas, and West Virginia [30].

Beginning in 1930 nationwide statistics from 48 states on the total number of tuberculosis cases were collected and reported to the national TB program of the U.S. Public Health Service (USPHS). Because of differences in case definitions or uniformity in reporting practices and the lack of complete reporting from all cities and states, interpretation of these surveillance data was difficult. As a result, surveillance data from the years 1930-1951 fluctuated from year to year [31].

In May 1951, for the first time in the United States, reporting standards of tuberculosis morbidity data were defined. In 1952, the first summary report of the Tuberculosis Program, Division of Special Health Services, USPHS was published. The second report published in 1953 was the first report that included reporting from all states, and it is commonly considered to be the first national report of TB cases utilizing a standardized format. All data were reported in aggregate form directly from the states to the National TB Control Program of the USPHS in the Annual Tuberculosis Report [32,33].

The first case definition included a designation of Group A, "active and probably active" cases, and Group B, "other reportable cases." Group A cases had bacteriological proof of TB or, in those without laboratory evidence, had other significant evidence of disease (e.g., characteristic chest radiograph or clinically active extrapulmonary TB). Group B included previously unreported tuberculosis cases such as those with a history of active disease or previous treatment within the past 5 years. Cases reported as Group B one year were not precluded from being reported as Group A cases in subsequent years. In 1953, 113,531 tuberculosis cases were reported in the United States with 88,919 (78%) classified as Group A [32].

In 1960, the National TB Control Program was transferred from the Public Health Service to the Communicable Disease Center, the precursor to CDC. In 1961, the National TB Control Program revised its recommendations on the reporting of tuberculosis cases. A recommendation that only active cases be counted to assess the incidence of tuberculosis was adopted by some states and became more widely used in 1962. It was also the first year that data reporting U.S. cases broken down by sex and age group became available. Not all new recommendations were applied uniformly by the states. A more complete reporting of cases based on the new recommendations was observed in 1963 [34].

From 1965 to 1980, TB skin test results for household and nonhousehold contacts of active cases were reported for a subset of states. By 1980, that number was 30 states and 25 cities of greater than 250,000 population [35]. A change in case counting criteria that began in 1975 rendered previously published surveillance data not directly comparable to subsequently published data. From 1975 on, cases formerly classified as reactivation TB were included in morbidity data. Additionally in 1975, detailed demographic and epidemiologic information on extrapulmonary cases was published [36].

In 1979, six states and three cities began reporting specific demographic, clinical, and TB risk factor data for each individual TB patient reported to the national program. All states transitioned to case-based reporting of TB surveillance data by 1985 [37,38]. In 1985, surveillance data was used to identify an unexpected number of TB cases above trends reported in previous years. Data from New York City and Florida suggested that acquired immunodeficiency syndrome (AIDS) may have played a role in the higher-than-expected number of cases. This report led to subsequent investigations in affected areas and resulted in increased focus on TB control in persons with HIV/AIDS, who were confirmed to be at increased risk of TB disease [39].

Current tuberculosis reporting in the United States

Tuberculosis surveillance in the United States has changed a great deal in depth and quality since its inception more than a century ago. These changes were driven by clinical knowledge of the disease, as well as the capabilities and infrastructure of states and the national TB program to collect, report, and analyze the data reported and to disseminate the information for public health use. All states, territories, and tribal governments now require designated health-care professionals to report confirmed cases of TB to local or state health departments [40,41]. Those required to report (e.g., physicians, laboratory personnel) vary by state and jurisdiction; and to whom they report can also vary slightly. Typically, all jurisdictions are required to report to a local or state health authority or both. Require-

ments for reporting of suspect cases vary widely by state. States also have legal requirements for local jurisdictions to maintain TB control programs and to screen, examine, and test suspect cases of TB [41].

TB surveillance carried out at the national, state, and local levels can help inform prevention and control efforts. Throughout the year, as part of the National Tuberculosis Surveillance System, all 50 U.S. states, as well as the District of Columbia, New York City, Puerto Rico, and other U.S.-affiliated areas in the Pacific and Caribbean, routinely report new cases of TB disease to CDC. The U.S.-affiliated areas in the Pacific and Caribbean are the Republic of the Marshall Islands, the Federated States of Micronesia, American Samoa, Palau, Guam, Northern Mariana Islands, Puerto Rico, and the U.S. Virgin Islands.

Starting in 2009, all reporting areas started the transition to National Electronic Disease Surveillance System (NEDSS)–compliant reporting systems. Before that time, a single electronic data system dependent on a dial-up modem; the Tuberculosis Information Management System (TIMS) was in place. The TIMS system often stood independently from other systems the reporting areas used and required dual entry of TB surveillance data. With the implementation of NEDSS-compliant systems, reporting areas use the same electronic systems for their own surveillance and reporting to CDC and other entities [42]. Reporting areas now supply their own NEDSS-compliant systems, either buying them commercially, building them, or using one of two CDC-built systems.

Reporting areas are able to submit their data throughout the year and can update older data at any time. Local jurisdictions report TB cases to their respective state health departments, who then forward data to CDC via their NEDSS-compliant electronic data systems. Data flow to a CDC central warehouse and then to the TB program at CDC. Data validation tables are run frequently to assess the completeness of the data. Error reports are generated and placed on a shared secure website that reporting areas can access through individual passwords. Surveillance staff from various reporting areas can access only their own reports and cannot view reports from other areas.

To assure uniformity and standardization of surveillance data, all TB programs in the United States report verified TB cases via the Report of Verified Case of Tuberculosis (RVCT) [43]. The RVCT collects

Table 14.2 Report of verified case of tuberculosis, Follow-up 1, and Follow-up 2 selected reporting variables.

Reporting section	Variable type	Variable name
RVCT	Unique identifier	State case number
RVCT	Demographic	Date of birth, sex, race, ethnicity, origin of birth, birth country, and county, city, and zip code of patient's residence
RVCT	Demographic	Pediatric TB patients
RVCT	Incidence and count	Report date, count date, and count status
RVCT	Clinical	Previous diagnosis of TB disease, site of TB disease, and vital status at TB diagnosis
RVCT	Clinical	Initial chest radiograph or other chest imaging study
RVCT	Risk factor	Immigration status at first entry to the United States, HIV status, homelessness status, resident of long-term care or correctional, injection, non-injection drug use, and excess alcohol use. Contact with MDR-TB patient, infectious patient, missed contact, incomplete treatment for latent TB infection, tumor necrosis factor alpha antagonist therapy, post–organ transplantation, diabetes mellitus, end-stage renal disease, and immunosuppression (not HIV/AIDS)
RVCT	Treatment	Date therapy started and initial drug regimen
Follow-up 1	Laboratory	Initial drug susceptibility test results, date isolate collected, specimen type, drugs tested, genotyping number, nucleic acid amplification test results, smear results for acid-fast bacilli (AFB), sputum or tissue culture results, and dates collected
Follow-up 2	Outcome	Sputum culture conversion
Follow-up 2	Outcome	Date therapy stopped, reason therapy stopped or never started, reason therapy extended beyond 12 months
Follow-up 2	Outcome	Type of outpatient health-care provider, directly observed therapy (DOT), and number of weeks on DOT
Follow-up 2	Outcome	Final drug susceptibility testing results, date isolate collected, specimen type, and drugs tested

Source: Centers for Disease Control and Prevention. Tuberculosis Surveillance Data Training. Report of Verified Case of TB (RVCT). Self-Study Modules. U.S. Department of Health and Human Services, CDC, Atlanta, GA: U.S. Department of Health and Human Services, CDC, 2009.

demographic, diagnostic, clinical, and risk-factor information on incident TB cases (Table 14.2). Extensive instructions and explanation of all variables accompanies the reporting form. A companion form, the Follow-up 1 (FU-1), records the date of specimen collection and results of the initial drug susceptibility test at the time of diagnosis for all culture-confirmed TB cases. Both the RVCT and the FU-1 form are submitted in the same calendar year that the patient is confirmed to have TB. The Follow-up 2 (FU-2) form collects outcome data on patient treatment and additional clinical and laboratory information. CDC requests that the FU-2 information be reported as soon as the patient

finishes treatment or as soon as care is terminated; however, reporting areas have up to 2 years following the reporting of the patient to submit these data.

Since 1993, the RVCT, FU-1, and FU-2 have been used to collect demographic and clinical information, as well as laboratory results for all reported TB cases in the United States (Table 14.2). The RVCT collects information about known risk factors for TB disease; and in an effort to more effectively monitor TB caused by drug-resistant strains, CDC also gathers information regarding drug susceptibility testing for culture-confirmed cases on the FU-2. Final drug susceptibility test results, results of sputum culture conversion, treatment delivery, and outcome and delivery of care for the patient (e.g., by health department, by private provider) are also reported on the FU-2. In 2009, eleven new variables were added to the RVCT. These are count status (see below), date of death and whether TB was a cause of death, the additional laboratory results of nucleic acid amplification and interferon gamma release assay, drug susceptibility testing results, genotyping data, chest computed tomography scans, and chest radiography. Other new variables included the primary reason for evaluation of TB disease and comorbid or epidemiologic conditions known to be risk factors for TB disease (e.g., diabetes mellitus, renal disease, immunosuppression not caused by HIV/AIDS, incomplete treatment for LTBI, known case contact of an infectious TB patient). On the FU-2, additional follow-up information is collected, including the reason for nonculture conversion, if the patient moved before therapy was completed and the new residence, the reason therapy was stopped or never started, or the reason therapy was extended beyond 12 months.

The state TB programs and CDC employ the concept of "count status" when determining if a TB case is to be included in the incidence count of a state, area, or the nation. The count status variable indicates if the patients are counted in the jurisdiction reporting them (e.g., patient resides in and was usually diagnosed with TB within the jurisdiction) or not counted. A noncounted case may be diagnosed, treated, or managed by the reporting jurisdiction, but does not meet NTSS criteria for counting by that jurisdiction (e.g., counted in another U.S. area, treatment initiated in another country, recurrent TB within 12 months after completing therapy). Until 2009, only counted cases were nationally reportable. Occasionally a local health department may begin or resume treatment on a patient diagnosed with TB outside their jurisdiction. Such a patient would normally be counted as an incident case in the locality where they were diagnosed. Since local health departments expend resources to care and follow these "uncounted" patients, it was decided in 2009 that health departments could report uncounted cases they managed along with any counted cases. "Uncounted" or "noncounted" cases do not contribute to the incident case rate in a given locality or jurisdiction, usually because treatment or diagnosis was initiated in another jurisdiction. Only counted, incident cases are tallied for the annual case rate reported by CDC. Reporting both counted and uncounted TB

cases allows a program to report a more accurate interpretation of their burden of care.

All reporting areas have the capability to submit verified cases of TB throughout the year. CDC encourages reporting areas to submit the RVCT as soon as a case of TB is confirmed. However, because of publication deadlines CDC calls for data on select variables from the previous year by the first week of February of the following year in order to publish preliminary data for World TB Day (March 24). By the first week of March of the following year, RVCT and FU-1 are required. After several months of cleaning and quality checks, the data are finalized for reporting and epidemiologic and programmatic analyses.

Tuberculosis surveillance data reporting and publication

All surveillance data collected should be intended for reporting or evaluation of program services. Surveillance data can be used (1) to monitor trends and respond to changes, (2) to guide planning of program activities, (3) to evaluate program effectiveness and impact of policy changes, and (4) to provide data for education and advocacy. The Division of TB Elimination at CDC reports aggregated TB surveillance data annually in *Reported Tuberculosis in the United States,* both in printed and online formats [4]. The annual report contains national case counts, crude incidence and mortality rates of TB, and the percentage change from the previous year for the number and rate of incidence. Incidence rates are also reported for states, New York City (which reports separately from the state of New York), the District of Columbia, and the U.S.-affiliated island nations.

TB data are stratified by race/ethnicity, age, sex, and geographic area to determine how various populations are affected. Data are also examined for other risk factors known to be associated with TB (e.g., birth in a country with high rates of TB or HIV infection, residence in correctional and long-term care facilities, homelessness, drug and alcohol abuse). The annual report is used widely by state and external partners, and selected data from the annual report are available for additional analysis via an interactive website [44]. Surveillance data are also published annually online in the form of a slide set that can be downloaded and used in presentations. In March of every year, to coincide with

World TB Day, CDC publishes an update on the status of TB epidemiology in the United States in the *Mortality Morbidity Weekly Report* (MMWR) [45–49]. World TB Day is commemorated on March 24 because that is the anniversary of the day that Robert Koch discovered the bacterium *Mycobacteria tuberculosis* as the cause of tuberculosis. The World TB Day MMWR article provides a forum in which CDC can describe the current epidemiology of the disease and showcase progress toward TB elimination in the United States. Recent articles have highlighted the growing majority of TB cases among foreign-born persons, the prevalence of TB among minority populations, and the unexpected decline in TB cases in 2009.

Quality, completeness, and timeliness of reporting

The CDC maintains a cooperative agreement with all reporting areas (states, territories, some large cities) that outlines the requirements for completeness, quality (accuracy), and timeliness of reporting of TB cases. In exchange for funding, the agreement requires reporting areas to maintain procedures for TB case detection and reporting and for ensuring completeness and quality of surveillance data [50]. Data collection is via the RVCT, which represents the minimum data elements for reporting to CDC. In an effort to promote completeness and quality of data, CDC frequently reports data received from TB programs back to program personnel through the NTSS report and the National Tuberculosis Indicators Project. Missing or inaccurate data items are linelisted by reported TB case, which enables state TB programs to easily identify where corrections are needed or where data were not received because of technical problems.

The National Tuberculosis Indicators Project (NTIP) is a secure Web-based monitoring system used to track the progress of TB control programs [51,52]. Fifteen high-priority program objectives are selected for NTIP; a subset of these are directed toward surveillance reporting, such as completion of treatment, known HIV status, and sputum culture conversion. TB programs can use NTIP data to track their progress toward program goals and to describe their performance and plans for improvement in their annual reports to CDC and stakeholders.

Few published reports exist on completeness and accuracy of RVCT data or on the completeness of TB case reporting. Most recently, in 2009, in response to an unprecedented decline in national TB cases, CDC investigated the completeness of reporting of TB cases and performed extensive case-finding audits in two states [53]. Thirty-six states reported declines in TB rates from 2008 to 2009, including Georgia and Pennsylvania, which experienced declines of 14.3% and 38.7%, respectively. The investigation reviewed paper and electronic records from state and local areas of verified and suspect TB cases, analyzed hospital discharge records for ICD-9 codes to identify possible TB-related hospitalizations, performed systematic queries of electronic data on specimens submitted to the public health laboratories, surveyed licensed private laboratories, and reviewed changes to surveillance and laboratory procedures used by the two TB programs. The report found two Georgia cases and six Pennsylvania cases that were not previously reported to their respective surveillance systems. The authors concluded that there was no evidence of surveillance artifacts or sufficient underreporting or underdiagnosis to account for the magnitude of the declines.

An earlier study evaluated the completeness and timeliness of TB case reporting in seven states during 1993 and 1994 [54]. The investigators reviewed 2711 records in laboratory data, death certificate records, hospital discharge records, pharmacy records, public insurance (Medicaid), and outpatient records. Only 0.5% (n = 14) of TB cases were previously unreported to public health authorities. Timeliness of reporting was less impressive, ranging from a median of 7 days to a median of 38 days following case detection. The percentage of cases reported within 3 days, as recommended by CDC, ranged from 1% to 34% among the seven state TB programs.

To evaluate the completeness and accuracy of individual RVCT data items, the California TB program sampled 594 TB cases reported in 1996 and 1997 [55]. The group performed medical record abstraction for 53 variables from the RVCT and compared the data abstracted from the patient's public health medical record to data reported to the state TB registry. Most (79.5%) of the RVCT categorical variables had at least 90% concordance between the medical record and the registry. The weighted absolute mean difference between the dates reported in the two systems ranged from 110.9 days for collection of the isolate for final susceptibility testing to 2.6 days for treatment start date. Similar results were found in a study conducted by CDC in 2006. Public health clinic records from the local health departments of Miami, Chicago, and the District of Columbia were abstracted on 94 TB patients who had completed treatment [56]. Abstracted data on 88 RVCT variables were compared to data received in the NTSS at CDC. At least 90% concordance was achieved on only 53% of the variables reviewed, mostly on demographic, as well as clinical and risk-factor variables. Most date variables were less than 50% concordant. Items such as the status of directly observed therapy for the patient could not be assessed because of nonstandard clinic recordkeeping practices. In 2009, to promote more accurate data capture for the newly revised RVCT, CDC developed an extensive training program to educate state and local TB surveillance staff on the definitions, standards, and procedures for reporting all variables on the RVCT [57].

Case study

Unexpected decline in TB rates, 2009

After analyzing preliminary national TB surveillance data from the 2009 reporting year, the Division of Tuberculosis Elimination at CDC discovered an unprecedented decline in TB case rates. The rate declined 11.4% from 4.2/100,000 in 2008 to 3.8/100,000 in 2009 in the preliminary data received [48]. It was the greatest decrease ever recorded for a single year and was the lowest recorded rate since TB surveillance began with full national coverage in 1953. An extensive analysis of the preliminary data showed that the decline of TB case rates occurred in nearly every population. Foreign-born and U.S.-born cases declined 9.0% and 15.8%, respectively. There were declines in every racial and ethnic group, ranging from 9.0% among non-Hispanic Asians to 15.2% among non-Hispanic whites. Culture-positive pulmonary TB cases declined 13.6% and culture-negative pulmonary TB cases declined 17.5% from 2008 to 2009. The unexpected decline in case rates could have meant fewer cases of TB were being diagnosed as a result of better TB control procedures, signaling a significant step toward TB elimination in the United States; however, it could also have been the result of population shift, underreporting, or underdiagnosis of disease. There had been notable

changes in the national surveillance system in the preceding year. Many states had begun the transition to using their own Web-based reporting systems and had adapted the revised RVCT. Some of the new state-built or commercial reporting systems lacked all the validation procedures that had been present in CDC's older reporting system (TIMS). As a result of the economic downturn in many states, there were anecdotal reports of reduction of TB staff in certain local areas. Because of these changes, CDC along with state TB programs embarked on an extensive investigation of case finding and program practices at the state and local level [48,58].

The investigators ruled out software system changes as the cause for the decrease in TB case rates. States that were using all types of computer software, including one of two new CDC-built systems, the traditional TIMS system, and state- or commercial-built systems, experienced declines. CDC-funded clinical mycobacteria laboratories reported receiving 5.9% fewer clinical specimens for TB testing from 2008 to 2009. The National Tuberculosis Controllers Association surveyed all 59 reporting areas for changes in surveillance, diagnostic laboratory procedures, and staffing. Among the 93% of TB program managers who responded to the survey, there was no indication that any of these changes led to the unexpected decline in cases. In fact, states that experienced staff reductions and reported at least 100 cases of TB showed less of a decrease in case counts than similar states that experienced no reductions in staff. In 10 high-burden counties across the nation no unreported cases were discovered. A detailed case-finding study in Pennsylvania and Georgia also failed to reveal substantial underreporting or underdiagnosis of TB cases [53]. A statistical analysis of monthly case counts for the past 10 years showed that there was a significant difference between observed and expected TB cases by treatment start date among U.S.-born and foreign-born cases. Foreign-born case counts experienced a significant decline starting in October 2007, and these decreases were consistent with trends seen in the foreign-born population as reported by the Census Bureau and those seen by the Department of Homeland Security among unauthorized immigrants to the United States [58]. The authors concluded that the observed decline in the 2009 TB case rate accurately reflected a true decline in the number of TB cases diagnosed in the United States.

STUDY QUESTIONS

1. Historically there have been many changes to the national reporting of TB surveillance data. What are some examples of how reporting changes affect surveillance trends?

2. What are the verification criteria for confirming a TB case? How are they hierarchical, and what are the three hierarchical levels?

3. What are counted and uncounted TB cases? How does count status relate to a state or county? What is the advantage of reporting uncounted TB cases by a reporting jurisdiction (e.g., state or county)?

4. Name four ways in which TB surveillance data should be used routinely.

5. Name methods that a TB program can use to assess the completeness and accuracy of their surveillance data.

6. Other than a real decline in TB cases, what are other possible causes for the unexpected decline in TB cases reported in 2009 [47]?

References

1. Hershkovitz I, Donoghue HD, Minnikin DE, et al. Detection and Molecular characterization of 9000-year-old *Mycobacterium tuberculosis* from a neolithic settlement in the Eastern Mediterranean. *PLoS ONE* 2008;**3**:e3426.

2. World Health Organization, Global Tuberculosis Report, 2012. World Health Organization, Geneva, Switzerland. 2012.

3. American Thoracic Society, Centers for Disease Control and Prevention, and Infectious Diseases Society of America. *Am J Respir Crit Care Med* 2005;**172**:1169–1227.

4. Centers for Disease Control and Prevention. *Reported Tuberculosis in the United States, 2011.* Atlanta, GA\: U.S. Department of Health and Human Services, CDC, October 2012.

5. Bennett DE, Courval JM, Onorato I, et al. Prevalence of tuberculosis infection in the United States population. The National Health and Nutrition Examination Survey, 1999–2000. *Am J Respir Crit Care Med* 2008;**177**:348–355.

6. World Health Organization. Tuberculosis fact sheet no. 104. October 2012. Available at http://www.who.int/mediacentre/factsheets/fs104/en/ (accessed April 2, 2014).

7. World Health Organization. TB/HIV Facts 2012–2013. 2014. Available at http://www.who.int/hiv/topics/tb/tbhiv_facts_2013/en/ (accessed April 4, 2014).

8. World Health Organization. Frequently asked questions about TB and HIV. 2014. Available at http://www.who.int/tb/challenges/hiv/faq/en/# (accessed April 4, 2014).

9. Centers for Disease Control and Prevention. Guidelines for prevention and treatment of opportunistic infections in HIV-infected adults and adolescents. *MMWR Morb Mortal Wkly Rep* 2009;**58**:1–198.

10. Burwen DR, Bloch AB, Griffin LD, et al. National trends in the concurrence of tuberculosis and acquired immunodeficiency syndrome. *Arch Intern Med* 1995;**155**:1281–1286.

11. Cantwell MF, Snider DE Jr, Cauthen GM, et al. Epidemiology of tuberculosis in the United States, 1983 through 1992. *JAMA* 1994;**272**:535–539.

12. World Health Organization. Tuberculosis MDR-TB & XDR-TB 2010 Report, Global Report on Surveillance and Response, 2010. Available at http://www.who.int/tb/features_archive/m_xdrtb_facts/en (accessed February 29, 2012).

13. Centers for Disease Control and Prevention. Notice to readers: Revised definition of extensively drug-resistant tuberculosis. *MMWR Morb Mortal Wkly Rep* 2006;**55**:1176.

14. Centers for Disease Control and Prevention. Tuberculosis Screening and Treatment Technical Instructions (TB TIs) using Cultures and Directly Observed Therapy (DOT) for Panel Physicians. Atlanta, 1991. Available at http://www.cdc.gov/immigrantrefugeehealth/exams/ti/panel/technical-instructions/panel-physicians/tuberculosis.html (accessed March 29, 2012).

15. Centers for Disease Control and Prevention. CDC Immigration Requirements: Technical Instructions for Tuberculosis Screening and Treatment Using Cultures and Directly Observed Therapy, October 1, 2009. Available at http://www.cdc.gov/immigrantrefugeehealth/pdf/tuberculosis-ti-2009.pdf (accessed March 27, 2012).

16. Liu Y, Weinberg MS, Ortega LS, Painter JA, Maloney SA. Overseas screening for tuberculosis in U.S.-bound immigrants and refugees. *N Engl J Med* 2009;**360**:23.

17. Centers for Disease Control and Prevention. Core Curriculum on Tuberculosis: What the Clinician Should Know, 5th ed. 2011.

18. Centers for Disease Control and Prevention, American Thoracic Society. American Thoracic Society and Centers for Cisease Control and Prevention diagnostic standards and classification of tuberculosis in adults and children. *Am J Respir Crit Care Med* 2000;**161**:1376–1395.

19. Centers for Disease Control and Prevention. Guidelines for preventing the transmission of *Mycobacterium tuberculosis* in health-care settings, 2005. *MMWR Recomm Rep* 2005; **54**(RR17):1–141.

20. Centers for Disease Control and Prevention. Updated guidelines for the use of nucleic acid amplification tests in the diagnosis of tuberculosis. *MMWR Morb Mortal Wkly Rep* 2009;**58**:7–10.

21. Centers for Disease Control and Prevention. Reference Laboratory, Division of Tuberculosis Elimination. Laboratory User Guide for U.S. Public Health Laboratories: Molecular detection of drug resistance (MDDR) in *Mycobacterium tuberculosis* complex by DNA sequencing (Version 2.0).

June 2012. Available at http://www.cdc.gov/tb/topic/laboratory/MDDRUsersGuide.pdf (accessed October 24, 2012).

22. Centers for Disease Control and Prevention. Guide to the Application of Genotyping to Tuberculosis Prevention and Control. 2012. Available at http://www.cdc.gov/tb/programs/genotyping/Chap1/Intro_2_Overview.htm (accessed August 22, 2012).

23. Centers for Disease Control and Prevention. Tuberculosis genotyping—United States, 2004–2010. *MMWR Morb Mortal Wkly Rep* 2009;**61**:723–725.

24. Dubos R, Dubos J. *The White Plague. Tuberculosis, Man and Society*. Boston, MA: Little Brown and Company; 1952.

25. Jacobs PP. Misleading mortality statistics on tuberculosis. Speech presented at the National Association for the Study and Prevention of Tuberculosis, Washington D.C., May 1912.

26. Cliff AD, Haggett P, Smallman-Raynor M, Stroup DF, Williamson GD. The importance of long-term records in public health surveillance: The US weekly sanitary reports, 1888–1912, revisited. *J Public Health Med* 1997;**19**:76–84.

27. Arana C The history of public health surveillance. *The Public Health Observer*. 2009. Available at http://publichealthobserver.com/public-health-articles/the-history-of-public-health-surveillance/ (accessed March 30, 2012).

28. Fox DM. Social policy and city politics: Tuberculosis reporting in New York, 1889–1900. *Bull Hist Med* 1975;**49**:169–175.

29. Linder FE, Grove RD (1947). Vital statistics rates in the United States 1900–1940. Table 20, Specific death rates for selected causes, by race, death registration states and each state, 1900–1940, every fifth year. Washington, D.C.: United States Government Printing Office.

30. Shryrock RH. *National Tuberculosis Association, 1904–1954. A Study of the Voluntary Health Movement in the United States*. New York: National Tuberculosis Association; 1957:96–106.

31. Lowell AM. *Tuberculosis in the United States. Monograph Series on Vital and Health Statistics*. Cambridge, MA: Harvard University Press; 1965:120–122.

32. Division of Chronic Disease and Tuberculosis. What is a reportable case of tuberculosis? *Public Health Rep* 1951;**66**:1291–1294.

33. Division of Chronic Disease and Tuberculosis. Reported tuberculosis morbidity and other data. U.S. Dept. of Health, Education, and Welfare, Public Health Service. PHS, 422, 1–6. 1954.

34. Division of Chronic Disease and Tuberculosis. Reported tuberculosis data. U.S. Dept. of Health, Education, and Welfare, Communicable Disease Center. PHS,638, 1–2. 1964.

35. Division of Tuberculosis Control. 1980 Tuberculosis in the United States. Centers for Disease Control and Prevention. HHS pub 83-8322: 21–26. 1983.

36. Center for Disease Control and Prevention. Tuberculosis Control Division. 1975 Tuberculosis Statistics: States and Cities. DHEW pub 77-8249: 1–6. 1976.

37. Centers for Disease Control. Tuberculosis Control Division. 1979 Tuberculosis in the United States. HHS pub 82-8322: 1–9. 1981.

38. Centers for Disease Control. Division of Tuberculosis Control. 1985 Tuberculosis Statistics: States and Cities. Centers for Disease Control. HHS pub 87-8249: 1–8. 1986.

39. Centers for Disease Control and Prevention. Tuberculosis–United States, first 39 weeks, 1985. *MMWR Morb Mortal Wkly Rep* 1985;**34**:625–627.

40. Centers for Disease Control and Prevention. Tuberculosis control laws—United States, 1993 Recommendations of the Advisory Council for the Elimination of Tuberculosis (ACET). *MMWR Morb Mortal Wkly Rep* 1993;**42**(RR-15):1–28.

41. Centers for Disease Control and Prevention. Tuberculosis Control Laws and Policies: A Handbook for Public Health and Legal Practitioners. The Centers for Law and the Public's Health. 2009. Available at http://tbcontrollers.org/docs/TBLawResources/TBControlLawsHandbook10012009.pdf (accessed April 2, 2014).

42. Centers for Disease Control and Prevention. National Electronic Disease Surveillance System. 2013. Available at http://wwwn.cdc.gov/nndss/script/nedss.aspx (accessed April 2, 2014).

43. Centers for Disease Control and Prevention. Tuberculosis Surveillance Data Training. Report of Verified Case of TB (RVCT). Self-Study Modules. U.S. Department of Health and Human Services, CDC, Atlanta, GA: U.S. Department of Health and Human Services, CDC, 2009.

44. Centers for Disease Control and Prevention. Online Tuberculosis Information System (OTIS), National Tuberculosis Surveillance System, United States, 1993–2009. U.S. Department of Health and Human Services (US DHHS), CDC WONDER On-line Database, February 2010. Available at http://wonder.cdc.gov/tb.html (accessed April 4, 2012).

45. Centers for Disease Control and Prevention. Trends in tuberculosis Incidence—United States, 2006. *MMWR Morb Mortal Wkly Rep* 2007;**56**:245–250.

46. Centers for Disease Control and Prevention. Trends in tuberculosis—United States, 2007. *MMWR Morb Mortal Wkly Rep* 2008;**57**:281–285.

47. Centers for Disease Control and Prevention. Trends in tuberculosis—United States, 2008. *MMWR Morb Mortal Wkly Rep* 2009;**58**:249–253.

48. Centers for Disease Control and Prevention. Decrease in reported tuberculosis cases—United States, 2009. *MMWR Morb Mortal Wkly Rep* 2010;**59**:289–294.

49. Centers for Disease Control and Prevention. Trends in tuberculosis—United States, 2010. *MMWR Morb Mortal Wkly Rep* 2011;**60**:333–336.

50. Centers for Disease Control and Prevention. U.S. Department of Health and Human Services, Centers for Disease Control and Prevention Tuberculosis Elimination and Laboratory, Cooperative Agreements, 2009, CDC-PS-10-1005, pp. 17–21.

51. Centers for Disease Control and Prevention. Fact Sheet: The National Tuberculosis Indicator Project (NTIP) Frequently Asked Questions (FAQ). 2012. Available at http://www.cdc.gov/tb/publications/factsheets/statistics/NTIPFAQs.htm (accessed April 1, 2012).

52. Centers for Disease Control and Prevention. Monitoring tuberculosis programs—National Tuberculosis Indicator Project, United States, 2002–2008. *MMWR Morb Mortal Wkly Rep* 2011;**59**:295–298.

53. Centers for Disease Control and Prevention. Assessment of declines in reported tuberculosis cases—Georgia and Pennsylvania, 2009. *MMWR Morb Mortal Wkly Rep* 2011;**60**: 338–342.

54. Curtis AB, McCray E, McKenna M, Onorato IM. Completeness and timeliness of tuberculosis case reporting: A multistate study. *Am J Prev Med* 2001;**20**:108–112.

55. Sprinson JE, Lawton ES, Porco TC, et al. Assessing the validity of tuberculosis surveillance data in California. *BMC Public Health* 2006;**6**:217–230.

56. Armstrong LR. Data validation pilot project. Quality Assurance Course, lecture, Centers for Disease Control and Prevention. August 2011.

57. Magee E, Tryon C, Forbes A, et al. The national tuberculosis surveillance system training program to ensure accuracy of tuberculosis data. *J Public Health Manag Pract* 2011;**17**: 427–430.

58. Winston CA, Navin TR, Becerra JE, et al. Unexpected decline in tuberculosis cases coincident with economic recession—United States, 2009. *BMC Public Health* 2011;**11**: 846–857.

Methods used in surveillance and data analysis

CHAPTER 15

Analysis and interpretation of surveillance data

Louisa E. Chapman and James N. Tyson

Centers for Disease Control and Prevention, Atlanta, GA, USA

Introduction

Analysis and interpretation of any surveillance data, including infectious disease surveillance data, faces six fundamental challenges. The first challenge is to understand the purpose and context of the specific surveillance system. The second challenge is to identify a baseline rate of observations and to recognize deviations from that baseline, including trends, clusters, and insignificant changes or surveillance artifacts. The third and fourth challenges are to interpret the meanings conveyed by these observations and to recognize the significance of these interpretations. The fifth challenge is to properly discern the degree of certainty that the available data can support regarding that interpretation. The last challenge is to communicate the observations (and the interpretation of their meanings, significance, and certainty) with clarity to the desired audience on a time table that enables meaningful action to be taken in response to the interpreted data.

Infectious disease surveillance is used to detect new diseases and epidemics, to document the spread of diseases, to develop estimates of infection-associated morbidity and mortality, to identify potential risk factors for disease, to facilitate research by informing the design of studies that can test hypotheses, and to plan and assess the impacts of interventions [1]. Surveillance for infectious diseases may focus on entities that are disease specific (e.g., laboratory confirmed *Vibrio cholerae* bacteria), syndromic (e.g., influenza-like illness), molecular (e.g., genotyping of polio virus [PV] to confirm a vaccine-derived origin), or proxies for the actual entities of interest (e.g., dead birds as a signal of possible West Nile virus spread). Regardless of the entity under observation, infectious disease surveillance involves the ongoing systematic collection, analysis, interpretation, and communication of information in a format that decision makers can easily interpret [1].

The origins of infectious disease surveillance can be traced to efforts by municipalities to enable early warning of decimating plagues. In 1662 in London, John Graunt published an analysis of bills of mortality compiled weekly since 1603. Graunt's analytic methods consisted primarily of counting and systematically categorizing entries, then comparing categories over defined times. Graunt's work predated the germ theory and was not a fully developed surveillance system, yet he described the periodicity of infectious diseases and demonstrated the value of converting numbers into rates to characterize the proportionate impact of plagues on a population and the value of contextual information for interpretation of surveillance data. Graunt's seventeenth century methods ("methids" as he called them) remain basic approaches to analysis and interpretation of infectious disease surveillance data today: (1) count entities and categorize them systematically; (2) when possible, link numerators with denominators to enable recognition of the proportionate impact of

Concepts and Methods in Infectious Disease Surveillance, First Edition. Edited by Nkuchia M. M'ikanatha and John K. Iskander.
Published 2014 by John Wiley & Sons, Ltd.

disease on populations; (3) examine data within the context of person, place, and time, using uniform time intervals; and (4) evaluate data for missing information or misattribution of cause, for duration of event impact, and for virulence of disease agents [2].

In America, Lemuel Shattuck analyzed Boston's vital statistics from 1810 to 1841 and proposed a public health infrastructure to gather health statistics at the state and local levels that anticipated modern public health surveillance functions [3–5]. As Superintendent of the General Register Office for England and Wales between 1838 and 1879, William Farr developed a system to routinely record official statistics, including specific causes of death, and compiled a "statistical nosology" which defined fatal disease categories to be used by local registrars. Farr routinely tabulated causes of death by disease, parish, age, sex, and occupation and was the first to compare mortality rates by occupation [6]. Between 1831 and 1866 cholera epidemics killed approximately 40,000 people in London. During these epidemics John Snow mapped the residences of those experiencing cholera deaths, proposed the then-radical hypothesis that people contracted cholera by drinking water contaminated with sewage, and famously interrupted the water supply to the population experiencing the highest mortality rate by removing the Broad Street pump handle (Figure 15.1) [7]. Statistical evidence collected by Farr linked the rate of deaths per thousand population with the water source and documented decreased mortality among customers of a company that relocated its intake above the tidal basin. As a result, public health engineering projects diverted sewage from water sources and ultimately eliminated cholera in industrialized countries [6].

U.S. statutes passed between 1850 and 1880 authorized the quarantine of vessels arriving from foreign ports to prevent epidemics. The 1878 Quarantine Act required publication of weekly international sanitary reports collected through the U.S. consular system [3–5].

Tavern keepers in the pre-Revolutionary American colony of Rhode Island were required to report contagious diseases among their patrons. In 1883, Michigan became the first U.S. state to require statewide reporting of certain infections to health officials [3–5]. Global disease surveillance data became more available when the Health Section of the League of Nations was established in 1923. By 1925, all U.S. states reported the incidence of pellagra and 23 communicable diseases. The United States began publishing domestic morbidity data in 1949 and added mortality data in 1952. During the 1950s and 1960s, the director of epidemiology at what is now the US Centers for Disease Control and Prevention (CDC), Alexander Langmuir, emphasized the use of systematic monitoring of disease in the population to inform action. U.S. national notifiable disease surveillance (see Chapter 3) assisted with elimination of endemic malaria and yellow fever and continues to be applied in disease elimination programs [3]. Langmuir described the basic tasks of the epidemiologist as "to count cases and measure the population in which they arise" [8]. In 1968 he wrote: "The one essential requirement for a surveillance system is a reasonably sophisticated epidemiologist who is located in a central position…who has access to information on the occurrence of communicable diseases…[and] power to inquire into and verify…facts… " [4].

As germ-theory science and abilities to link disease outcomes to both etiologic agents and risk factors for infection have progressed, analysis and interpretation efforts have become more meaningful and increasingly complex. Yet surveillance remains most effective when it is simplest. The foundation laid by Graunt's seventeenth century "methids," the progressive development over the nineteenth and twentieth centuries of systematic data collection and improved data definitions, the addition of mapping as an analytic tool, and the continual twentieth century emphasis on translation of surveillance data into disease-elimination action inform current standards of practice for surveillance analysis and interpretation. Early twenty-first-century innovations attempt to recognize syndromes and aberrations in states of disease when patients first present for care and to move communication of those patterns closer to the time of presentation [9]. Twenty-first-century public health demands technological tools that enable "real-time" information delivery.

Challenge 1: understand the purpose and context of surveillance systems

Surveillance data may come from widely different systems with different specific purposes. It is essential that the purpose and context of any specific system be understood before attempting to analyze and interpret

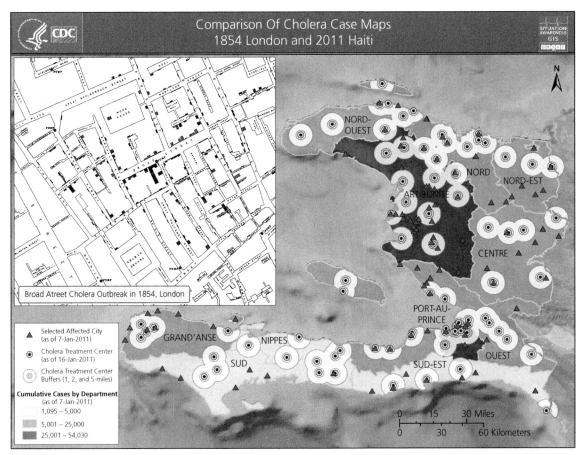

Figure 15.1 This map is adapted from CDC Situation Awareness unit surveillance maps of Haiti, 2011. It identifies affected cities and treatment centers based on the best publically available data at the time and illustrates walking buffers around the treatment centers. The map superimposes information from CDC; the National Cholera Monitoring System; Haiti's Ministry of Public Health and Population (Ministère de la Santé Publique et de la Population, MSPP); MSPP's Division of Epidemiology, Laboratory and Research (Direction d'Epidémiologie, de Laboratoire et de Recherches, DELR); Haiti's National Public Health Laboratory (Laboratoire National de Sante de Publique, LNSP) (case data); the United Nations Stabilization Mission in Haiti (MINUSTAH) (Department boundaries); and the Pan-American Health Organization (PAHO) (cholera treatment center) as of January 2011 onto a base layer developed from NASA [30]. John Snow's hand-drawn map of the residences of fatal cholera cases associated with the Broad Street pump in London in 1850 is inset. This figure illustrates the utility of integrating surveillance data into visualization products (specifically maps), of handheld computing devices for transmission of georeferenced surveillance data, and of spatial analysis combined with satellite imagery to assess risk factors. Source: Left image adapted from Snow, John. On the Mode of Communication of Cholera, 2nd edition. London: John Churchill, New Burlington Street, England, 1855. Reproduced with permission of Ralph R. Frerichs, University of California, Los Angeles School of Public Health Department of Epidemiology. Right image developed by Brian Kaplan with the CDC GRASP unit and with the Situational Awareness Unit of the Centers for Disease Control and Prevention Emergency Operations.

the surveillance data produced by that system. It is also essential to understand the methodology by which the surveillance system collects data. Is the data collected actively or passively? Is the surveillance system new or longstanding? Is the surveillance system freestanding or integrated into a larger system of data collection?

Challenge 2: identify baselines and recognize deviations

The most fundamental challenge for analysis and inter-pretation of surveillance data is the identification of a baseline. A baseline identifies the range of the normal

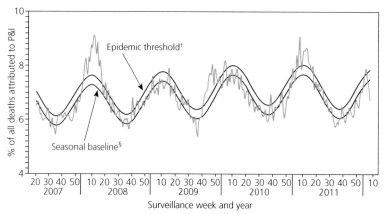

* For the reporting week ending February 11, 2012.
† The epidemic threshold is 1.645 standard deviations above the seasonal baseline.
§ The seasonal baseline is projected using a robust regression procedure that applies a periodic regression model
  to the observed percentage of deaths from P&I during the preceding 5 years.

Figure 15.2 Percentage of all deaths attributable to pneumonia and influenza (P&I) by surveillance week and year—122 U.S. Cities Mortality Reporting System, United States, 2007–2012. This graph illustrates the periodicity of influenza infection and the seasonal range of associated baseline observations, the utility of time series forecasting, the determination of epidemic thresholds, and the potential for mathematical models to contribute to the scientific basis for public health policy. Source: Adapted from [10]. Centers for Disease Control and Prevention.

or expected rate of occurrence for the entity under surveillance and provides the measure against which changes in status can be recognized. The baseline may be a series of single points but more often encompasses a range of values. For infections characterized by seasonal outbreaks, the baseline range will vary by season in a generally predictable manner as shown for influenza (Figure 15.2) [10]. The comparison of observations to the baseline range allows characterization of the impact of intentional interventions or natural phenomenon and determination of the direction of change. As an example, Reye's syndrome is a rare, but often fatal, syndrome of pediatric hepatic failure that was associated with common childhood febrile illnesses such as influenza and chickenpox through the 1960s. Figure 15.3 illustrates the progressive impact on the prevalence of Reye's syndrome in the United States of field investigations that raised suspicion that aspirin use in children might be a risk factor, of publication of a Surgeon General's advisory recommending against the use of aspirin to treat febrile childhood illnesses, and of regulatory action requiring changes in the labels of aspirin-containing medications (Figure 15.3) [11].

Resource investment in surveillance often occurs in response to a newly recognized disease (e.g., Hantavirus

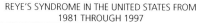

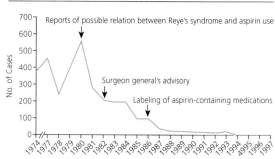

Figure 15.3 Number of reported cases of Reye's syndrome in relation to the timing of public announcements of the epidemiologic association of Reye's syndrome with aspirin ingestion and in relation to the labeling of aspirin-containing medications. Source: Adapted from [11] to illustrate the value of time series plotting and of context for interpretation.

Pulmonary Syndrome in 1993); a suspected change in the frequency, virulence, geography, or risk population of a familiar disease (e.g., introduction of West Nile virus into North America in 1999); or following a natural disaster (e.g., monitoring for gastrointestinal illness among Haitians displaced by the 2010 earthquake). In these situations, no baseline data are available against which to judge the significance of data collected under newly implemented surveillance. Baselines may be altered by changes in surveillance methods or by attention received by a surveillance system (e.g., publicity associated with a high-profile case) which may also alter the number of cases reported to the system. Neither new surveillance methods nor publicity reflect real changes in the state of nature, but both complicate determination of what should constitute the baseline against which apparent deviations are judged for significance. When uncommon entities are under surveillance, what may appear to be erratic variation in incidence may merely reflect the inherent instability of small number observations within a baseline range.

Standardize observations

A first step in analysis is to assess whether the methods used for data collection were precisely defined and standard throughout data collection. Differences in data collection methods may result in apparent differences in disease occurrence between geographic regions or over time that are merely artifacts resulting from variations in surveillance methodology. Data should be analyzed using standard periods of observation (e.g., by day, week, decade). It may be helpful to examine the same data by varied time frames. An outbreak of short duration may be recognizable through hourly, daily, or weekly grouping of data but obscured if data are examined only on an annual basis. Conversely, meaningful longer-term trends may be recognized more efficiently by examining data on an annual basis or at multiyear intervals.

Ensure precise case definitions

Surveillance systems may collect information on precisely defined or more vaguely defined disease entities. Surveillance design often utilizes case definitions that identify suspected, probable, and confirmed cases. Suspected cases may meet a general syndromic or clinical case definition; probable cases would fulfill the requirements for the suspected case definition plus meet more specifically defined criteria; and confirmed cases would fulfill the requirements for the probable case definition with the addition of the presence of a pathognomonic finding, a positive confirmatory laboratory test or other defining criteria. For example, the World Health Organization cholera case definition of "acute watery diarrhea,

with or without vomiting, in a patient aged 5 years or more" might be used as a suspected case definition during a field investigation; the addition of "who resides in an administrative department affected by cholera" might convert it to a probable case; and confirmation of *Vibrio cholerae* in stool would convert it to a confirmed case. If the surveillance system design has not already categorized data collected in this manner, sorting the observations into suspect, probable, and confirmed cases should be an early step in analysis. Doing so allows analysis of the data as a whole and of the three levels of cases.

Analyze denominator data

The meaning and significance of numerator data (e.g., the number of cases of colitis caused by overgrowth of the enteric bacteria *Clostridium difficile* observed in a municipality this week and the same week 1 year ago) become more clear when numerators can be associated with denominators (e.g., the number of residents of the municipality this week and the same week 1 year ago). A doubling of the number of cases of *C. difficile* colitis in the municipality over the course of 1 year appears alarming. It ceases to alarm if the population under observation has also doubled, resulting in a stable rate of disease. If the numerator has doubled but the denominator has remained stable, additional contextual observations may be informative. Correlation of this increase with the rate of antibiotic use or the predominant class of antibiotic prescribed may suggest a potential for public health action (i.e., intervention to influence antibiotic prescribing patterns).

An early approach to analysis of infectious disease surveillance data was to convert observation of numbers into observations of rates. Describing surveillance observations as rates (e.g., number of cases of measles per 10,000 population over a defined time period) standardizes the data in a way that allows comparisons of the impact of disease across time and geography and among different populations, which identifies the comparative impact of different infectious agents on a population (e.g., deaths per 10,000 population due to measles compared to the mortality rate per 10,000 from tuberculosis).

Ensure systematic presentation

Organization of data into line listings (a list of one observation per line) or tables were approaches used by

Graunt in 1662 to describe mortality from plagues [2] and are approaches used by CDC in the U.S. National Notifiable Disease Surveillance System (NNDSS) database in 2012 [12]. Line listings or systematic tables allow characterization of data by temporal occurrence and by number of cases. The percentage change per interval of time can be calculated, and variations in the rate of change can be recognized.

Compare observations over time

A usual and early step in surveillance data analysis is to compare current against historic observations for a similar period of time. This can be accomplished by development of a time series—a sequence of observations measured at successive time intervals preferentially spaced uniformly over time. The temporal ordering of observations allows recognition of the direction of change in the observation values over time, but also of the temporal pace of change and whether deviations are random or patterned.

Surveillance observations of infectious diseases in the pre-vaccine era, including those by Graunt in the 1600s, reveal a periodicity to epidemics of infectious diseases. This periodicity resulted from the occurrence of a major epidemic leading to widespread herd immunity among survivors, followed by a period of steady accumulation of susceptible individuals within the population, followed again by major epidemics that occur when an infectious agent is reintroduced into a population that has accumulated a large enough population of susceptibles to sustain transmission. This periodicity is illustrated in Figure 15.4 using measles as an example [13].

Use visual display of data

Plotting a time series of surveillance observations is often the easiest way to recognize characteristics of the data. Deviations from baseline over time may exhibit periodicity; that is, patterns of deviation may repeat themselves with regularity. Simple line or bar graphs reveal changes in rates of occurrence of disease over time (Figure 15.3) [11], including seasonal periodicity (Figure 15.2) [10] or periodicity related to the accumulation and immunization of susceptibles in the population (Figure 15.4) [13]. The use of both vertical axes can allow the comparison of two time series in one graph, or as in Figure 15.4, the comparison of observa-

tions graphed on a linear scale (left-hand axis) to those same observations graphed on a logarithmic scale (right-hand axis) [13]. When the data covers a large range of values, logarithmic scales reduce a wide range of values to a more manageable scale.

In the mid-nineteenth century, John Snow's "ghost map" (Figure 15.1, inset) identified water supplied by the Broad street pump as a risk factor for cholera [7]. Today geographic information system mapping is increasingly used to develop visual displays of infectious disease data that enable temporal and spatial recognition of disease spread and provide insight into risk factors. A CDC Situation Awareness unit surveillance map of Haiti shown in Figure 15.1 illustrates the "walking buffers," the areas surrounding treatment centers within which access to care is likely to improve survival.

Analyze aberrations

Understanding the sensitivity and specificity of surveillance systems is important. Reporting to surveillance systems may be active or passive. Epidemiologists must keep this in mind when assessing apparent changes in surveillance data. The first step in analysis of an unusual increase in observations reported through a surveillance system is to question whether the incidence of disease or the sensitivity of surveillance or both have increased. Statistical methods based on tests of randomness have been applied to infectious disease surveillance data for the purpose of analysis of aberrations. Methods include adaptations of quality control charts from industry; Bayesian, cluster, regression, time series, and bootstrap analyses; and application of smoothing algorithms, simulation, and spatial statistics [1,14].

While statistical analysis can be applied to surveillance data, the use of statistics for this purpose is often limited by the nature of surveillance data. Populations under surveillance are often not random samples of a general population, and may not be broadly representative, complicating efforts to use statistics to estimate morbidity and mortality impacts on populations. The ability to extrapolate outcomes of analyses to other populations may be limited, and standard errors may not be calculable. Incomplete reporting of demographic data also limits analytic options [1].

When separate surveillance systems observe the same disease entity using different case definitions and data

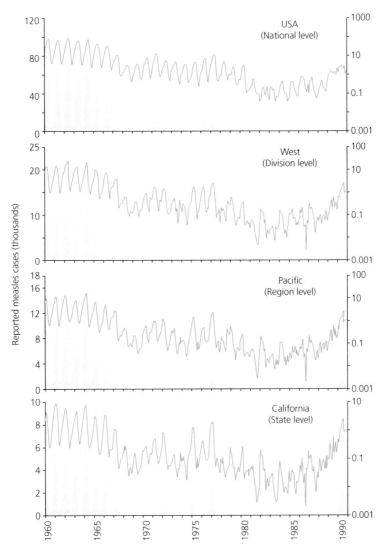

Figure 15.4 Monthly measles time series for the United States, 1960–1990, at (top to bottom) four descending spatial scales: the United States, the West Division, the Pacific Region, and the state of California. Source: Adapted from [13] to illustrate the periodicity of infectious and vaccine preventable diseases, the impact of diminishing numbers of observations or regional bias in data collection on analysis, the use of both vertical chart axes to allow comparison of two time series, the use of solid bar charts (left-hand axis) vs. line traces (right-hand axis), and of the same data plotted using linear (left-hand axis) and logarithmic (right-hand axis) scales.

collection methods, demographic analytic approaches have been used to assess the completeness of coverage of the separate systems. These include the Chandrasekar-Deming method and the Lincoln-Peterson Capture-Recapture method, which are used to estimate the total number of cases and the confidence interval, respectively [15,16].

Time series forecasting and regression methods have been fitted to mortality data series to forecast future epidemics of seasonal diseases, most commonly influenza, and to estimate the excess associated mortality. Time series forecasting uses a model to predict future values based on previously observed values. Influenza is characterized by predictable seasonal outbreaks estimated to be responsible for 3,000–49,000 deaths annually in the United States. Farr quantified the impact of the 1847–1848 influenza epidemic in London by estimating excess mortality [6]. The U.S. CDC currently uses weekly data reported to the 122 Cities Mortality Reporting System to monitor influenza-associated mortality in near real time. Excess mortality is defined in this system by using the ratio of pneumonia and influenza deaths to all deaths. A robust regression method applies a periodic regression model to the observed percentage of deaths attributed to pneumonia and influenza during the preceding 5 years to project an expected baseline for the current season. When the upper bound of the 95% confidence interval around this baseline is exceeded for 2 or more consecutive weeks (the defined epidemic threshhold for influenza associated deaths), then excess influenza-associated deaths are estimated by subtracting the number of deaths attributable to pneumonia and influenza predicted by the baseline death ratio for that week from the numbers actually observed (Figure 15.2) [17]. The contributions of earlier versions of these models to the scientific basis for vaccine recommendations are among the earliest applications of use of mathematical models to guide public policy [18,19].

Employ molecular analysis

The late twentieth century development of polymerase chain reaction (PCR) and other genetic laboratory techniques have made possible characterization of infectious agents at the genomic and protein sequence levels. Genetic sequencing of pathogens associated with cases enables very precise defininition of relationships among agents and, thus, the ability to confirm or refute common sources of infection.

As an example, the Global Poliovirus Laboratory Network uses PCR to identify polioviruses by serotype and whether they are vaccine-related or wild. PCR is further used to screen for genetically divergent vaccine-related polio viruses (called "vaccine-derived polio viruses" or VDPVs) of public health importance and to assign wild isolates to specific genotypes within a serotype. All wild polio viruses and VDPVs are routinely sequenced in the ~900-nucleotide VP1 region to address key epidemiologic questions such as (1) the genetic relationships among isolates (determines epidemiologic linkage among cases), (2) the genetic diversity among

isolates, (3) the estimated dates of VDPV emergence or wild polio virus importation, (4) the source of imported polio viruses, (5) the main pathways of transmission, and (6) the extent and duration of surveillance gaps (as indicated by the frequency and magnitude of gaps in the sequence dataset). Sequence data can be used as a high-resolution surveillance tool because the poliovirus genome evolves at a rapid and nearly uniform rate of 1% nucleotide substitutions per year (equivalent to 1–2 nucleotide substitutions per week over the entire 7,450-nucleotide poliovirus genome). Most of the genetic changes do not affect key biological properties, but the rapid nucleotide sequence evolution rate serves as a "molecular clock" useful for establishing the dates of important epidemiologic events [20].

Challenges 3, 4, and 5: interpretation of meaning, significance, and degree of certainty

Recognition of each deviation from baseline necessitates determination of the meaning and significance of that deviation. An apparent increase in incidence of disease may represent the onset of an epidemic in the population under surveillance, variation within a normal range of baseline activity or an artifact. Changes in surveillance methodology such as a change in case definition of the entity under surveillance, the application of a more sensitive laboratory assay for diagnosis, or the stimulation of "passive" reporting due to publicity associated with the entity under surveillance can also result in deviations from the baseline range in the absence of any meaningful change in the underlying state of disease in the population. A failure to appreciate the context of data collection in these instances would result in a misinterpretation of the meaning or significance of the observations.

The appropriate interpretation of data from most surveillance systems is as much of an art as a statistical or scientific challenge. In a lecture at the University of Lille, France, in 1854, Louis Pasteur famously declared, "In the fields of observation, chance favors only the mind that is prepared" [21]. This is never more true than in efforts to interpret and discern the significance of surveillance data. The most critical tool for the analysis and interpretation of surveillance data remains an engaged, prepared and critical mind, properly positioned to investigate circumstances associated with data collection. The more information an epidemiologist has about the purpose of the surveillance system, the people who perform the reporting, and the circumstances under which the data are collected and conveyed through the system, the more likely it is that the epidemiologist will interpret the data correctly.

Characterize person, place, and time

Traditional analysis of epidemiological data has stressed the characterization of person, place, and time. The demographic characteristics of age, sex, and race or ethnicity have become standard components of data collection. Analysis of surveillance data including these personal characteristics has identified disparities in health status among subpopulations that may point to risk factors for disease [14].

Define epidemic thresholds

To assist in the timely use of surveillance data, epidemiologists often define "epidemic thresholds" or "response thresholds" for conditions of intense scrutiny or predictable intermittent signficance (e.g., seasonal influenza). Defining such thresholds is technically difficult and often results from a combination of statistical efforts to assess whether departures from historical trends constitute meaningful changes combined with policy decisions on what level of deviation requires action to protect public health. It is an exercise in interpretation of the *significance* rather than of the *meaning* of surveillance data. Since 1962 CDC has determined that there is excess pneumonia and influenza mortality, likely due to influenza, when the observed proportion of deaths attributed to pneumonia and influenza exceeds the seasonal baseline (referred to as the "epidemic threshhold") for two consecutive weeks, as identified by a cyclical regression model fitted to a time series of weekly deaths reported by sentinel U.S. cities (Figure 15.2) [10,17].

Ascertain degree of certainty

When deviations from baseline are recognized and appear to represent real changes rather than artifactual observations and when an interpretation of their meaning and significance has been made, it remains necessary to assess the degree of certainty the available data can support regarding that interpretation. In con-

trolled studies, case and control populations can be compared, and therefore statistical analyses may be applied to define the probability that differences observed are significant and do not represent chance. The degree of confidence that can be placed in those findings can be defined. The ability to use statistics to determine significance of findings in surveillance data is more limited. When a large volume of data is available, an easy empiric certainty regarding significance can often be determined (Figure 15.2). For rare diseases, certainty regarding substantial variation is harder to achieve. Small numbers are inherently unstable. If 1 week of surveillance identifies one case of disease, three cases during the following week triples the incidence and might trigger concerns regarding an epidemic. However, if in 1 year of observation between one and five events are observed per week, the initial tripling was likely meaningless. Alternatively, a full year of weekly observations ranging between no cases and one per week would indicate that three observations in a week do have significance. The power to discern meaningful differences is also affected by the size of the population under surveillance and the frequency of the condition among that population.

Challenge 6: communicate for public health action

The last challenge in analysis and interpretation of infectious disease surveillance data is to communicate the interpreted significance of that data to the right audience with clarity and on a time table that enables meaningful response action. The transnational scope of disease control activities and access to new tools has increased expectations regarding the rapid availability of information during crises.

Local, state, and federal public health authorities, legislatures, and other decision makers depend on surveillance data to enable evidence-based public policy decisions. When the need arises, decision makers must have ready access to interpreted information. To maximize utility, surveillance data must be assessed and interpreted regularly. "Communicating with clarity" entails clearly communicating not merely conclusions based on the available data, but also the degree of confidence in those conclusions that the data can support.

Evolving approaches to disease detection, analysis, and interpretation

Public health crises such as the 2010 introduction of cholera into Haiti highlight the need to find increasingly rapid methods to acquire, analyze, interpret and communicate information. Increases in the information response cycle (i.e., the more rapid availability of accurate interpreted data in response to information needs) can strengthen the capacity for public health response (Figure 15.1).

The pace of the information response cycle becomes especially critical during public health emergencies. Technological advances in communication tools and the almost instantaneous availability of electronic information enable an information response cycle that exceeds that achievable using traditional surveillance methods. The advent of applied Web-enabled information sharing and dynamic visualization technologies has made possible nearly simultaneous communication and analysis of information from disparate sources. These technologies allow public health professionals who are geographically distant from each other to effectively collaborate, in near real time, on analyses of mutual interest [22,23].

Snow's nineteenth century map demonstrated the utility of integrating public health data into a visualization product (Figure 15.1) [7]. The twenty-first-century ability to electronically layer information from multiple sources onto a display and to manipulate that data using geospatial and temporal analyses, and modeling techniques can enable epidemiologists to make contextual sense of disparate information [22–26]. Manipulation of layers of data allows experts to apply practical knowledge and intuition in ways that may identify patterns or generate novel insights. Real-time visualization of developing information superimposed over baseline observations on Web-enabled maps can provide contextual understanding that may be critical to response decisions in rapidly evolving situations.

Ubiquitous access to Internet-capable computing devices provides opportunity to leverage the "wisdom of crowds" and the Internet to conduct surveillance [27]. Public health professionals are attempting to determine how data obtained from standard surveillance sources can be amplified through association with crowd-sourced information, which may include photos, videos, text, or audio observations of, for instance, damage to critical infrastructure during a natural disaster that may impact sanitation or water supplies. The challenge is to recognize which open-source, social-media, and crowd-sourced data can serve as reliable disease indicators.

In the absence of formal traditional surveillance systems, the rapid, organized capture of information about events that may represent risk to the health of the public has been termed "event-based surveillance." Relevant events may include mass gatherings, natural disasters, outbreaks or individual cases of unidentified disease, unexplained deaths, or rumors circulating in a community in which no formal surveillance is conducted. Event-based surveillance, which has been advocated for detection of emerging infections [28], is based on the capture of unstructured descriptions and ad-hoc reports (which may include rumors) of human disease events (e.g., clustering, unusual cases) but also of events that may represent exposures that are potentially hazardous to human health, such as disease in animals and suspected environmental contamination. Event reports may be transmitted through established routine reporting channels but also through informal channels such as media reports and reports from health workers and nongovernmental organizations. This approach contrasts to surveillance systems characterized by routine collection of data with predefined case definitions and action thresholds. However, both approaches attempt to develop systematic databases that enable recognition of deviations from steady states and support interpretation of the significance of those deviations for human health. Event-based surveillance is particularly effective in detecting disease outbreaks in countries with weak public health surveillance systems [28,29].

Wider use of privately owned computing devices is one potentially transformational approach to providing critical information faster during crisis situations. Technologies that enable the use of handheld computing devices (e.g., smart phones) for surveillance purposes can be anticipated to continue to evolve and to contribute to dramatic advancements in the speed and manner of information flow. New ways of rapidly detecting unusual patterns in disease surveillance data are continually being explored. Recent initiatives have explored whether an increase in transactions involving specific medications or a shift in the pattern of chief complaints by persons presenting for outpatient health care could enable more timely detection of changes in the health status of populations [9]. The challenge for surveillance professionals is to harness that information in a manner that leads to proportionate increases in directing the speed and effectiveness of public health responses.

Case studies

U.S. National Notifiable Disease Surveillance System, 2012

The U.S. NNDSS collects information from state and territorial health departments on more than 70 notifiable diseases [12]. Reporting is usually passive, and completeness varies depending upon the disease and the reporting source. The recognition of a disease and the degree of reporting completeness may be influenced by the availability of diagnostic facilities, control measure presence, public awareness, and the resources and priorities of state and local health officials. Changes in surveillance methods may cause changes in disease reporting, independent of alterations to the true incidence of a disease [12,14].

Weekly, MMWR posts on the Internet 3 tables and a figure containing U.S. state health department notifica-

tions of provisional NNDSS case counts. NNDSS Table I provides provisional case counts of infrequently reported notifiable diseases (<1,000 cases during the prior year) for the current week and cumulatively for the current year. To allow comparisons that enable recognition of deviations from baseline, the table also presents the 5-year weekly average (calculated by adding the incidence counts for the current week, the 2 weeks preceding the current week, and the 2 weeks following the current week, for a total of 5 preceding years) and the total cases reported for each of the previous 5 years [12]. The figure depicts the ratio of provisional current reports of selected notifiable diseases to historic data using an aberration detection algorithm. Data exceeding a defined threshold are identified using a hatched bar (Figure 15.5) [12].

Cholera: London 1850 and Haiti 2010

In 1850 Snow's "ghost map" demonstrated clustering of deaths from cholera among households that drew water from the Broad Street well. Snow removed the pump handle and published his hypothesis that cholera was transmitted via polluted water (Figure 15.1) [7].

In January 2010, a magnitude 7.0 M_w earthquake disrupted infrastructure and left more than 1 million

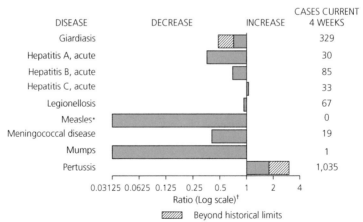

* No measles cases were reported for the current 4-week period yielding a ratio for week 16 of zero (0).
† Ratio of current 4-week total to mean of 15 4-week totals (from previous, comparable, and subsequent 4-week periods for the past 5 years). The point where the hatched area begins is based on the mean and two standard deviations of these 4-week totals.

Figure 15.5 Selected notifiable disease reports, United States; comparison of provisional 4-week totals April 21, 2012, with historical data. Note that no measles cases were reported for the reporting week illustrated in this figure. This graph illustrates the utility of ratios and log scales for visualizing surveillance data, of the comparison of current to historic data, and of defined thresholds for interpretation of significance. Adapted from [12], Centers for Disease Control and Prevention.

Haitians homeless. In October 2010, Haitian officials were notified of unusually high numbers of patients from Artibonite and Centre departments who had acute watery diarrhea and dehydration. The Haitian National Public Health Laboratory isolated *Vibrio cholerae* from stool specimens obtained from patients in the affected area.

In the United States, the CDC Situation Awareness Unit used satellite imagery to produce surveillance maps that visualized the spatial relationships between the locations of initial cholera cases and the Artibonite River. Coordinates of new cases, of cholera treatment centers, and of other entities of interest were transmitted electronically by emergency responders in Haiti using "smart phones." Spatial analysis used terrain, slope, road networks, walking impediments, average walking speed, and other factors to realistically estimate the catchment area in which the probability of survival of afflicted residents might be improved through easier access to care. These "walking buffers" surrounding treatment centers were overlaid on a virtual globe, immediately visualizing gaps in healthcare access among populations at risk. Sharing this information through public websites enabled rapid coordinated effort by response groups on the ground in Haiti to establish new treatment facilities at locations that best served the populations at most risk (Figure 15.1).

valuable tool for analysis and interpretation of infectious disease surveillance observations.

In the context of public health practice, a key value of surveillance data is not just in the observations from the surveillance system but also in the fact that these data often stimulate action to collect better data, usually through field investigations. Field investigations may improve understanding of risk factors that were suggested by the surveillance data itself. Often, field investigations triggered by surveillance observations lead to research studies such as case control comparisons that identify and better define the strength of risk factors. The outcome of such studies may, in turn, help to guide public health control measures.

Acknowledgments

The authors thank Lawrence B. Schonberger, MD, for mentoring in the art and science of infectious disease surveillance analysis and interpretation; Olen Kew for bringing precision and clarity to the description of how molecular biology informs surveillance; Mehran Massoudi, PhD, for critical reviews; and Brian Kaplan and the CDC Geospatial Research, Analysis and Service Program (GRASP) for development of Figure 15.1.

Conclusions

Despite proliferation of new systems and methodologies, the fundamental conceptual challenges for the analysis and interpretation of any surveillance data remain the same. The initial challenge is to understand the purpose and context of the system through which observations were collected. The second challenge is to recognize a baseline and deviations including trends and clusters. The next set of challenges involves interpretation of the meaning of these observations, determination of the significance of that meaning, and application of judgment regarding the degree of confidence in that interpretation. The last challenge is to clearly communicate with the appropriate audience on a time course that enables effective and responsive action. The disciplined application of a prepared mind remains the most

STUDY QUESTIONS

1. Why is identification of baseline values the most fundamental challenge for analysis and interpretation of surveillance data?
2. What are three possible explanations for observed changes in surveillance data incidence?
3. What is the advantage of translating surveillance observation numbers into rates?
4. How can a time series, including time series forecasting, be used to interpret the significance of surveillance observations?
5. What are several characteristics of surveillance data that may limit the ability to use statistical methods for analysis?
6. What are several characteristics that complicate interpretation of the significance of apparent clustering identified through surveillance data?

References

1. Thacker SB, Berkelman RL, Stroup DF. The science of public health surveillance. *J Public Health Policy* 1989;**10**: 187–203.

2. Graunt J. *Natural and Political OBSERVATIONS Mentioned in a following Indes, and made upon the Bills of Mortality.* Printed by Tho:Roycroft, for John Martin, James Allestry, and Tho:Dicas, at the Sign of the Bell in St. Paul's Churchyard, London, MDCLXII. Rendered into HTML format by Ed Stephan 25 January, 1996. Available at http://www.edstephan.org/Graunt/bills.html (accessed April 7, 2014).

3. Langmuir AD. The surveillance of communicable disease of national importance. *N Engl J Med* 1963;**288**:182–192.

4. Langmuir AD. Evolution of the concept of surveillance in the US. *Proc R Soc Med* 1971;**64**:681–684.

5. Cliff AD, Haggett P, Smallman-Raynor MR, Stroup DF, Williamson GD. The importance of long-term records in public health surveillance: The US weekly sanitary reports, 1888–1912, revisited. *J Public Health Med* 1997;**19**: 76–84.

6. Langmuir AD. William Farr: Founder of modern concepts of surveillance. *Int J Epidemiol* 1976;**5**:13–18.

7. Snow J. *On the Mode of Communication of Cholera*, 2nd ed. London: John Churchill, New Burlington Street, England; 1855. Available at http://www.ph.ucla.edu/epi/snow/snowbook.html (accessed April 7, 2014). Developed for the University of California, Los Angeles School of Public Health Department of Epidemiology website by Ralph R. Frerichs.

8. Langmuir AD. The territory of epidemiology: Pentimento. *J Infect Dis* 1987;**155**:349–358.

9. Bradley CA, Rolka H, Walker D, Loonsk J. BioSense: Implementation of a national early event detection and situational awareness system. *MMWR Syndr Surveill Suppl* 2005; **54**:11–19.

10. Centers for Disease Control and Prevention. Update: Influenza activity—United States, 2000–2011. *MMWR Morb Mortal Wkly Rep* 2012;**61**:123–8.

11. Belay ED, Bresee JS, Holman RC, et al. Reye's syndrome in the United States from 1981 through 1997. *N Engl J Med* 1999;**340**:1377–1382.

12. Centers for Disease Control and Prevention. National Notifiable Disease Surveillance System (NNDSS) webpage. 2014. Available at http://www.cdc.gov/osels/ph_surveillance/nndss/phs/infdis2011.htm (accessed April 7, 2014).

13. Cliff AD, Haggett P, Smallman-Raynor MR, Stroup DF, Williamson GD. The application of multidimensional scaling methods to epidemiological data. *Stat Methods Med Res* 1995;**4**:102–123. Available at http://smm.sagepub.com/content/4/2/102 (accessed April 7, 2014).

14. Thacker SB, Stroup DF. Future directions for comprehensive public health surveillance and health information systems in the US. *Am J Epidemiol* 1994;**140**:383–397.

15. Chandra Sekar C, Deming WE. On a method for estimating birth and death rates and the extent of registrations. *J Am Stat Assoc* 1944;**44**:101–115.

16. Cormack RM. The statistics of capture-recapture. *Oceanogr Mar Biol Ann Rev* 1968;**6**:455–506.

17. Thompson WW, Shay DK, Weintraub E, Brammer L, Cox N, Anderson LJ, Fukuda K. Mortality associated with influenza and respiratory syncytial virus in the United States. *JAMA* 2003;**289**:179–186.

18. Eickhoff TC, Sherman IL, Serfling RE. Observations on excess mortality associated with epidemic influenza. *JAMA* 1961;**176**:776–782.

19. Langmuir AD, Henderson DA, Serfling RE. The epidemiological basis for the control of influenza. *Am J Public Health Nations Health* 1964;**54**:563–571.

20. World Health Organization, Centers for Disease Control and Prevention. Tracking progress toward global polio eradication—Worldwide, 2009–2010. *MMWR Morb Mortal Wkly Rep* 2011;**60**:441–445.

21. Pasteur L. Speech delivered at Douai on December 7, 1854, on the occasion of his formal inauguration to the Faculty of Letters of Douai and the Faculty of Sciences of Lille). Reprinted In: Vallery-Radot P, ed. *Oeuvres de Pasteur*, Vol. 7. Paris: Masson and Co.; 1939:131.

22. Centers for Disease Control and Prevention. User Defined Situation Awareness, a CDC SA-GRASP Mapping Application. 2014. Available at http://emergency.cdc.gov/situationawareness/NaturalHazards/Interactive/index.html (accessed April 7, 2014).

23. Centers for Disease Control and Prevention. Situation Awareness webpage. 2013. Available at http://emergency.cdc.gov/situationawareness/ (accessed April 7, 2014).

24. National Oceanic and Atmospheric Administration. National Weather Service, National Hurricane Center. 2013. Available at http://www.nhc.noaa.gov/gtwo_atl.shtml (accessed April 7, 2014).

25. United States Geological Survey. Volcano Hazards Program. 2013. Available at http://volcanoes.usgs.gov/ (accessed April 7, 2014).

26. National Oceanic and Atmospheric Administration. National Weather Service Flood Map. 2014. Available at http://water.weather.gov/ahps/ (accessed April 7, 2014).

27. Eysenbach G. Infodemiology and infoveillance: Framework for an emerging set of public health informatics methods to analyze search, communication and publication behavior on the internet. *J Med Internet Res* 2009;**11**(1):e11.

28. World Health Organization. Western Pacific Region. A Guide to establishing event-based surveillance. 2008. ISBN 978 92 9061 321 3 (NLM Classification: WA 110) WHO Regional Office for the Western Pacific, Manila,

Phillipines. Available at http://www.wpro.who.int/entity/emerging_diseases/documents/docs/eventbasedsurv.pdf (accessed June 12, 2012).

29. World Health Organization Western Pacific Region. A guide to establishing event-based surveillance. 2008. Available at http://www.wpro.who.int/emerging_diseases/ documents/docs/eventbasedsurv.pdf (accessed April 7, 2014).

30. Stockli R, Vermote E, Saleous N, Simmon R, Herring D. The Blue Marble Next Generation—A true color earth dataset including seasonal dynamics from MODIS. 2005. Published by the NASA Earth Observatory.

CHAPTER 16

Global surveillance for emerging infectious diseases

Jennifer B. Nuzzo

UPMC Center for Health Security, Baltimore, MD, USA

Introduction

By the middle of the twentieth century, sharp declines in mortality associated with infectious diseases in the United States prompted optimistic views about conquest of infectious agents among medical and public health leaders [1,2]. This short-lived optimism was replaced by new threats, including emergence of human immunodeficiency virus/acquired immunodeficiency syndrome (HIV/AIDS) and reemergence of drug-resistant tuberculosis [3].

During the last 15 years, several high profile outbreaks have led to calls for enhanced surveillance for infectious diseases. These incidents included the deliberate dissemination of anthrax in the United States during 2001, the rapid spread of severe acute respiratory syndrome (SARS) caused by a novel coronavirus in 2003, the emergence and ongoing zoonotic transmission of highly pathogenic H5N1 avian influenza, and the global pandemic of influenza A/H1N1 in 2009. Each of these events demonstrated the ongoing health risks posed by infectious diseases. Each of these events was associated with significant social and economic consequences felt on a global scale. As a result, there have been increasing efforts to improve infectious disease surveillance around the world.

This chapter focuses on approaches to global surveillance including attributes for indicator-based and event-based systems, outbreak response systems, and key developments including the new International Health Regulations. The increased contributions of nontraditional sectors in surveillance (e.g., the agencies responsible for security are discussed) and current challenges, including insufficient capacity to detect diseases, are highlighted.

Overview of surveillance

Definition of terms

Historically, the term "disease surveillance" has been used to refer to the systematic collection and evaluation of data pertaining distribution and trends of incidence of morbidity and mortality within a population [4]. Disease surveillance is not a single act, but rather a series of actions in a multistep process. The general phases of action that occur in the process disease surveillance are illustrated in Figure 16.1.

Traditionally, surveillance has been the purview of governmental public health agencies and has focused on a predefined list of diseases or conditions, referred to as indicator-based surveillance. The continued emergence of new infectious disease threats, including the potential deliberate use of biological agents as weapons, has led to changes in the practice of infectious disease surveillance. Event-based surveillance is generally used to detect or monitor rare, new, or otherwise unusual events. These systems are not usually tied to a specific disease, and may use strategies like news media scans for reports of undiagnosed outbreaks in rural villages. Events identified via these types of surveillance systems may require an epidemiological investigation to determine whether an event should be of concern to public health authorities. Guidelines from the World Health

Concepts and Methods in Infectious Disease Surveillance, First Edition. Edited by Nkuchia M. M'ikanatha and John K. Iskander.
© 2015 John Wiley & Sons, Ltd. Published 2015 by John Wiley & Sons, Ltd.

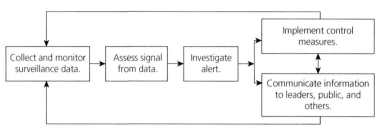

Figure 16.1 General phases of activity that occur during disease surveillance.

Organization (WHO) state that event-based surveillance is useful in areas where there are weak traditional indicator-based disease surveillance capacities. A more detailed comparison of indicator- and event-based surveillance is shown in Table 16.1.

In recent years, a new term, biosurveillance, has been adopted, particularly among those in the U.S. policy community, to describe the broad set of activities involved in monitoring data that may be directly or indirectly related to the health status of plants, animals, or humans in order to improve the abilities to detect, recognize, report, and respond to disease threats [5]. Biosurveillance may include traditional indicator-based disease surveillance approaches and may also include systems that monitor nonhuman or nondisease endpoints. In the United States, for example, the BioWatch program uses air sensors to monitor for the presence of pathogens that may be associated with bioterrorism.

Architecture of systems for global surveillance and outbreak response

The primary responsibility for global surveillance belongs to individual countries. Within countries, the entities responsible for carrying out surveillance vary. For example, the United States has a federated system of disease surveillance, in that individual states have primary responsibility for conducting disease surveillance. States report disease surveillance data to the Centers for Disease Control and Prevention (CDC) on a voluntary basis, as discussed in detail in Chapter 3. In other countries, disease surveillance activities are more centralized [6]. For example, in many countries that have national healthcare systems, a national health agency receives disease reports directly from healthcare facilities.

Typically, surveillance activities are indicator-based, organized around specific diseases or conditions, such as HIV or tuberculosis. Increased interest in detecting emerging infectious disease outbreaks and other "unknown" events has prompted increased adoption of event-based surveillance systems. Once a new disease emerges and is recognized, countries may implement dedicated indicator-based surveillance activities. For example, some countries now maintain dedicated surveillance systems for West Nile virus and H5N1 (avian) influenza.

The recognition of outbreaks typically begins with the recognition and reporting of an unusual case or cases of disease or an unusual pattern of illness within a community (e.g., a rare pathogen, unusual frequency or severity of known disease). Reports are often received from astute clinicians or laboratories. Public health authorities may decide to investigate reports to determine whether they are credible or whether they warrant further action. Outbreaks that appear to be credible and that may have international public health significance must be reported to the WHO (see section on International Health Regulations). Countries may then decide to take action or request assistance from the WHO or other countries.

The increasing frequency of disease outbreaks that have spread across national borders has led to the development of multicountry surveillance networks. Some countries have formed agreements and partnerships with their geographic neighbors for the purposes of improving their individual and collective abilities to detect, investigate, and respond to disease outbreaks and epidemics. Countries that participate in surveillance networks typically agree to share disease outbreak information and to collaborate in efforts to control disease spread. They may also share technical methods and other resources that can enhance disease surveillance practices in countries within the network. In some cases, the sharing and joint analysis of

Table 16.1 Comparison of key attributes and components of event-based and indicator-based surveillance.

	Event-based surveillance	Indicator-based surveillance

Case definitions	• Definitions can be used to help guide reporting.
	• Definitions are broad, such as a cluster of deaths in the same village during the same time period.
	• Definitions are more sensitive than those used in indicator-based surveillance.
		• Diseases and syndromes have a case definition that may include one or all of the following:
		  ○ clinical presentation,
		  ○ characteristics of people affected, and/or
		  ○ laboratory criteria.
		• Definitions are more specific than those used in event-based surveillance.

Timeliness	• All events should be reported to the system immediately.	• Data are usually reported each week or month. • Some diseases and syndromes may be immediately notifiable. • Even where electronic reporting exists, a delay often remains between case identification and when data aggregated are reported to the system by a health facility. • Where laboratory criteria are included in the case definition, a further delay in reporting may occur.
Data/Information	• The data format is not predefined. • For each event as much information as possible is collected and recorded. • Designated staff collecting the information attempt to obtain key pieces of information (i.e., time, place, person) to assist with event confirmation and assessment.	• Data are aggregated for each disease/syndrome. • Data format is predefined and may include a breakdown by demographic or other variables (i.e., number of cases 0–4 and >5 years of age).
Reporting structure	• Loose structure • Reports are unstructured and can enter the system at any time. • Forms are used to capture the event information, but the format is sufficiently flexible to collect qualitative and quantitative data. • A unit/team is designated to triage, confirm, and assess each reported event and trigger a response, as appropriate.	• Clearly defined • Reporting forms are used by reporting units to pass information through the system often on predefined days of the week or month. • Zero reporting is often used. • A unit/team is designated to analyze the surveillance data at regular intervals.
Reporting units	• Open, sometimes undefined (i.e., the general public can report directly to the system)	• Facility-based, closed
Trigger for initial action	• A report that is confirmed and assessed as a potential risk to public health	• Predefined thresholds
Analysis	• Rapid risk assessment	• Predefined intervals (weekly, monthly)
Response	• Immediate • The response to an event is built into the surveillance system.	• May be delayed as a result of the time taken to collect and analyze data • The response to an outbreak is built into the surveillance system.

Source: Adapted from *A Guide to Establishing Event-based Surveillance*. Available at http://www.wpro.who.int/emerging_diseases/documents/docs/eventbasedsurv.pdf. Reprinted with permission of WHO.

surveillance data across a network have contributed to a more complete understanding of the nature of the outbreak [7,8].

Multicountry disease surveillance networks now exist in many parts of the world, such as the Middle East, Southeast Asia, Southern Africa, Southeastern Europe, and East Africa. Examples include the following [9]:

- The Mekong Basin Disease Surveillance (MBDS) network, which includes Cambodia, Southern China, Lao PDR, Myanmar, Thailand, and Vietnam, works to improve surveillance and response to outbreaks of H5N1, cholera, and Dengue hemorrhagic fever. MBDS members have worked together to provide post-disaster relief, for example, during the aftermath of Cyclone Nargis in Myanmar in May 2008.
- The Middle East Consortium on Infectious Disease Surveillance (MECIDS) includes public health experts and ministry of health officials from Israel, the Palestinian Authority, and Jordan. The network has worked to improve regional surveillance for foodborne disease by providing training and by developing standard procedures and a common platform for data sharing and analysis. The network is significant in that its members have had success in finding common ground across borders of countries in conflict.
- The Southern African Centre for Disease Surveillance (SACIDS) includes disease experts from Tanzania, Mozambique, Zambia, the Democratic Republic of Congo, and South Africa. Network members work to improve their capacity to detect, identify, and monitor infectious diseases affecting humans and animals. The network has also partnered with a number of nongovernmental institutions, including Sokoine University of Agriculture (SUA), the Royal Veterinary College, and the London School of Hygiene and Tropical Medicine, to promote sharing of knowledge and resources such as diagnostic equipment and laboratories equipped for biocontainment. The East African Integrated Disease Surveillance Network (EAIDSNet) is a regional, intergovernmental collaborative initiative of the national health and agriculture ministries and the national health research and academic institutions within East Community partner states (Kenya, Uganda, Tanzania, Rwanda, Burundi). The network activities are aimed at enhancing surveillance and response to diseases in humans and animals with the East African partner states.

Key developments in approaches to global surveillance

2005 revision to International Health Regulations

Countries have a long had an obligation to conduct surveillance for infectious diseases and to share information about outbreaks with the international community. The International Health Regulations (IHR) codify the measures that countries must take to limit the international spread of disease while ensuring minimum interference with trade and travel. Formally adopted by the 22nd World Health Assembly in 1969, the history of the IHR dates back to discussions in an international sanitary conference in 1851 [10]. For much of their existence, the focus of the IHR has been to require countries to report to the WHO the occurrence of any cases of a short, defined list of diseases, such as cholera or plague.

In 2005, the IHR were significantly revised, in part because of experience during the 2003 SARS outbreak. Global perception that SARS was worsened by China's lack of communication about the outbreak raised questions about the effectiveness of the existing IHR and prompted calls for the regulations to be updated and strengthened.

The current IHR contain several provisions aimed at strengthening global surveillance. For example, states that are party to IHR are obligated:

- to strengthen and maintain surveillance to detect and assess whether events that may constitute a public health emergency of international concern (PHEIC);
- to notify WHO within 24 hours of all events that qualify as PHEIC, and after notification, submit pertinent data (e.g., laboratory results); and
- to the extent possible, to collaborate with other countries in detection and response to events covered under IHR.

Additionally, IHR grants WHO the authority to consider unofficial reports of disease outbreaks. The rationale for this provision is based on the observation that unofficial reports that an outbreak was occurring in China circulated for months before SARS was officially recognized by any government. At the time, WHO was not able to publicly comment or respond to the reports until it received official notice from the affected country [11]. Under the revised IHR, WHO and other countries can now take better advantage of newer event-based surveillance systems, such as the Public Health Agency of Canada's Global Public Health Intelligence Network (GPHIN) [12] and the U.S. government's Project Argus [13], both of which scan news sources worldwide looking for reports of potential disease outbreaks.

Increasing interest in surveillance for security purposes

Concerns about biological terrorism have raised the profile of infectious disease surveillance in the United States and around the globe [14]. Following the terrorist attacks on the World Trade Center in New York City, the CDC issued a recommendation that healthcare providers and public health practitioners maintain heightened surveillance for any patterns of illness that may be associated with a deliberate release of a biological agent [15]. In October and November of that same year, 22 people were infected and five people died when letters containing powdered anthrax spores were mailed to individuals in Florida, New York, and Washington, D.C. [11]. These events emphasized the connection between global surveillance and security. The conduct of public health surveillance to detect any deliberate release of biological agents is not new: In 1951, the CDC founded the Epidemic Intelligence Service because of concerns about biological warfare arising from the Korean War [12]. Public health practitioners were also instrumental in investigating an outbreak of salmonellosis that was caused when a religious group in The Dalles, Oregon, deliberately contaminated salad bars in the hope of influencing local elections by incapacitating voting members of the community [13].

Security communities recognized the relevance of global surveillance to their goals of protecting the political, economic, and military well-being of nations [16]. Improving global surveillance for biological terrorism and emerging infectious diseases is now a major focus of the U.S. Department of Defense's (DoD) threat reduction programs [17]. DoD spends more on global health surveillance than any other U.S. governmental agency [18].

Increased adoption of syndromic surveillance systems

Interest in improving the detection and monitoring of biological attacks and other infectious disease outbreaks has led to increased adoption of new approaches to disease surveillance, such as syndromic surveillance [19]. The initial objective of syndromic surveillance was to increase the speed with which outbreaks or clusters of diseases were detected by examining different types of data that may be associated with changes in health status and are likely to be available sooner than data from traditional reporting sources . Data sources that have been tapped for syndromic surveillance range from volume-of-sales data on over-the-counter medicines to workplace or school absenteeism. New York City, which was among the first to adopt syndromic surveillance methods, implemented a "drop-in" surveillance system in 2001 that monitors data on visits to emergency departments [20].

According to a 2008 survey of U.S. health departments, 88% of respondents reported that they employ syndromic-based approaches as part of routine surveillance [21]. As health departments have gained experience with syndromic surveillance, the way in which these approaches are used has evolved. Whereas the initial objective of syndromic surveillance was to obtain earlier detection of outbreaks than was possible with traditional public health surveillance methods, the focus of these efforts has largely shifted to monitoring the pace and progress of infectious disease outbreaks and other events that may impact public health [22].

Increased availability of electronic health information

The expansion of the Internet and mobile communication technologies has also had considerable impact on the practice of surveillance. For example, the diffusion of mobile phones into remote areas of the world has also created possibilities for enhanced disease reporting and outbreak detection. As of 2011, close to 6 billion cellular phones were active worldwide, which corresponds to a penetration of 86% of the world's population [23]. Mobile phones have been used to expedite the reporting of diseases among members of Peru's Navy [24] and to increase the detection of animal disease outbreaks in Sri Lanka [25].

In addition to helping to improve communication with existing public health surveillance systems, mobile communications and Internet-based tools are making new types of health data available. One of the earliest examples of Internet-based surveillance is ProMED, which was founded in 1993 to provide early warning of emerging infectious disease outbreaks [26]. ProMED scans, translates, and reviews global news reports for evidence of potential outbreaks. It has grown over time to include more than 60,000 subscribers in over 185 countries [27]. ProMED is credited with having provided some of the earliest indications of the start of the 2003 global SARS outbreak [28,29].

Some researchers are investigating whether other sources of Internet-based data, such as Internet searches and social media streams, can provide meaningful indication of disease outbreaks. A commonly cited example is Google.org Flu Trends, which analyzes search-engine queries to detect increases in occurrence of influenza-like illness within geographic locations [30]. Others have investigated whether Twitter status updates can be mined and analyzed in order to detect outbreaks and better understand the burden of disease in communities [31,32]. The concept behind these approaches is that infected individuals may search for or share information about their disease status before they seek medical care. In this sense, these approaches are not unlike syndromic surveillance in that that they seek to detect outbreaks using nonclinical data available before the cause of illness is determined.

Crowd sourcing can further supplement existing surveillance efforts, as was demonstrated during investigation of the 2011 *Escherichia coli* O104:H4 outbreak in Germany. After a team of scientists from Germany and China sequenced the outbreak strain, they released sequence data into the public domain [33]. Within 24 hours, volunteer bioinformaticians on four different continents had assembled the entire genome and, a day later, had assigned the genome to an existing sequence type. There have also been efforts to tap the "wisdom of the crowds" to participate directly in surveillance. For example, Web-based systems can enable members of the public to report that they are experiencing symptoms that may be consistent with foodborne illness along with information about foods they consumed prior to onset of symptoms [34]. Participatory epidemiology approaches are also being developed for influenza. Flu Near You—a program being developed by HealthMap of Children's Hospital Boston, the American Public Health Association, and the Skoll Global Threats Fund—recruits individuals who report on a weekly basis whether or not they are experiencing influenza-like illness [35].

Development of surveillance efforts to predict future disease threats

In recent years there has been an increasing interest in developing surveillance methods that can help to predict the emergence of pathogenic threats to humans before these pathogens can cause significant disease in humans. Most approaches are rooted in the observation that the vast majority of human pandemics have been caused by animal pathogens that have developed the ability to infect human hosts (e.g., SARS, H5N1, H1N1, Ebola, Marburg, Nipah, Hendra, and HIV). One common approach involves the monitoring of high-risk human populations for the emergence of new pathogens (e.g., monitoring of bushmeat hunters may have led to early recognition of Ebola virus). Researchers seek evidence that a particular novel pathogen is becoming more likely to infect humans, which may indicate the potential to spread beyond the high-risk population. This approach requires an understanding of the social and behavioral patterns that make populations uniquely vulnerable to specific infections.

In 2009, the U.S. Agency for International Development launched a multiyear program to preempt (or combat at their source) newly emerging diseases of animal origin that could threaten human health [36]. The global Emerging Pandemics Threat (EPT) program has funded five related projects aimed at improving the surveillance, diagnosis, investigation, and response to disease outbreaks of zoonotic potential. One project, PREDICT, involves a 5-year research effort to improve disease surveillance in wildlife and people located in areas deemed to be disease "hot spots" (i.e., places where social and environmental conditions favor zoonotic disease transmission).

Remaining challenges

Inadequate laboratory capabilities and clinical expertise to detect diseases

Development of accurate and reliable diagnoses of illnesses is a fundamental challenge in global surveillance. Clinical specimen collection, analysis, and laboratory confirmation of the etiology of disease outbreaks are important components of any disease surveillance system [37]. In many areas of the world, however, insufficient diagnostic capacity leads to no or faulty diagnoses, inappropriate treatments, and disease misreporting. For example, surveillance for malaria is challenged by a common reliance on clinical symptoms for diagnosis, which has been shown to be a poor predictor of actual infection [38,39]. In light of these realities, WHO, the Institute of Medicine, and other organizations and expert groups have concluded there is a need for the development of tools that can improve the speed and accuracy and reduce the costs of diagnosing infectious diseases [40–45].

The reliance on laboratory testing to provide accurate diagnosis of many diseases, such as cholera or yellow fever, has consequences for surveillance. In many countries, the functioning of public health laboratories is compromised because of lack of funding, personnel, and equipment. A WHO report indicates that more than 60% of laboratory equipment in countries with limited resources is outdated or not functioning [46]. Even when there is sufficient laboratory capacity, laboratory-based diagnosis of disease can also be slow, delaying detection of outbreaks. For example, it can take more than a month to determine whether a patient is infected with drug-resistant strains of tuberculosis.

A number of government agencies and international organizations are working to accelerate the development of infectious disease diagnostics in order to improve global surveillance and therefore global health. In 2009, the U.S. National Security Council (NSC) identified enhanced detection of infectious diseases as a priority goal for improving national security. The NSC called on U.S. government agencies to work with international partners to improve the capacity to diagnose infectious diseases [47]. The U.S. President's Emergency Plan for AIDS Relief also includes provisions to promote the development and acquisition of infectious disease diagnostics [48]. Organizations such as WHO and the Foundation for Innovative New Diagnostics have prioritized clinical diagnostic technology procurement, regulation, and training for high-burden, but underdiagnosed, diseases such as tuberculosis [49]. Two of the fourteen Grand Challenges in Global Health—an initiative led by the Gates Foundation—call for the development of new tools for diagnosing infectious diseases and for assessing the health status of populations [50].

These efforts have helped to support the development of new approaches for diagnosing infectious disease. Rapid, point-of-care diagnostic tests that confirm infection more quickly than traditional laboratory tests are now available for identification of pathogens that causes hepatitis B and HIV, among others. It has been suggested that molecular-based diagnostic tests, which do not require the culturing of organisms, may reduce the cost of building and maintaining laboratories that handle live agents [51]. One concern is that rapid diagnostic tools may not provide accurate and adequate informa-

tion to guide appropriate response [52,53]. For example, during the 2009 H1N1 influenza pandemic, rapid point-of-care flu tests, which have become increasingly used in diagnosis and management of influenza, were prone to high levels of false-negative results [54,55]. Such performance limitations put increasing pressure on clinical and public health laboratories [56]. There is also an effort to develop multi-analyte diagnostics that can analyze patient samples for the specific gene sequences or protein signatures of multiple pathogens simultaneously [57]. Some have argued that the ability to test for multiple pathogens in a single-patient sample could be useful during outbreaks. For example, a multi-analyte test might have expedited the detection of a yellow fever outbreak that occurred in Uganda in 2010. Having not seen a case of yellow fever in Uganda for decades, health officials had a low clinical suspicion for yellow fever and misdiagnosed patients first with the Ebola virus and then with plague [58].

Shortages of trained personnel

A lack of adequate numbers of skilled public health personnel who are well trained to work either in diagnostic laboratories or as epidemiologists poses significant challenges to efforts to improve global surveillance [59]. A number of programs exists to train individuals in the fields of laboratory diagnostics, epidemiology, veterinary medicine, and biosafety. Successful training programs also enhance the management and analytic abilities of in-country surveillance professionals. Two such efforts are the CDC's Field Epidemiology Training Program (FETP) and Field Epidemiology Laboratory Training Program (FELTP). Started in 1980, the FETP and FELTP programs were modeled after the CDC's Epidemic Intelligence Service [60]. The 2-year training FETP program provides in-country personnel with classroom and field instruction in epidemiology, communications, economics, and management. Individuals in the FELTP programs train in these areas, as well as in laboratory-based surveillance.

Disincentives for reporting

From the perspective of an individual nation, there are few incentives to report an outbreak of a disease to the international community. Rather, the decision to report diseases may result in adverse consequences—significant drops in tourism and trade, closings of borders, and other measures that the IHR are supposed to prevent. Such was the case during the 2009 influenza A/H1N1 pandemic, which represented one of the first tests of global cooperation under the revised IHR. Though the international community generally lived up to their IHR requirements [61], as Katz and Fischer pointed out, there were some notable exceptions [62]. At the onset of the pandemic, WHO issued clear recommendations that countries should not ban imports, close borders, or restrict travellers to contain the outbreak at national borders. Despite these recommendations, a number of countries pursued these measures, which caused undue economic harm to other nations [63].

The geographic distribution of most infectious disease outbreaks suggests that much of the burden of global surveillance falls on countries with limited resources, where the availability of trained personnel, diagnostic laboratories, and funding required to support surveillance may be lacking [63,64]. Yet without adequate surveillance, these countries can fall prey to "inaccurate reports and rumors [which] can rapidly lead to social disruption nationally and unwarranted panic internationally" [65]. As a result, some countries have begun to push back against current approaches to global surveillance. For example, in 2007, Indonesia announced that it would no longer share clinical H5N1 influenza specimens with international laboratories after learning that an Australian pharmaceutical company developed an H5N1 vaccine based on a sample that was originally isolated in Indonesia [66,67]. Indonesia's health officials were concerned that those samples would be either developed into vaccines that Indonesia (a nation clearly affected by avian influenza) could not afford or patented by vaccine companies.

Inadequate integration of animal and human health surveillance

Improving global surveillance will also require better integration of animal health data with systems for human health surveillance. Zoonoses, or diseases that can transmit between humans and animals, have been responsible for nearly two-thirds of infectious disease outbreaks that have occurred since 1950 and more than $200 billion in worldwide economic losses in the last 10 years [52]. Despite the significant economic and health threats caused by these diseases, worldwide capacity for surveillance of zoonotic diseases is insufficient [52].

Two key barriers block improvement of zoonotic disease surveillance. First, there are inadequate levels of political support for zoonotic surveillance in the United States and in other countries. Many countries maintain separate agencies that are responsible for human and animal health. These agencies typically do not have surveillance for zoonoses within their mission; and, as a result, they may be reluctant to lead national efforts to integrate surveillance at the interface of human and animal health. Second, there is often insufficient funding available to conduct surveillance in areas critical to detection of zoonoses, such as surveillance for diseases in wildlife and pets. For example, despite documented outbreaks in which humans have been infected by their pets (e.g., the zoonotic outbreak of monkeypox in Wisconsin that began in Gambian rats that were imported as pets), there exist few programs for surveillance of diseases with zoonotic diseases associated with pets.

Despite these barriers, some efforts to improve the integration of human and animal health surveillance have been developed. For example, the Canadian Science Centre for Human and Animal Health, a state-of-the-art BSL-4 laboratory in Winnipeg that is jointly operated by the Public Health Agency of Canada and the Canadian Food Inspection Agency, was created to better integrate human and animal surveillance through the co-location of animal and human health laboratories [68]. ArboNET, a national system for the surveillance of arboviral diseases in the United States, is another program that attempts to link human and animal health surveillance. Developed by the CDC after the first cases of West Nile Viruses in the Western Hemisphere occurred in New York City in 1999 [69], ArboNET transmits data from virologic testing of mosquito and bird populations to human and animal health authorities to help guide programs for mosquito control and public health risk communication [52].

Information barriers between public health agencies and other sectors

The increasing use of electronic health records (EHRs) may have important implications for surveillance. Rapid access and mining of EHRs can help to facilitate the detection and management of disease outbreaks. For example, hospital-based surveillance was critical in obtaining an early understanding of the clinical severity of the 2009 influenza A/H1N1 pandemic. In the United States, the lack of direct digital connections between healthcare clinics and laboratories is seen as a major impediment in the timeliness and completeness of disease reporting [70]. Recent efforts by governments to develop and implement automated methods to extract data from EHRs and to communicate with surveillance agencies may be important steps in detecting and managing outbreaks [71,72].

A number of recent outbreaks have also demonstrated the need for integration of nonhealth data into existing surveillance efforts. For example, private sector supply chain and inventory data proved useful in identifying the contaminated sources responsible for the 2011 *E. coli* outbreak in Europe and the 2008 *Salmonella* Saintpaul outbreak in the United States [73,74]. Following the 1984 outbreak of salmonellosis in Oregon, information from law enforcement helped to determine that the outbreak was deliberate and not the result of an ill food handler, as public health authorities had initially suspected [75,76]. Unfortunately, in many places exchange of information between public health agencies and other entities happens largely on an ad-hoc basis. In the United States, Congress tried to address this problem in 2007 with passage of legislation that calls on the Department of Homeland Security to develop a National Biosurveillance Integration Center (NBIC) to coordinate biosurveillance across the federal government [77]. However, implementation of NBIC has been slow [78].

Conclusion

The continued emergence of new pathogens and the occurrence of several high-profile outbreaks have led to increasing efforts to improve surveillance across the globe. Over the last few decades, there have been significant changes in the way in which infectious disease surveillance is practiced. New regulations and goals for infectious disease surveillance have given rise to the development of new surveillance approaches and methods and have resulted in participation by nontraditional sectors, including the security community. Though most of these developments have positively shaped global surveillance, there remain key challenges that stand in the way of continued improvements. These include insufficient diagnostic capabilities and lack of trained staff, lack of integration between human and animal-health surveillance efforts, disincentives for countries to report disease outbreaks, and lack of information exchange between public health agencies and

other sectors that are critical for surveillance. To ensure continued commitment to global surveillance goals, the international community must work to address these remaining challenges.

STUDY QUESTIONS

1. Describe the major differences between event-based and indicator-based surveillance Give an example of when each approach would be useful.
2. How does biosurveillance differ from traditional disease surveillance? Provide an example of a biosurveillance system that was developed after 2001.
3. In what major ways did the 2005 revisions to the International Health Regulations change global surveillance for emerging infectious diseases? Give an example of an event that may be considered a Public Health Event of International Concern.
4. How do syndromic surveillance approaches differ from traditional disease surveillance? How has thinking about the primary objectives of syndromic surveillance changed over time?
5. Give an example of how nonhealth information may be useful for conducting surveillance for emerging infectious disease outbreaks?
6. Describe at least two of the remaining challenges facing global surveillance. How are these likely to hinder the world's ability to detect or respond to outbreaks of emerging infectious diseases?

References

1. Sigerist HE. *The Great Doctors: A Biographical History of Medicine*. New York: W. W. Norton; 1933.
2. Armstrong GL, Conn LA, Pinner RW. Trends in infectious disease mortality in the United States during the 20th century. *JAMA* 1999;**281**(1):61–66.
3. Pinner RW, Teutsch SM, Simonsen L, Klug LA, Graber JM, Clarke MJ, Berkelman RL. Trends in infectious diseases mortality in the United States. *JAMA* 1996;**275**(3): 189–193.
4. Langmuir AD. The surveillance of communicable diseases of national importance. *N Engl J Med* 1963;**268**:182–192.
5. White House. Homeland Security Presidential Directive/HSPD 21. 2007 Oct 18. Available at http://www.fas.org/irp/offdocs/nspd/hspd-21.htm (accessed July 12, 2012).
6. Morse SS. Global infectious disease surveillance and health intelligence. *Health Aff (Millwood)* 2007;**26**(4):1069–1077.

65. Cash R, Narasimhan V. Impediments to global surveillance of infectious diseases: Consequences of open reporting in a global economy. *Bull World Health Organ* 2000;**78**(11): 1358–1367.

66. Aglionby J. Indonesia agrees to share bird flu samples. Financial Times, 2007 Feb 16. Available at http://www.ft.com/cms/s/0/4d1995ae-bdf1-11db-bd86-0000779e2340.html#axzz1HMPuxbjf (accessed July 12, 2012).

67. Irwin R. Indonesia, H5N1, and global health diplomacy. *Glob Health Governance* Spring 2010;**3**(2).

68. Public Health Agency of Canada. National Microbiology Laboratory Report of Accomplishments. 2008. Available at http://www.nml-lnm.gc.ca/new-nouv/rapport-report-eng.htm (accessed July 12, 2012).

69. Lindsey NP, Staples JE, Lehman JA, Fischer M. Surveillance for human West Nile virus disease—United States, 1999–2008. *MMWR Surveill Summ* 2010;**59**(2):1–17.

70. National Biosurveillance Advisory Subcommittee. Improving the Nation's Ability to Detect and Respond to 21st Century Urgent Health Threats: First Report of the National Biosurveillance Advisory Subcommitee. 2009 Apr. Available at http://www.avma.org/atwork/NBASreport072209.pdf (accessed July 10, 2012).

71. Toner E, Nuzzo J, Watson M, et al. Biosurveillance where it happens: State and local capabilities and needs. *Biosecur Bioterror* 2011;**9**(4):321–330.

72. International Society for Disease Surveillance. Final Recommendation: Core Processes and EHR Requirements for Public Health Syndromic Surveillance. 2011 Jan. Available at http://www.syndromic.org/uploads/files/ISDSRecommendation_FINAL.pdf (accessed July 12, 2012).

73. European Food Safety Authority. Tracing Seeds, in Particular Fenugreek (*Trigonella foenum-graecum*) Seeds, in Relation to the Shiga Toxin-Producing *E. coli* (STEC) O104:H4 2011 Outbreaks in Germany and France. Parma, Italy. EFSA/ECDC Joint Rapid Risk Assessment 2011. Available at http://www.efsa.europa.eu/en/supporting/doc/176e.pdf (accessed July 12, 2012).

74. Pew Charitable Trusts. Lessons to Be Learned from the 2008 Salmonella Saintpaul Outbreak. Pew Charitable Trusts' Produce Safety Project. 2008 Nov. 17. Available at http://www.pewtrusts.org/uploadedFiles/wwwpewtrustsorg/Reports/Produce_Safety_Project/produce_safety_salmonella.pdf (accessed July 12, 2012).

75. Carus S. Working Paper: Bioterrorism and Biocrimes: The Illicit Use of Biological Agents since 1900. 2001 Feb. Available at http://www.ndu.edu/centercounter/full_doc.pdf (accessed July 12, 2012).

76. Ill handlers suspected in Oregon food poisonings. New York Times October 21, 1984. Available at http://www.nytimes.com/1984/10/21/us/ill-handlers-suspected-in-oregon-food-poisonings.html (accessed July 10, 2012).

77. Implementing Recommendations of the 9/11 Commission Act of 2007 (9/11 Commission Act). Pub. L. 110-53. Available at http://intelligence.senate.gov/laws/pl11053.pdf (accessed July 12, 2012).

78. United States Government Accountability Office. Efforts to Develop a National Biosurveillance Capability Need a National Strategy and a Designated Leader. Report to Congressional Committees. 2010 Jun. Report No. GAO-10-645. Available at http://www.gao.gov/new.items/d10645.pdf (accessed July 12, 2012).

CHAPTER 17

Infectious disease surveillance and global security

David L. Blazes[1] and Sheri Lewis[2]

[1] *Uniformed Services University of the Health Sciences, Bethesda, MD, USA*
[2] *Johns Hopkins University Applied Physics Laboratory, Columbia, MD, USA*

Introduction

Current state of global, regional and national disease surveillance

The World Health Organization (WHO) serves as the universally recognized steward for global health with a mandate from the United Nations (UN) and all 195 member states to coordinate global health efforts including disease surveillance and outbreak detection and response [1]. The WHO relies on numerous tools to implement its mission, including binding treaties such as the International Health Regulations (IHR) [2]. The new guidelines were significant in that they increased the visibility of public health within the greater global foreign policy and diplomatic communities. Despite unanimous agreement to comply with the IHR, most UN member countries do not yet have the capability to detect, analyze, report, and respond to an outbreak of a disease with the potential to spread globally, commonly referred to as a Public Health Emergency of International Concern (PHEIC) [2]. To date, only 30 member states have claimed the full capacity to comply with the IHR [3].

In 2000, WHO created an operational response unit called the Global Outbreak Alert and Response Network (GOARN) with the primary goal of improving global health security [3]. The WHO itself does not possess the numbers of technically trained personnel that would be required to meet this goal, so it relies on a voluntary network of institutions and personnel organized through the GOARN operational framework. The GOARN works to prevent the international spread of epidemics by assuring that the correct technical expertise is provided to a location in need in a timely fashion helping to build sustainable response capacities on the local level. Members of the GOARN include laboratory networks, scientific institutions in UN member states, surveillance networks, UN organizations such as UNICEF, and medical nongovernmental organizations such as Medecins sans Frontieres. The GOARN has established Guiding Principles that describe expectations for preparedness and response to epidemics, as well as procedures that attempt to standardize operations. The GOARN network has demonstrated its effectiveness in responses to over 50 events in 40 countries, including the SARS epidemic, H5N1 avian influenza outbreaks, and several cholera outbreaks around the world [4].

The WHO's headquarters is located in Geneva, Switzerland, but many public health activities are delegated to regional offices. These regional offices are: the Regional Office for the Americas, also known as the Pan-American Health Organization (PAHO), in Washington, DC, United

Concepts and Methods in Infectious Disease Surveillance, First Edition. Edited by Nkuchia M. M'ikanatha and John K. Iskander.
Published 2014 by John Wiley & Sons, Ltd.

States; the Regional Office for Europe (EURO) in Copenhagen, Denmark; the Regional Office for Southeast Asia (SEARO) in New Delhi, India; the Western Pacific Regional Office (WPRO) in Manila, Philippines; and the Regional Office for Eastern Mediterranean (EMRO) in Cairo, Egypt [1]. The capability of these regional offices depends on the commitment of the countries in the region and their relationship with WHO headquarters.

A limited number of organizations with financial resources and regional governance structures that allow for such activities also conduct regional disease surveillance. Among these are the European Center for Disease Prevention and Control (ECDC) and the Asia Pacific Economic Council's Emerging Infections Network (APEC EIN) [5,6]. The ECDC was established in 2005 by the European Union to strengthen defenses against contagious infectious diseases in Europe through comprehensive disease surveillance and early response to potential threats. In addition to surveillance and response activities, ECDC provides timely and relevant data and technical expertise to the Europe Union countries. The ECDC was crucial in the response to the recent outbreak of *Escherichia coli* O1:O4 that led to hemolytic uremic syndrome in Europe because of contaminated food. Other regional networks such as APEC EIN are less formalized and more narrowly focused on emerging infections and their impact on trade [6].

Role of the military in global infectious disease surveillance

Other organizations with longstanding interest in disease surveillance are the world's militaries. Timely detection of new diseases and epidemics is important to for protection of service members. It is also a key requirement for global public health security, increasingly recognized as crucial to stability. Timely detection of disease outbreaks requires adequate infectious disease surveillance, the ability and willingness to report to global public health authorities, and a meaningful mechanism for providing response to control an outbreak. The global presence of militaries in support of peacekeeping or strategic missions makes these requirements even more relevant for the military, especially when reporting of potential disease outbreaks among personnel in a foreign country is required. Additionally, military, government, and nongovernmental personnel

dispatched around the world have a special responsibility to prevent the spread of contagious diseases through their travels. In the past, militaries have inadvertently contributed to the spread of infectious diseases, including influenza during the 1918–1919 pandemic and, more recently, cholera in Haiti [7]. Because of this reality and the recognized responsibility to the overall public health, militaries continue to make significant contributions to global infectious disease surveillance efforts, often in direct support of the IHR mission [8]. As discussed later in this chapter, the United States Department of Defense supports development of electronic systems to facilitate disease reporting within partner host countries [9].

U.S-based global disease surveillance

Global Disease Detection Program
The Centers for Disease Control and Prevention (CDC) has a major role in disease surveillance and response throughout the world. Initially charged with a domestic responsibility, CDC over time has developed an increasingly global presence. The Global Disease Detection Program and Emergency Response (GDDER), begun in 2004, is CDC's lead initiative for developing and strengthening global capacity to rapidly detect, accurately identify, and promptly contain emerging infectious disease and bioterrorist threats that occur internationally [10]. The GDDER was created to "mitigate the consequences of a catastrophic public health event, whether by an intentional act of terrorism, or the natural emergence of a deadly infectious virus" [10].

CDC approaches its mission of improving global health security through building cooperative partnerships. The GDDER program was designated as the first WHO Collaborating Center for Implementation of International Health Regulations, National Surveillance and Response Capacity [10]. In this role, the GDDER program partners with Ministries of Health, WHO, and already established CDC programs to improve core public health capacities in developing countries targeting early identification and control of emerging infectious diseases. Some of these established programs include the influenza surveillance network, field epidemiology and laboratory training programs emerging infections and zoonotic disease surveillance, laboratory

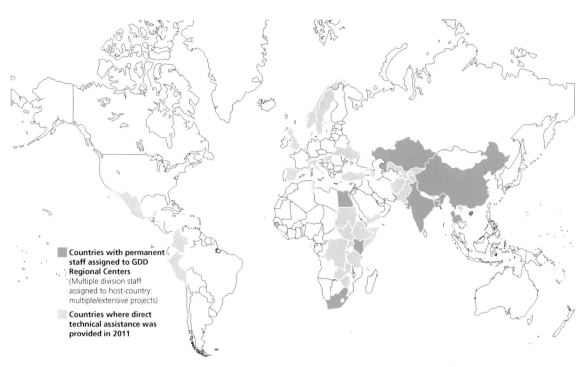

Figure 17.1 CDC Global Disease Detection and Response network. Source: http://www.cdc.gov/globalhealth/gdder/gdd/regionalcenters.htm. Centers for Disease Control and Prevention.

strengthening and capacity building, and risk communication and emergency response.

The GDDER program has centers throughout the world that are located in places where their expertise may be maximally leveraged by the host countries and regions (Figure 17.1). Centers are currently located in Bangladesh, China, Egypt, Georgia, Guatemala, Kazakhstan, Kenya, India, South Africa, and Thailand. Several of these grew from existing CDC activities. For example, the laboratory in Guatemala was founded in 1978 as a parasitic diseases research center. Other GDDER centers have built strategic partnerships such as with the International Centre for Diarrheal Disease Research in Bangladesh (ICDDR, B) and the Naval Medical Research Unit 3 (NAMRU-3) in Cairo, Egypt. The most recent GDDER sites include collaborations in China and South Africa, two additional hot spots in terms of emerging infectious diseases. Sites are chosen in close consultation with the host countries and WHO; new sites are planned but their realization depends, largely, on availability of funding.

Over the period 2006–2011, the GDDER regional centers have responded to more than 900 outbreaks around the world. Provided at the request of the host government, this support is especially important for countries with limited resources or in countries experiencing outbreaks caused by dangerous pathogens such as Ebola virus, Marburg virus, SARS, or Nipah virus. In 2011, the GDD program was responsible for detecting seven pathogens new to their region and three organisms that were new to the world [10].

Much of the value of the GDDER program is realized through building public health capacity in host countries. Since 2006, over 65,000 public health officials had been trained, including 74 graduates of the prestigious Field Epidemiology Training Program (FETP).

Global Emerging Infections Surveillance and Response System

The U.S. Department of Defense (DoD) created the Global Emerging Infections Surveillance and Response

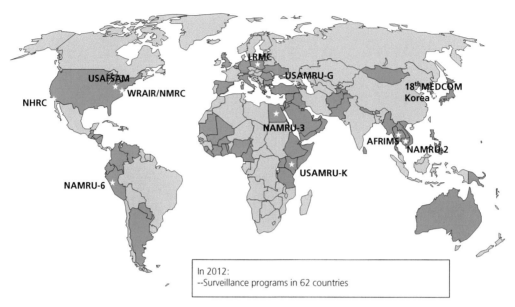

Figure 17.2 DoD Global Emerging Infections Surveillance network.

System (GEIS) in 1997, soon after a presidential decision directive (PDD-7) mandated that all agencies within the government increase capabilities to detect and respond to global emerging infectious diseases [11]. Through this program, the DoD created a global network based on regional surveillance efforts utilizing DoD overseas medical research laboratories that had been working with host countries for decades on infectious diseases of common interest. These laboratories work side by side with host country scientists in Egypt, Cambodia, Peru, Thailand, Kenya, and numerous other countries. (Figure 17.2). For example, the Naval Medical Research Unit Three (NAMRU-3) based in Cairo, Egypt, was first established to confront typhus during World War II. Over the ensuing decades, the success of NAMRU-3 in this initial control program led to broad infectious diseases research and surveillance initiatives that were mutually beneficial to both countries.

One mission of the GEIS program is to develop, implement, support, and evaluate an integrated global emerging infectious disease (EID) surveillance and response system. Protection of U.S. and allied service members is also a strategic focus. Equally important and well aligned with its primary focus of global public health security is the recognition that adequate health allows for country-level security and, thus, contributes to regional stability—one of the stated strategic goals of the DoD and the U.S. government [12]. By 2012, the GEIS network included 33 partners in 76 countries (Figure 17.2). Key partners continued to be the five DoD overseas research laboratories, each of which has numerous collaborations in their respective regions in Southeast Asia, Africa, the Middle East, and Latin America. The GEIS program has also supported reference laboratories that develop and test diagnostic assays for deployment overseas in addition to conducting disease surveillance in military and nonmilitary associated populations within the United States.

Today, medical research laboratories established by U.S. military are vital to infectious disease surveillance efforts in host countries. Despite political and social strife during the past 60 years, NAMRU-3 remains active in face of infectious disease threats such as avian influenza (influenza A/H5N1). The U.S. Army Medical Research Unit–Kenya (USAMRU–K) has also collaborated in surveillance efforts with national ministries of health and defense for over four decades. The collaborative research partnerships in each of these settings have been responsible for numerous scientific discoveries concerning emerging and tropical infectious diseases, including the isolation of novel pathogens, the first description of artemesinin-resistant Plasmodium falciparum, and several reference strain contributions to Northern and Southern hemisphere influenza vaccines (including the seed strain for the 2009 influenza A/H1N1 virus) [11].

Case studies

Influenza surveillance

Influenza is one of the leading causes of annual morbidity and mortality from respiratory infections globally, accounting for up to 500,000 deaths per year throughout the world [13]. It is the pandemic potential from genetically shifted novel strains, however, that drives the interest in monitoring influenza infections. The 1918 influenza pandemic caused more deaths than any other pandemic in recorded history, with some authors estimating that over 50 million deaths occurred worldwide [14]. The most recent pandemic occurred in 2009 but it did not result in a significant increase in mortality.

Global Influenza Surveillance and Response System
Coordinated global influenza surveillance has been conducted since 1952 through WHO [15]. In 2013, the Global Influenza Surveillance and Response System (GISRS) consisted of six WHO Collaborating Centres, four Essential Regulatory Laboratories (ERLs), and over 140 institutions in more than 100 countries (Figure 17.3). Influenza samples are collected through various sampling schema that depend on the public health systems of individual WHO member states. These

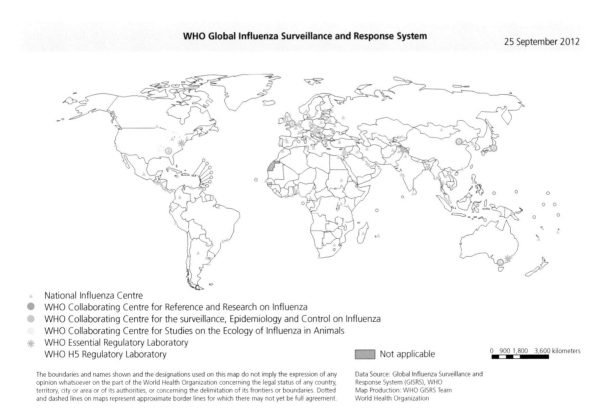

Figure 17.3 WHO's Global Influenza Surveillance and Response System map. *Based on UN M49 classification of developing/developed countries. Source: Reproduced with permission of WHO. http://gamapserver.who.int/mapLibrary/Files/Maps/GISRS_20130425_1.png.

samples are processed at one of the National Influenza Centers (NICs), and isolates are then forwarded to one of the WHO Collaborating Centers for further analysis and comparison with other isolates from the region and around the globe. The scale of genetic (genotypic) and antigenic (phenotypic) differences among the influenza strains indicates the potential for pandemic spread. Any novel viruses discovered are considered for inclusion in the annual influenza vaccine preparations.

The global influenza virus surveillance process occurs on a continuous basis throughout the year. Vaccine preparations are updated annually, with each vaccine typically including one strain of influenza A/H3N2, one influenza A/H1N1, and one influenza B. Distinct Northern and Southern hemisphere vaccine preparations may be offered, depending on the expected circulating influenza strains and the seasonality of the respective temperate regions. In addition to vaccine strain selection, the GISRS monitors burden of illness related to influenza-like illness (ILI) and severe acute respiratory infections (SARI), as well as influenza virus susceptibility to medications such as oseltamivir.

The Department of Defense GEIS program

The DoD GEIS program in collaboration with CDC identified the first four cases of the pandemic 2009 influenza A/H1N1, conducted influenza A/H1N1 diagnostic training in over 40 countries, and assisted in the first diagnosis of the virus in 14 countries [10]. These efforts are facilitated through partnerships with the host countries. As mentioned above, one of the key components of both the GDDER and GEIS programs is their emphasis on building capacity at the host-country level, which includes the support of NICs.

Challenges in influenza surveillance

Influenza surveillance is not without controversy. There has been concern that sharing data and viral isolates from disease surveillance activities has not resulted in equitable benefits for countries with limited resources (mainly with respect to access to vaccines and antiviral medications) commensurate with their contributions [16]. This concept of viral sovereignty has undermined trust and transparency and, thus, global disease surveillance and global public health security. A recent major

diplomatic impasse lasted for 4 years, during which time several countries did not share viral isolates with the GISRS. At the May 2011, the World Health Assembly, a Pandemic Influenza Preparedness (PIP) framework for influenza virus sharing, benefits sharing, and standard material transfer agreements was drafted and agreed upon (WHA 60.28) by key member states, industry partners, and the WHO [17]. There remain underlying issues regarding institutionalization of data and sharing of samples but at present, all 195 member states theoretically contribute to the GISRS.

Electronic disease surveillance

The state of electronic disease surveillance has changed drastically worldwide since the late 1990s. The advent of both the Internet and mobile health (mHealth) technologies has enabled the public health community to collect and transmit data much more readily than in the past. This new capacity, although groundbreaking for public health professionals, has also come with challenges. For example, now that the public health community has more data available to them, methods must be developed to collect, store, analyze, and disseminate this data in a timely, efficient manner. These very issues have presented numerous hurdles in the developed world and are more acute in resource-limited countries.

Prior to the terrorist attacks in the United States on September 11, 2001, electronic disease surveillance systems were in the early stages of development, with the CDC and many health departments relying on short-term, drop-in surveillance for large events and mass gatherings. These systems were labor intensive and often required personnel in emergency departments to examine patient logs at recurring intervals for a set period of time before and after events in order to provide data to public health officials. Given this process, these types of systems were not sustainable for extended periods.

Electronic Surveillance System for the Early Notification of Community-based Epidemics

Today, most health departments in the United States rely on electronic systems that acquire process, analyze, and visualize validated data sources such as emergency department chief complaints, physician diagnosis data, over-the-counter medication sales, and poison control center data for assessing community health. One such system is the Electronic Surveillance System for the Early Notification of Community-based Epidemics (ESSENCE), which is currently in use by many U.S. state and local health departments, by the U.S. military, and the U.S. Veterans Health Administration [18].

Early Warning Outbreak and Response System

During the early years of system development and adoption in the developed world, similar efforts were underway in countries with fewer resources. The Early Warning Outbreak and Response System (EWORS) was developed in conjunction with one of the U.S. Navy overseas labs for use in a number of Southeast Asian countries. This system was based in civilian urban hospitals and required clinicians to identify patients with possible infectious diseases and to manually complete a questionnaire. These questionnaires were then entered into an on-site computer and transmitted via email to a central EWORS hub. In Peru, with the assistance of the regional U.S. Navy lab, the Peruvian Navy developed a surveillance system that relies on providers using a phone to enter patient information via an interactive voice response (IVR) system. Both of these systems were instrumental in the evolution of electronic disease surveillance systems in that they highlighted the potential of such systems and identified areas where technology could vastly improve the process [19].

The biggest limitations to the development and sustainment of electronic disease surveillance systems, particularly in resource-limited countries, are the ease with which data are collected, accessed, and used by public health officials. Systems that require large amounts of resources, whether that is in the form of the workforce or information technology (IT) infrastructure, will not be successful in the long term. Successful systems run on existing hardware that can be maintained by modestly trained IT professionals and are easy to use by end users in public health [20].

Suite for Automated Global Electronic bioSurveillance System

To develop a successful system, careful consideration must be paid to data collection, analysis and visualization, information sharing, and system evaluation. One system that has developed a "toolkit" approach is the Suite for Automated Global Electronic bioSurveillance System (SAGES) based upon the civilian ESSENCE system. One or more SAGES tools may be used in concert with existing surveillance applications, or the SAGES tools may be used en masse for an end-to-end biosurveillance capability. This flexibility allows for the development of an inexpensive, customized, and sustainable disease surveillance system. The ability to assess anomalous disease activity rapidly may lead to better compliance with IHR (2005) [21].

Data can be as simple as raw text of individual patient encounters and as complicated as information gathered by way of detailed analysis or end user interpretation [22]. In countries with reliable Internet connectivity and sophisticated healthcare and inventory systems, data can be acquired through mechanisms such as Health Level 7 (HL-7), secure file transfer protocol (sFTP) or email [23]. In countries with limited resources, there is a need to capture data from remote settings that lack these means of data transfer. Therefore, it is imperative to utilize mobile collection platforms, such as cell phones, which are ubiquitous throughout much of the world (Figure 17.4). The complexity of data collection via cell phones will depend on infrastructure. For example, in areas lacking high penetration of smart phones, a simple texting protocol can be utilized. In areas where smart phones are readily accessible, one may opt to use forms via the phone. These forms can be submitted via short message service (SMS); the use of forms minimizes the potentials for error. One area that requires additional consideration is the security of data transmitted via SMS. Although patient privacy laws vary greatly throughout the world and personally identifiable information is not currently being collected in most systems of this type, there can be sensitivities based on the organization using the data and the type of diseases under surveillance [20].

Practical considerations for electronic surveillance systems

Once data are collected, they should be aggregated, analyzed, and presented in a way that allows the end user to determine quickly whether additional actions are warranted. Use of algorithms can further facilitate statistical anomalies that alert end users, at predefined

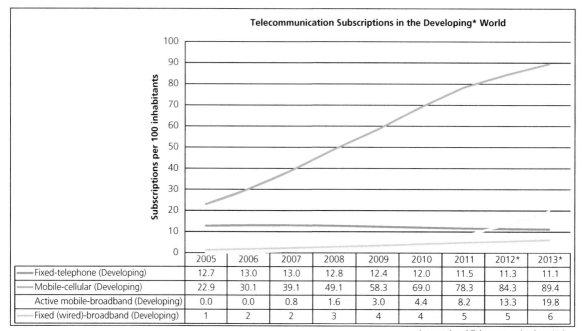

Figure 17.4 Mobile penetration in resource-limited settings. Source: Adapted from International Telecommunications Union. *Key Global Telecom Indicators for the World Telecommunication Service Sector*. http://www.itu.int/en/ITU-D/Statistics/Documents/statistics/2013/ITU_Key_2005-2013_ICT_data.xls (accessed January 23, 2014).

time intervals, of potential problems that require further investigation. Indeed, many automated systems now allow end users to directly query their data and determine whether there are concerns. For example, if a novel respiratory condition, such as SARS, emerges, the system end user can query for a particular case definition, run detection algorithms, and determine whether further investigation is warranted [23]. Many algorithms are available for analysis of data collected by a variety of systems including the open source CDC Early Aberration Reporting System (EARS) and SAGES. Visualization is just as important as the alerting components of a system. Feedback from users has demonstrated that visual data presentation (e.g., with time series, charts, maps, and line listings) is important in understanding a given situation. It also allows end users to share such information with the decision makers and public health colleagues in neighboring jurisdictions or countries. Typically, decision makers would be public officials authorized to approve public health response measures. Capabilities that aid in information sharing includes the ability to export data into other file type such as map images as pictures and data listings as spreadsheet [21].

Once a system has been operational for a period, it is very important to evaluate the system to ensure it is working as intended and is assisting the public health end users in doing their jobs as efficiently as possible. Factors to consider include the frequency of data dropouts, the amount of time it takes for people in the field to input the data, and the time required to maintain the supporting IT infrastructure. Ideally, the system will also aid in improving public health outcomes by enabling public health officials to identify and respond to a potential outbreak earlier than they would have otherwise.

Challenges in disease surveillance for global security

Achieving comprehensive disease surveillance on a global scale is a complex proposition. The challenges are myriad and include local, national, regional, and global issues. Governance of a global disease surveillance system is complex, especially as the WHO faces fiscal constraints and a fluctuating global leadership role [24]. To meet the requirements for IHR compliance with the ultimate goal of optimizing global public health security, public health practitioners at all levels must understand these challenges. [25].

Global public health has increasingly been recognized as a foreign policy concern, and this has introduced a new set of power brokers into the public health arena including those normally associated with diplomacy, public policy, economics, and national security [26]. The newly added dimensions of politics and security sometimes engender perceptions of "intelligence gathering" on the part of WHO and other agencies. Some have decried this "securitization of public health," citing this as unnecessary and potentially damaging to public health efforts. This perspective, however, has been central to the WHO since its inception, with its constitution stating that the "health of all peoples is fundamental to the attainment of peace and security" [2]. The IHR framework supports global health security with less emphasis on borders and more on cooperative action where needed[27]. Through effective global disease surveillance, timely detection of outbreaks, and appropriate response to control the spread of epidemics, the outcome of "global health" is thereby a significant component of "global security."

Knowledge is power; and when knowledge has the potential to impact national or international affairs, data sharing may become difficult. This became clear with the cessation of influenza virus sharing with GISRS by several countries with limited resources. Complete and transparent data sharing is likely an unobtainable ideal. It is more likely that countries would share some information after data analysis to meet their moral obligation

to the international community. However, in some countries, public health have expressed reluctance in compliance with IHR citing common but less-contagious diseases as higher priorities [28].

Because of the potential for rapid spread of contagious disease, effective disease surveillance should ideally be comprehensive. Unfortunately, this is hardly feasible in many countries with limited resources. Under Article 44 of the IHR, developed countries have an obligation to assist lesser developed member states with obtaining and maintaining the necessary capabilities. Sustainability of these surveillance capabilities once established is a key consideration; and successful solutions will likely include novel methods of financing such as cost sharing between donor countries, industry, and host-country governments. Standardization of surveillance data is also challenging. Ideally, both epidemiologic and laboratory data related to disease surveillance will be comparable among member states, but standardization of these data is not without controversy. Each member state has specific laws and requirements that are dependent on availability of funding and access to technology. Efforts through Article 44 of IHR are attempting to improve sustainability of surveillance through improving standardization [3].

Finally, having a well-trained public health workforce remains an obstacle to optimal surveillance in many countries. Efforts to improve this "human" capacity include programs such as the CDCs FELTP, as well as shorter training programs in outbreak management [29].

Conclusions

Maintaining global health security is a complex and challenging endeavor—one that affects all citizens of the world. The persistent threats to public health security from all continents mandate that each country contribute to the common good through efforts such as health surveillance. All sectors of society from doctors and scientists to the military and politicians must play a role in these surveillance efforts, which will likely include traditional epidemiologic methods and novel techniques, such as the use of mobile phones, for reporting and genetic sequencing of outbreak-related strains.

STUDY QUESTIONS

1. Give an example a global disease surveillance system coordinated by the World Health Organization, and describe briefly how this system contributes to public health response to outbreaks.

2. Briefly describe the role of the United States Department of Defense in global surveillance.

3. Identify and briefly describe two examples of electronic surveillance systems.

4. Give an example of a practical limitation in implementation of electronic disease surveillance systems in settings with limited resources, and discuss a possible solution.

5. Public health emergencies (e.g., pandemics) are global threats to security. What are some of the arguments for and against this perspective?

6. Sustainability is always a concern for externally funded public health programs. In your own opinion, what are some of the reasons why medical research laboratories established by US military (e.g., in Egypt and Kenya) have remained active for decades?

References

1. World Health Organization. World Immunization Week 2014: Know, Check, Protect. 2014. Available at http://www.who.int (accessed March 1, 2013).

2. World Health Organization. The International Health Regulations (2005). World Health Organization, June 2007. Available at http://www.who.int/ihr/en (accessed August 2, 2011).

3. Chungong S. Update on global IHR implementation and extensions. Presented at IHR AFRO Regional meeting, Lusaka, Zambia. December 2012.

4. World Health Organization. Global Outbreak Alert & Response Network. 2014. Available at http://www.who.int/csr/outbreaknetwork/en/ (accessed February 22, 2013).

5. ECDC. Mission. 2014. Available at http://www.ecdc.europa.eu/en/aboutus/mission/pages/mission.aspx (accessed April 18, 2014).

6. Kimball AM, Horwitch C, O'Carroll P, et al. APEC Emerging Infections Network: Prospects for comprehensive information sharing on emerging infections within the Asia Pacific Economic Cooperation. *Emerg Infect Dis* 1998;**4**(3):472.

7. Enserink M. Haiti's cholera outbreak. Cholera linked to U.N. forces, but questions remain. *Science* 2011;**332**(6031): 776–777.

8. Johns MJ, Blazes DL, Fernandez J, Russell KL, Chen DW, Loftis R. The US military and the International Health Regulations (2005): Perceptions, pitfalls and progress toward implementation. *Bull World Health Organ* 2011;**89**: 234–235.

9. Lewis SL, Feighner BH, Loschen WA, et al. SAGES: a suite of freely-available software tools for electronic disease surveillance in resource-limited settings. *PLoS ONE* 2011;**6**(5): e19750.

10. Centers for Disease Control and Prevention. Global Disease Detection and Emergency Response Activities at CDC 2012. Center for Global Health. Centers for Disease Control and Prevention. Atlanta, Georgia. August 2012. Available at http://www.cdc.gov/globalhealth/GDDER/pdf/gdder_report2012.pdf (accessed February 28, 2013).

11. Russell KL, Rubenstein J, Burke RL, et al. The Global Emerging Infection Surveillance and Response System (GEIS), a U.S. government tool for improved global biosurveillance: A review of 2009. *BMC Public Health* 2011;**11**(Suppl 2):S2.

12. Chretien JP, Gaydos JC, Malone JL, Blazes DL. Global network could avert pandemics. *Nature* 2006;**440**(7080): 25–26.

13. World Health Organization. Immunizations, Vaccines and Biologicals—Influenza. 2008. Available at http://www.who.int/immunization/topics/influenza/en/index.html (accessed March 14, 2013).

14. Johnson NP, Mueller J. Updating the accounts: Global mortality of the 1918–1920 "Spanish" influenza pandemic. *Bull Hist Med* 2002;**76**:105–115.

15. World Health Organization. Influenza: Surveillance and Monitoring. 2014. Available at http://www.who.int/influenza/surveillance_monitoring/en/ (accessed March 14, 2013).

16. Franklin N. Sovereignty and international politics in the negotiation of the avian influenza Material Transfer Agreement. *J Law Med* 2009;**17**(3):355–372.

17. Sixtieth World Health Assembly (Resolution WHA 60.28). May 2011. Available at http://apps.who.int/gb/ebwha/pdf_files/WHA60/A60_R28-en.pdf (accessed August 2, 2011).

18. Lombardo J, Burkom H, Elbert E, et al. A systems overview of the Electronic Surveillance System for the Early Notification of Community-based Epidemics (ESSENCE II). *J Urban Health* 2003;**80**(2 Suppl 1):i32–i42.

19. Chretien JP, Blazes D, Glass JS, et al. Surveillance for emerging infection epidemics in developing countries: EWORS and Alerta DISAMAR. In: Lombardo J, Buckeridge D, eds. *Disease Surveillance: A Public Health Informatics Approach*. Hoboken, NJ: Wiley; 2007:367–396.

20. Campbell TC, Hodanics CJ, Babin SM, et al. Developing open source, self-contained disease surveillance software applications for use in resource-limited settings. *BMC Med Inform Decis Mak* 2012;**12**:99.

21. Loschen WA. Methods for information sharing to support health monitoring. *Johns Hopkins APL Tech Dig* 2008;**27**(4): 340–346.

22. Wojcik R, Hauenstein L, Sniegoski C, Holtry R. Obtaining the data. In: Lombardo J, Buckeridge D, eds. *Disease Surveillance: A Public Health Informatics Approach.* Hoboken, NJ: Wiley World Telecommunication/ICT Indicators Database 2012 (16th Edition); 2007:367–396.

23. Begier EM, Sockwell D, Branch LM, et al. The National Capital Region's Emergency Department syndromic surveillance system: Do chief complaint and discharge diagnosis yield different results? *Emerg Infect Dis* 2003;**9**(3): 393–396.

24. Frenk J, Moon S. Governance challenges in global health. *N Engl J Med* 2013;**368**:936–942.

25. Quandelacy T, Johns MJ, Meynard JB, Lewis S, Montgomery JM, Blazes DL. The role of disease surveillance in

26. Fidler D The rise and fall of global health as a foreign policy issue. *Glob Health Governance* Spring 2011;**IV**(2). Available at http://www.ghgj.org (accessed August 3, 2011).

27. Fischer J, Kornblet S, Katz R. The International Health Regulations (2005): Surveillance and Response in an Era of Globalization. Stimson Center Global Health Security Program Report. June 2011.

28. Soto G, Araujo-Castillo RV, Neyra J, et al. Challenges in the implementation of an electronic surveillance system in a resource-limited setting: Alerta in Peru. *BMC Proc* 2008;**2**(Suppl 3):S4.

29. Lescano AG, Salmon G, Pedroni E, Blazes DL. Outbreak response training: What can realistically be done before the next pandemic? *Science* 2007;**318**(5850):574–575.

achieving IHR Compliance by 2012. *Biosecur Bioterror* 2011;**9**(4):408–412.57.

CHAPTER 18

Implementation of the National Electronic Disease Surveillance System in South Carolina

Eric Brenner

South Carolina Department of Health and Environmental Control, Columbia, SC, USA

Background: organization of public health in South Carolina

In South Carolina, a single agency, the Department of Health and Environmental Control (DHEC) is responsible for public health at the statewide level, and county health department (CHD) level. In South Carolina, unlike a number of other states, the CHD staff in all 46 counties are also DHEC employees. Most often, each county (or large municipality) has its own independent health department, and the state health department assumes an indirect role for coordination (see Chapter 3). One of the largest organizational units within DHEC is the Bureau of Disease Control. As shown in Table 18.1, this bureau is comprised of several divisions, each of which has traditionally maintained its own disease surveillance system. Most of this chapter will focus on surveillance systems used by the Division of Acute Disease Epidemiology (DADE), but advantages and disadvantages of combining all systems used by other disease control programs into a single system will also be discussed.

Surveillance versus surveillance systems

Discussions regarding adoption of a new surveillance system may sometimes semantically cloud essential distinctions between the terms "surveillance" and "surveillance system." Concepts of surveillance are discussed in various sections of this book. Surveillance broadly refers to the core function of public health practice focused on monitoring trends in reportable diseases for purposes of program planning and evaluation, and identification of disease outbreaks requiring a public health response. However, the term "surveillance system" may be used not only to describe the detailed operational and administrative manner in which particular surveillance activities are carried out, but also more narrowly to refer to a computer software system which supports surveillance activities. It must be emphasized that adoption of a new surveillance software system does not in and of itself imply any changes in a jurisdiction's legal basis or requirements for public health surveillance, its list of officially reportable diseases, or broad objectives and functions. Nonetheless, as will be discussed in this chapter, some features of a software system may offer opportunities to improve or expand the surveillance process, thus improving the surveillance system itself.

Historical perspective: the NETSS era

The National Electronic Telecommunications System for Surveillance (NETSS) was used by the majority of public health jurisdictions in the United States throughout much of the 1990s [1]. NETSS was built around early

Concepts and Methods in Infectious Disease Surveillance, First Edition. Edited by Nkuchia M. M'ikanatha and John K. Iskander.

Table 18.1 Divisions of the DHEC Bureau of Disease Control with responsibilities related to disease surveillance and control.

Division	Primary Function	Information system used in the 1990s
Division of Tuberculosis Control	Surveillance and control of tuberculosis	TIMS (Tuberculosis Information Management System)
Division of HIV and STD Control	Surveillance and control of HIV and STDs	HARS (HIV-AIDS Reporting System STD-MIS (STD Management Information System)
Division of Acute Disease Epidemiology (DADE)	Surveillance and control relating to ~60 reportable conditions, including vaccine preventable diseases, vector-, food-, and waterborne infections, meningococcal infections, potential bioterrorism agents, etc.	NETSS (National for National Electronic Telecommunications System for Surveillance)

DOS-based versions of Epi Info, a widely used software developed by the Centers for Disease Control and Prevention (CDC) for analysis of surveillance and other epidemiologic data [2]. Advantages of the NETSS system were its extremely low cost, ease of installation, and ease of use. Surveillance jurisdictions received troubleshooting assistance through the CDC Help Desk and the CDC-provided system updates. Typically, no in-house information technology (IT) support was required. Nevertheless, surveillance systems experienced several technical difficulties during the NETSS era:

1. **System fragmentation:** Surveillance data were fragmented into several incompatible systems (see Table 18.1) that lacked interoperability. Further, these systems, each of which had been designed separately, were built on different technical and software platforms and sometimes even ran on different operating systems.

2. **Slow data flow and double data entry:** Transmission of data from NETSS systems within jurisdictions was largely paper-based and thus inefficient and often delayed. For example, a positive laboratory test for a reportable disease, often already computerized in a hospital's own laboratory computer system, might then be transcribed by hand onto an official DHEC paper reporting form and mailed to DHEC. Upon receipt, the same information would then be entered by hand into the NETSS database in a DHEC computer.

3. **Older technologies:** Though the Internet was well established by 2000, NETSS was not Web based; rather, it relied on stand-alone, personal computer

(PC)–based software built on technologies that were typically 10 years or more old.

Beginning of the NEDSS era

By the late 1990s, it had become clear both at the CDC and in many state health departments that a more modern approach to surveillance informatics was needed. The CDC, in consultation with numerous partners, initiated efforts to modernize the nation's disease control surveillance systems [3–6], via an initiative that came to be known as the National Electronic Disease Surveillance System (NEDSS). NEDSS was not conceived of as a software system, but rather as a set of technical standards on which any number of NEDSS-compatible systems could then be based. Although many details of individual software applications might vary from jurisdiction to jurisdiction, standardization of multiple features across jurisdictions' systems was essential to ensure that data transmitted to the CDC from surveillance sites could easily be merged into a single standardized national surveillance data stream. For example, though the look and feel of data entry screens might vary from state to state, coding schemes used to specify names of specific diagnostic tests important for surveillance purposes (e.g., immunological assays to diagnose measles or hepatitis B) would be standardized across states, as would be the technical specifications for construction of the electronic messages sent from states to CDC. Early NEDSSS standards proposed that system architecture elements should:

- be Web-browser based,
- be built on an integrated relational database,
- emphasize secure data storage and transmission,
- use HL-7 messages between computers, and
- be written using accepted contemporary programming practices.

Funding early state preparations for NEDSS

Because of the complexity of the emerging NEDSS specifications, it was clear that states would need both time and financial assistance to transition from NETSS to NEDSS. CDC thus arranged an initial 3-year series of funding cycles during which states could apply for grant funds needed to begin their internal NEDSS planning process. These initial cycles (2000–2002) were funded via federal-state collaborative funding mechanisms involving the Council of State and Territorial Epidemiologists (CSTE), then the CDC Epidemiology and Laboratory Capacity (ELC) grant and federal bioterrorism grants.

Options for deployment of NEDSS-compatible software systems

States with IT resources could opt to develop systems that were compatible with NEDSS. States lacking significant IT expertise contracted with private IT companies or, as South Carolina did, chose to adopt the NEDSS-based system (NBS) provided by CDC. The NBS was developed by the CDC and made available at no cost to interested states. States selecting this option became known as "NBS states" and by the mid-2000s these numbered nearly 20. Epidemiology and IT staff from these states soon began to share system information and technical tips and tricks with one another via email and periodic conference calls. This shared experience was especially important early on, as the NBS package initially delivered to states typically required extensive customization and IT infrastructure preparation before deployment was possible.

Early administrative and technical challenges

In South Carolina, DADE initially faced considerable technical challenges associated with customization and deployment of the NBS. DHEC disease control professionals, though experienced with public health surveillance, consultation, and outbreak investigation, had not previously needed to manage a large complex IT project, and at that time DADE did not have a professional IT team of its own. Consequently, DADE initially opted to use CDC NEDSS grant funds to contract with a private IT company with expertise in development, customization, and deployment of large complex relational databases. By 2002, there were five major partners in the project:

1. DHEC's DADE group, who would be the end users of the software
2. CDC's own NEDSS-team
3. The private IT contractor employed by CDC to develop the system
4. The private IT group hired by DHEC to customize the system and make it operational
5. DHEC's own Bureau of Information Services (BIS)

Though the BIS did not have sufficient staff to manage the NBS customization and deployment effort, it did have considerable experience with complex relational databases, and as the unit charged with broad oversight over informatics for the entire agency, it played a strong technical advisory role and was consulted regarding all major decisions.

NEDSS technical characteristics

The technical specifications of the NBS run to several hundred pages but a few points merit mention:
- **NBS database structure:** While NETSS was built in what was largely a flat-file data structure (using in some instances a small number of additional related tables), in contrast the NBS was built upon a large complex relational database structure consisting of approximately 150 related tables (Box 18.1) [7,8].
- **NBS database platform:** The NBS was designed to run on only one of two major commercial relational database systems: Oracle or the Microsoft SQL-Server. At DHEC, the decision was made was made to use MS SQL-Server, software which eventually came to be used for other agency data systems as well.
- **Other NBS software requirements:** The servers that run the NBS use a specialized version of Windows called Windows-Server In addition the NBS uses its

Box 18.1 Flat files and relational databases: a primer

Databases organize data into structured tables that provide a standardized way of entering, accessing, and updating data. A *flat file* is a single table in which data are organized into rows and columns. Each row represents a single record, and each column contains data for a single variable (e.g., LAST_NAME, FIRST_NAME). Students new to data management are often familiar with spreadsheet software that, because it presents cells organized into rows and columns, can conveniently be used to set up a flat file. A true relational database is composed of a few or even dozens of separate tables that are related to one another through special *key fields*. Though relational databases are more complex to design, they are typically more flexible and offer numerous technical advantages. The difference between surveillance systems built on flat files and those structured as relational databases can be understood through a simple example.

A flat file surveillance system might have one row for each reported case and one column for each variable pertaining to the case (e.g., LAST_NAME, FIRST_NAME, ADDRESS, DATE_OF_BIRTH, SEX, DIAGNOSIS, REPORT_DATE). Let us imagine, however, that a particular person has had several diseases and thus has several entries (rows) in the flat file. For example, the patient may have been diagnosed with hepatitis B one year, hepatitis C the next, HIV 2 years later, and tuberculosis 3 years after that. In a flat file, the first five variables of these case reports would have had to be entered four different times. This would constitute not only a waste of data entry time but would also provide multiple opportunities for data entry errors or inconsistencies (e.g., having the DATE_OF_BIRTH entered once as 3/7/1980 and another time as 7/3/1980). Suppose that between diagnosis with HIV and diagnosis with tuberculosis, the patient had changed his address. At that point the addresses for the first three entries would thus be incorrect, and the address corrections would have to be made to the previous three disease reports in order to update the flat file. This example shows that the attractive apparent simplicity of a flat file structure may obscure problematic issues in data management.

To avoid such difficulties, a relational database approach to the example given above might have a table called PERSONS and another table called REPORTS. The PERSONS table might contain information about the person himself, such as LAST_ NAME, FIRST_NAME, ADDRESS, DATE_OF_BIRTH, SEX, along with a unique identifier field which might be called PERSON_ID. The REPORTS table could then simply have three fields: PERSON_ID, DIAGNOSIS, and REPORT_DATE. The key field PERSON_ID provides an unambiguous way to link the two tables. The basic identifying information (LAST_NAME, FIRST_NAME, DATE_OF_ BIRTH, SEX) is found in the PERSONS table. Any changes, such as to an address, are entered a single time.

This simple example illustrates some of the potential advantages of relational database structures. A special challenge to database designers is to determine how complex to make the table structure. A design with dozens of tables can offer both theoretical and practical advantages; however, the database may then suffer from performance issues, require a database specialist to maintain and update it, and may pose difficulties for health department end users who are accustomed to accessing, manipulating, and analyzing flat file data. Any proposed surveillance system software design may bring financial, operational, and other trade-offs all of which must be taken into account when selecting one system design or set of features over another. In public health, it is essential that IT-savvy epidemiology and management staff participate in system design discussions along with the IT professionals, so that program and end-user requirements are not overlooked.

Finally, note that in the Microsoft Office software suite, Excel is commonly used to manage data organized as a flat file, whereas Access is a tool that can be used to create more complicated relational database structures. In the world of large databases, especially those accessed simultaneously by multiple users, more complex server-based software (e.g., Microsoft's SQL Server, IBM's DB2, or ORACLE) are typically used. These software systems must be managed by computer professionals, but the perspectives of epidemiologists should be discussed during the system design phase.

own licensed version of SAS (a commonly used statistical analysis software platform) to perform certain internal data manipulations. Finally, the NBS has also used several smaller specialized utilities for internal messaging and other technical tasks.
- **NBS hardware requirements:** At DHEC the NBS hardware configuration called for a set of four servers. This set of servers which actually run the NBS are referred to as the "production servers." Additional four-server sets are maintained for development (e.g., when programmers are working on new features), for testing newly developed modules or upgrades supplied by CDC, and for end-user training purposes. Thus, at DHEC the overall system requirement for running the NBS was for four sets of four servers.

- **NBS data extraction:** As mentioned previously, the NBS stores data in a complex relational structure involving dozens of tables. Though this data architecture is optimal from the point of view of consistency and quality of data entry and efficient storage, this data structure does not provide simple data access to health department end-users such as epidemiologists, medical officers, or nurse consultants. For example, a user might simply wish to obtain a list of all salmonella cases reported from a particular county in a particular year characterized by week or month of onset, municipality, zip code, or sex and age group. NBS data reside in tables referred to collectively as the Operational Data Store (ODS). Extracting even the simple line list of cases described above would be time consuming, even for an IT professional proficient in advanced programming. Accordingly, the NBS also maintains a reporting database (RDB) that contains essential case information (current as of the end of the previous work day) in a single flat-file structure. Thus users typically extract data or run reports from the RDB rather than from the ODS. Data can be easily extracted from the RDB in a format that can be opened with Excel spreadsheet software or standard statistical software as needed.
- **Data migration and entry:** The technical term for moving data from an old system to a new system is "data migration." An early question in the NEDSS era was whether it would be possible to migrate data from the old NETSS Epi Info system over to the new NBS. The possibility was studied extensively; but, as migration from the NETSS flat-file structure into the highly relational NBS structure (with its stringent rules regarding use of standardized codes and reference tables) would have been exceedingly complex, it was decided to retain the old NETSS data separately. Analyses of data that span the NETSS and NEDSS eras are thus done by extracting data from the two systems, renaming codes and variables as needed to achieve data consistency, and merging old and new data in a neutral software environment such as Excel, Epi Info, EpiData, or SAS.

In the 1990s, data entry for NETSS was performed at the DHEC central office by one full-time employee and one backup employee. Once the Web-based NBS was deployed, data entry was decentralized. Within DHEC, case reports and laboratory test results are now entered at the regional level, typically by either the regional disease surveillance and response coordinator (often a public health nurse) or by administrative support staff. DHEC has now trained and granted NBS data entry access to nearly 200 users based in dozens of hospitals, private laboratories, free-standing medical clinics, and other institutions. Hospital users typically work either in infection control (e.g., infection preventionists) or in the microbiology laboratory.

Hospital and private reference laboratories receiving specimens from South Carolina patients may choose to configure their own laboratory information management systems (LIMS) so that these can transmit positive test results for reportable diseases directly to the NBS via the Internet. Such direct electronic links greatly speed up the transmission to DHEC of laboratory results of public health importance. For diseases such as pertussis or hepatitis A, for which provision of post-exposure prophylaxis to high-risk contacts should be administered as promptly as possible, the hours or sometimes even days saved in this manner may prevent the occurrence of secondary cases.

Resources for NBS users

To this point we have emphasized IT and technical issues relating to NEDSS and the NBS. However, details regarding software systems, no matter how modern and sophisticated, should not obscure the essential role played by timely and informed professional leadership in all aspects of the surveillance process. Indeed, such informed human participation may paradoxically be of greater importance in this era of NEDSS. For example, in each DHEC health region, electronically captured case reports or laboratory test results are placed in an electronic queue within the NBS for review. A well-trained regional DHEC staff member must review the report to determine what further public health action may be needed. Although DHEC had formed local "Epi teams" even in the NETSS era, funding was not then available to support full-time epidemiologists to thoroughly investigate all cases and reports. Coincidentally with the advent of the NEDSS initiative, federal funds became available to states to support local staff needed to exploit the enhanced surveillance and investigation capabilities made possible by NBS. As DHEC progressively deployed the NBS throughout its regional offices in 2003–2004, several systems to support users were developed. These included (1) NBS training programs conducted both centrally and at the regional level, (2) establishment of a telephone help desk available during working hours to aid users facing technical problems with the software, and (3) creation of a newsletter distributed electronically to all users that contained information regarding NBS system updates and tips and tricks for problem solving related to the many features of the NBS.

Case counting and notifications to CDC

Details of case investigations, as recorded in the NBS, also provide information as to whether the case in question meets the standard CDC case definition for public health surveillance [9]. Even though the initial report and subsequent investigation may have been carried out and data entered at the county level, the final determination as to which cases entered into the NBS should or should not be counted are made through final review by DHEC at the state level. Though even suspect cases warrant local public health investigation, only those cases which meet the CDC criteria as confirmed or probable cases are submitted via the NBS HL-7 messaging service to the CDC where they will then be counted as incident cases at the national level.

Demonstrated benefits of the NBS

From the start, most NBS users intuitively felt that the new system brought improved promptness and completeness of notifiable disease case reporting. In 2008, when DHEC had been using the NBS for nearly 5 years, analysis of the agency's experience presented at the national Public Health Information Network conference in Atlanta confirmed:

- an increase in number of system users to 26 in the central office, 40 in public health regions, and 234 providers in 42 facilities;
- a five-fold increase in the number of monthly laboratory reports captured electronically compared to the previous manual data entry era; and
- increased timeliness of laboratory reporting, with reduction of the average delay from laboratory testing to disease reporting from 23 days for mailed disease report cards, to 6 days for provider data entry and 1.4 days for electronic laboratory reporting.

Summary

The transition from NETSS to the NBS during this past decade was a necessary step for DHEC. Like many transitions, this one carried both advantages and disadvantages (Table 18.2). Some of the complex administrative,

Table 18.2 Advantages and disadvantages of adoption of NBS.

Advantages	Disadvantages
Decentralization of data entry: Shared workload; data entry is closer to the actual source of information.	**Cost:** NBS-associated costs borne by CDC and/or by states that have adopted the system have amounted to many millions of dollars over the past decade.
Electronic laboratory reporting: Significant reduction in data entry load; allows rapid assignment of lab results, requiring investigation to the appropriate person; identifies cases that might otherwise have not been reported.	**Complex design:** The NBS relational database with over 120 tables is extraordinarily complicated; requires full-time IT staff to support the SQL database and the multiple servers on which the system runs.
Enhanced communication between public health and medical providers: On-site NBS training. Help Desk consultations and distribution of the NBS newsletter contribute to building active collaborative partnerships. Subsequent strengthening of surveillance activities thus go beyond only what the software does.	**System complexity leads to frequent system downtime:** IT staff must simply reboot the system or further troubleshoot to identify problem.
Allows some site-specific customization of data entry: For example, the addition of condition-specific questions such as for varicella and West Nile virus.	**Difficult for many end users to extract data for common epidemiology queries:** Customizable report options are not simple to use. Ad-hoc data extraction and analysis require expertise in informatics.

Box 18.2 Tips for collaborating with a software design team.

1. No matter how extensive your basic Excel spreadsheet skills are, you should improve these by reading an intermediate-to-advanced book. Become fluent regarding theory and use of Excel functions like pivot tables, "what-if" analyses, The Solver, and more.
2. Learn to use CDC's Epi Info at least at an intermediate level.
3. Learn a programming language. A good language with which to start might be one of the variants of BASIC such as Microsoft's Visual Basic or Liberty BASIC.
4. Ask to attend a meeting of the IT team that develops and maintains your software systems. Afterwards discuss the meeting with one of the programmers and then with the project manager.
5. Learn key IT terminology related to the data systems that you use regularly. Examples may include "requirements" and "business rules." Ask for definitions or explanations when unfamiliar terms are used.

financial, and technical challenges that had to be overcome to make this transition have been outlined in this chapter. Lessons learned include:

- There is a need for health department epidemiologists to gain at least general insight into how IT consultants approach software system design. This understanding can permit them to contribute the essential end-user perspective of the working epidemiologist at all stages of IT project development and deployment (Box 18.2)
- There is a need for disease control units to have ready access to IT professionals who are familiar with software systems used in infectious disease surveillance and control.
- There is a value in using, wherever possible, public domain software tools (e.g., the newest releases of Epi Info) and economical software system design. Together, these programs may allow public health to achieve most of the functionality offered by high-end commercially designed software, perhaps at a fraction of the cost. Savings realized on complex software system development and maintenance might then be allocated to provide additional epidemiology staff to work on the front lines of case investigation and other disease prevention and control activities.

STUDY QUESTIONS

1. What are some of the key advantages of modern electronic systems used to report and manage infectious disease surveillance data? Are there any disadvantages?
2. Why is it important for epidemiologists and other disease control professionals to have a working knowledge of information technology and software design? What additional computer skills can be of benefit to infectious disease surveillance personnel?
3. Read one or more of the articles relating to public health informatics [see references 10–13]. Discuss each article from the perspective of an IT professional, an epidemiologist, and a public health program manager.

References

1. Centers for Disease Control. National Electronic Telecommunications System for Surveillance—United States, 1990–1991. *MMWR Morb Mortal Wkly Rep* 1991;**40**(29): 502–503.
2. CDC's Epi Info Page. Available at http://www.cdc.gov/epiinfo (accessed April 28, 2014).
3. National Electronic Disease Surveillance System Working Group. National Electronic Disease Surveillance System (NEDSS): A standards-based approach to connect public health and clinical medicine. *J Public Health Manag Pract* 2001;**7**(6):43–50.
4. Centers for Disease Control and Prevention. Status of state electronic disease surveillance systems—United States, 2007. *MMWR Morb Mortal Wkly Rep* 2009;**58**(29):804–807.
5. Centers for Disease Control and Prevention. State electronic disease surveillance systems—United States, 2007 and 2010. *MMWR Morb Mortal Wkly Rep* 2011;**60**(41): 1421–1423.
6. NEDS/NBS. Available at http://wwwn.cdc.gov/nndss/script/nedss.aspx (accessed April 28, 2014).
7. Hernandez MJ. *Database Design for Mere Mortals: A Hands-On Guide to Relational Database Design*, 3rd ed. Boston: Addison Wesley; 2013.
8. Hock-Chuan, Chua. A Quick-Start Tutorial on Relational Database Design. 2010. Available at http://www.ntu.edu.sg/home/ehchua/programming/sql/Relational_Database_Design.html (accessed August 5, 2013).
9. Centers for Disease Control and Prevention. History of Case Definitions. 2013. Available at http://wwwn.cdc.gov/nndss/script/casedefHistory.aspx (accessed April 23, 2014).

10. Savel TG, Foldy S, Centers for Disease Control and Prevention. The role of public health informatics in enhancing public health surveillance. *MMWR Surveill Summ* 2012;**61**(Suppl):20–24.

11. Heisey-Grove DM, Church DR, Haney GA, Demaria A Jr. Enhancing surveillance for hepatitis C through public health informatics. *Public Health Rep* 2011;**126**(1):13–18.

12. Dixon BE, Grannis SJ. Why "what data are necessary for this project?" and other basic questions are important to address in public health informatics practice and research. *Online J Public Health Inform* 2011;**3**(3):1–9.

13. Wells S, Bullen C. A near miss: The importance of context in a public health informatics project in a New Zealand case study. *J Am Med Inform Assoc* 2008;**15**(5):701–704.

CHAPTER 19

Practical considerations in implementation of electronic laboratory reporting for infectious disease surveillance

Richard S. Hopkins[1] and Nkuchia M. M'ikanatha[2]

[1] *Department of Epidemiology, University of Florida, Gainesville, FL, USA*
[2] *Pennsylvania Department of Health, Harrisburg, PA, USA*

Introduction

A primary objective in infectious disease surveillance through case reports is to trigger an appropriate public health response so that further illness can be prevented and public fears allayed [1]. Increasing timeliness and completeness of reporting are essential to achieving these objectives. Reporting to public health agencies of laboratory results indicative of the presence of a case of a reportable disease has been an important surveillance method in most states since the 1980s; 49 states had at least some laboratory reporting requirements by 1999 [2]. During the past decade, increasingly widespread use of electronic information systems by clinical laboratories enabled public health officials to receive these reports much more quickly, completely, and accurately [3]. By mid-2013, 54 of the 57 jurisdictions responsible for conducting surveillance (48 state and six large local health departments) were receiving at least some laboratory reports through electronic laboratory reporting (ELR) (Figure 19.1). Participation of clinical laboratories in ELR, however, remains suboptimal. Based on a 12-month estimate, approximately 62% of 20 million reports were submitted to the 54 public health jurisdictions via ELR in 2013 [4].

To enhance public health surveillance, ELR is included in the recent federally led initiative to transform healthcare delivery through incentives for meaningful use of ELR [5]. These incentives are expected to accelerate adoption of ELR by hospital laboratories. Implementation of ELR, however, is complex; a recent evaluation

of the status of deployed ELR systems suggests a need for improvements in integrating data for diseases that have a high volume of laboratory reports (e.g., sexually transmitted diseases) [4]. This chapter focuses on the practical considerations for implementation of ELR including the development process and potential practical challenges. As an illustrative example, the chapter discusses experiences and lessons learned in implementation of ELR in Florida.

The role of clinical laboratories in surveillance

Case definitions for nationally notifiable diseases

The role of clinical laboratories in infectious disease reporting has evolved over time, and it became increasingly important after the 1990 adoption of public health surveillance case definitions for nationally notifiable diseases by the Council of State and Territorial Epidemiologists (CSTE) in collaboration with the Centers for Disease Control and Prevention (CDC). Case definitions established uniform criteria, including specific laboratory criteria, for classifying (e.g., probable or confirmed) and counting cases consistently across jurisdictions [6].

Laboratory criteria are essential in some (e.g., meningococcal disease; hepatitis A, B, and C; salmonellosis; tuberculosis; gonorrhea; and campylobacteriosis) but not all surveillance case definitions. Diseases and con-

Concepts and Methods in Infectious Disease Surveillance, First Edition. Edited by Nkuchia M. M'ikanatha and John K. Iskander.

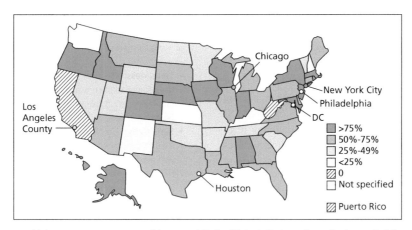

Figure 19.1 Percentage of laboratory reports received by 57 public health jurisdictions through electronic laboratory reporting in the United States in 2013. The jurisdictions include 50 states, the District of Columbia, Puerto Rico, and five cities. As of July 31, 2013, a total of 54 of the 57 jurisdictions were receiving at least some laboratory reports through ELR. Source: Centers for Disease Control and Prevention, *Morbidity and Mortality Weekly Report*. September 27, 2013;62(38);797–799.

ditions under public health surveillance change with clinical knowledge, advances in laboratory diagnostic technology, and changes in infectious disease incidence, as do case definitions. The CSTE annually adds or subtracts diseases from the list of Nationally Notifiable Diseases [7] and updates case definitions through position statements considered and adopted by its members [8]. For example, the HIV/AIDS surveillance case definition, first published in 1997, has undergone multiple revisions in response to improvements in diagnostic methods (see Chapter 12 for detailed discussion on HIV/AIDS including the evolution of the case definition).

Although each jurisdiction has its own list of reportable diseases, CSTE encourages all jurisdictions to submit data on nationally notifiable diseases to CDC's National Notifiable Diseases Surveillance System (NNDSS) [7]. The data in NNDSS allows public health jurisdictions to monitor their progress in meeting objectives for programs funded through CDC Epidemiology and Laboratory Capacity for Infectious Diseases (ELC) Cooperative Agreement. ELC grants support programs that focus on specific areas (e.g., foodborne diseases), and they support infrastructure for conducting surveillance. These grants are awarded to all jurisdictions that directly report data to NNDSS, and the local health departments in the six largest cities (e.g., Los Angeles County and Philadelphia) [9]. (See Chapter 3 for a fuller description of NNDSS and national, state, and local public health surveillance systems.) Studies conducted

in jurisdictions that were leaders in requiring electronic laboratory reporting in the late 1990s document an increase in timeliness and completeness of case reporting when compared to passive reporting by physicians and laboratories [10,11].

Mandatory reporting by clinical laboratories

For decades, public health officials have recognized the need to mandate disease reporting from a variety of sources. For example, an evaluation of a communicable diseases surveillance system in Vermont in the mid-1980s identified a need to mandate reporting by clinical laboratories. Aware of possible misinterpretation, the study cautioned that mandatory reporting by clinical laboratories would not "eliminate physician's legal responsibility to report disease" [12]. Comprehensive surveys conducted since the mid-1990s by the Council of State and Territorial Epidemiologists indicate that most diseases designated as nationally notifiable are reportable in most NEDSS jurisdictions by both clinical laboratories and physicians. For example, in 2010 laboratory evidence of anthrax was reportable in all 50 states and the District of Columbia; laboratory evidence of *Chlamydia trachomatis* infection was reportable in 50 of these 51 jurisdictions; cyclosporiasis in 41; and babesiosis in 17 [13].

Public health reporting requirements vary by jurisdiction. Some provide a single list with distinct requirements for healthcare providers and clinical laboratories, whereas others have a separate list of requirements for clinical laboratories [14,15]. These requirements explicitly specify a timeframe for reporting specified conditions. Maryland's list, for example, includes a category for conditions that necessitate immediate reporting (e.g., *Bacillus anthracis*) and a category for other conditions that are reportable within one working day (e.g., *Listeria monocytogenes*). In addition to an explicit requirement for immediate reporting by telephone for specified conditions (Figure 19.2), Oregon law requires clinical laboratories that report an average of >30 records per month to the local public health authority to submit data through ELR.

For specific diseases, many jurisdictions require that laboratories submit an isolate or a specimen to the state public health laboratory for confirmation and additional characterization. Wyoming, for example, requires that clinical laboratories submit isolates or other appropriate material indicative of certain conditions specified on a list of reportable diseases and conditions [16]. To facilitate surveillance and epidemiological investigations, laboratories are often required to include patient information (e.g., first and last name, date of birth, sex, home address) in their case reports. Additional information includes type of specimen (e.g., stool, urine, blood), collection date, test performed, and results. Details about the submitting provider (e.g., name and address) are also required. Some jurisdictions make information on what is reportable easily accessible by providing confidential case report forms on their websites [17].

Benefits and challenges in implementation of electronic laboratory reporting

Electronic laboratory reporting benefits to surveillance

Attributes of surveillance systems are described in detail in the *Updated Guidelines for Evaluating Public Health Surveillance Systems* [18]. ELR can result in increased

---

Box 19.1 Potential benefits of ELR on selected attributes of surveillance systems.

- **Timeliness:** Electronic reports generally arrive several days earlier than conventional paper reports. Receiving timely test results allows early initiation of public health response.
- **Sensitivity:** Fully implemented, systems are at least as sensitive as conventional reporting systems. ELR sensitivity varies by disease, but it is typically higher than paper-based reports for diseases that are otherwise inconsistently reported (e.g., salmonellosis) [10].
- **Positive Predictive Value:** Laboratory reports for cases of diseases diagnosed by laboratory tests that have low rates of false positives (e.g., culture for enteric organisms) will have high positive predictive value. In addition, reduction in manual data entry errors can result in more accurate case reports.
- **Acceptability:** Stakeholders accept well-thought-out systems that among other characteristics communicate expectations on what diseases are reportable and technical specifications [20].
- **Flexibility:** Adding new reportable laborataory findings, data fields, or test codes can be done if IT support for both reporters (clinical laboratory) and surveillance system users is in place.

---

timeliness, sensitivity, positive predictive value, and acceptability (Box 19.1). When implemented effectively, ELR should result in more rapid reporting of cases requiring public health action and should facilitate tracing of contacts and provision of antimicrobial prophylaxis. Based on evidence from deployed systems, electronic case reports arrive approximately 4 days earlier than those from a paper-based system [10]. The benefits of receiving timely test results, however, depend on the necessity to initiate public health response. For example, if positive test results of organisms typically associated with outbreaks (e.g., *Salmonella* species) are received in a timely manner, this can trigger

---

Figure 19.2 Poster used in Oregon to disseminate a list of conditions reportable by clinical laboratories. Immediately reportable conditions are highlighted with a telephone icon. Source: http://public.health.oregon.gov/DiseasesConditions/ CommunicableDisease/ReportingCommunicableDisease/Pages/index.aspx. Reproduced with permission of Oregon Division of Public Health.

☻ Report by phone immediately, day or night. New reportables are highlighted.
◐ Report within 24 hours.
    NOTE: Those items below without a symbol next to them require reporting
    within one local public health authority working day.
🔬 Forward isolate (aliquot or subculture) to the Oregon State Public Health Laboratory.

BACTERIA
Bacillus anthracis [5] ☻ 🔬
Bordetella pertussis
Borrelia
Brucella
Campylobacter
Chlamydia trachomatis
Chlamydophila psittaci
Clostridium botulinum ☻
Clostridium tetani
Corynebacterium diphtheriae [5] ☻ 🔬
Coxiella burnetii
Ehrlichia/Anaplasma
Enterobacteriaceae family isolates
that are non-susceptible to
carbapenem antibiotics and meet
the OHA case definition [5, 14] 🔬
Escherichia coli (Shiga-toxigenic) [6] 🔬
Francisella tularensis [5] ☻ 🔬
Grimontia hollisae [5] 🔬
(formerly *Vibrio hollisae*)
Haemophilus ducreyi
Haemophilus influenzae [5,7] ◐ 🔬
Legionella
Leptospira
Listeria monocytogenes [5] 🔬
Mycobacterium bovis [5] 🔬
Mycobacterium tuberculosis [5] 🔬
Mycobacterium, other
(non-respiratory only)
Neisseria gonorrhoeae

Neisseria meningitidis [5,7] ◐ 🔬
Rickettsia
Salmonella [5] 🔬
Shigella [5] 🔬
Treponema pallidum
Vibrio cholerae [5] ☻ 🔬
Vibrio, non-cholerae [5] 🔬
Yersinia pestis [5] ☻ 🔬
Yersinia, non-pestis [5] 🔬

FUNGI
Cryptococcus [5] 🔬

PARASITES
Babesia
Cryptosporidium
Cyclospora
Giardia
Plasmodium
Taenia solium [8]
Trichinella

PRION DISEASES
Creutzfeldt-Jakob disease
(CJD) and other prion illnesses

VIRUSES
Arboviruses [1, 13]
Arenaviruses [10] ☻
Filoviruses [10] ☻
Hantavirus

Hepatitis A [9] 🔬
Hepatitis B [9] 🔬
Hepatitis C
Hepatitis D (delta)
Hepatitis E
Hemorrhagic fever viruses [10] ☻
HIV infection and AIDS
Influenza, novel strain [11] ☻
Measles (rubeola) ☻
Mumps
Polio ☻
Rabies ☻
Rubella ☻
SARS-coronavirus ☻
Variola major (smallpox) ☻
West Nile
Yellow fever ☻

OTHER IMPORTANT REPORTABLES
Any "uncommon illness of potential
public health significance" [1]

Any outbreak of disease [1]

Results on all blood lead testing
should be reported within seven
days unless they indicate lead
poisoning, which must be reported
within one local health department
working day. [12]

All CD4 counts and HIV viral loads

FOOTNOTES
1. Oregon Revised Statute 433.004; Oregon Administrative Rule 333-018
   (http://arcweb.sos.state.or.us/pages/rules/oars_300/oar_333/333_018.html)
2. Refer to www.healthoregon.org/diseasereporting for a list of local health departments, reporting FAQs, and more details
   about what to report. When in doubt, report.
3. ORS 433.004 and OAR 333-018-0013 (http://arcweb.sos.state.or/us/pages/rules/oars_300/oar_33/333_018.html);
   Manual for Mandatory Electronic Laboratory Reporting (www.healthoregon.org/elr)
4. ORS 431.262; OAR 333-018 (http://arcweb.sos.state.or.us/pages/rules/oars_300/oar_333/333_018.html);
   OAR 333-026-0030 http://arcweb.sos.state.or.us/pages/rules/oars_300/oar_333/333_026.html)
5. Isolates must be forwarded to the Oregon State Public Health Laboratory (phone: 503-693-4100).
6. All confirmed or suspect isolates of *E. coli* O157, and all non-O157 Shiga-toxin-positive broths,
   must be forwarded to the Oregon State Public Health Laboratory (phone: 503-693-4100).
7. Report only isolates from normally sterile sites (e.g., neither sputum nor throat cultures).
8. Report cysticercosis and all undifferentiated *Taenia* spp. (e.g., eggs in stool O & P).
9. IgM-positive HAV and HBV serum specimens must be forwarded to the Oregon State Public Health Laboratory.
10. Hemorrhagic fever caused by viruses of the filovirus (e.g., Ebola, Marburg) or arenavirus
    (e.g., Lassa, Machupo) families are reportable.
11. Influenza A virus that cannot be subtyped by commercially distributed assays.
12. "Lead poisoning" means a blood lead level of at least 10 micrograms per deciliter.
13. Any other arthropod-borne viruses, including, but not limited to California encephalitis, Colorado tick
    fever, Dengue, Eastern equine encephalitis, Heartland virus, Kyasanur Forest, St. Louis encephalitis.
14. See CRE poster (OHA 8578) for further information.

OHA 8576 (Rev. 04/2014)

Table 19.1 Calculation for sensitivity and predictive value positive for a surveillance system.

Detected by surveillance	Condition present		
	Yes	No	
Yes	True positive A	False positive B	A + B
No	False negative C	True negative D	C + D
	A + C	B + D	Total

Note: Sensitivity = A/(A + C); predictive value positive (PVP) = A/(A + B).
Source: Adapted from Table 3 in German RR, Lee LM, Horan JM, et al. Centers for Disease Control and Prevention, *Morbidity and Mortality Weekly Report*. July 27, 2001; 50(RR13): 1–35.

an investigation. ELR also provides documentation for conditions that are reportable by telephone (e.g., *Listeria monocytogenes*) [14].

Increased sensitivity in this context refers to the ability of the system to ensure that reports are made for all positive test results (Table 19.1). When fully implemented, ELR systems are at least as sensitive as conventional paper-based systems [19,20]. Sensitivity is significantly higher for reports received through ELR for those diseases whose diagnosis requires laboratory testing (e.g., *Chlamydia trachomatis*) [11]. In addition, ELR systems typically result in higher positive predictive value (PPV). This concept in surveillance means that reported cases are more likely to represent true cases (Table 19.1). ELR systems can have high PPV for diseases that have laboratory tests that are specific with only rare false positives (e.g., culture for enteric organisms) [21]. Additionally, reduction in manual data-entry errors increases accuracy of case reports [19].

Resource needs and challenges in implementation of electronic laboratory reporting

For clinical laboratories with automated information systems that offer electronic services such as order entry forms and results reporting to providers, ELR can be relatively inexpensive. The cost for software to extract

reportable conditions from an existing system was estimated at $40,000 in Indiana [22], which would be reasonable given the relatively high cost of laboratory information systems. In some cases, however, data extraction and messaging with an existing laboratory information system may be difficult. Building an information system to capture reportable conditions from a wide of array of test types (e.g., microbiology, virology, parasitology) is a challenge for small clinical laboratories in hospitals. Typically, ELR messages must comply with specific information technology (IT) standards [23]. To offset the cost of participation in ELR, including cost for complying with these standards, qualified hospital facilities can take advantage of monetary incentives available through the EHR Incentive Program to offset the cost of adapting ELR [5].

In addition to monetary costs, clinical laboratories may encounter other barriers to implementation of ELR. Clinical laboratories may be unaware of reporting requirements, specifically what and how to report. To address this well-known barrier, jurisdictions provide guidance for electronic laboratory reporting [24]. Experience from New York City and elsewhere, however, suggests that in addition to guidance, there is a need for regular communication between public health officials and individuals who are responsible for reporting in clinical laboratories [20]. Transfer of electronic messages with reportable disease data can also present a practical challenge to clinical laboratories. Although approaches used to submit electronic data to public health authorities vary, laboratories are expected to comply with criteria set by public health authorities in each jurisdiction. Typically, laboratories identify reportable conditions in their test catalog and then map them into standard codes acceptable to the respective public health jurisdiction (Box 19.2). The codes used are typically LOINC and SNOMED, which respectively refer to Logical Observation Identifiers Names, Codes, and Systematized Nomenclature of Medicine [25,26]. Receipt of nonstandardized data is one of the main reasons for delays in automated processing of ELR cited by public health jurisdictions [27]. Recently, an ELR working group created an updated reportable condition–mapping table to facilitate extraction of LOINC and SNOMED codes for nationally notifiable diseases by clinical laboratories [28].

Public health authorities often require that laboratories submit data as messages that comply with an

Box 19.2 Practical steps in implementation of ELR.

Preparatory phase

1. Identify the reportable conditions in your facility's test catalog.
2. Map reportable tests to LOINC and SNOMED codes accepted by applicable public health authority.
   ⇒ These codes are extracted by disease listing from the Reportable Condition Mapping Table (RCMT) available at: http://www.phconnect.org/group/rcmt/forum/topics/rcmt-download.
3. Ensure that your information system can produce a message compliant with an up-to-date HL7 ELR Version (most current as of 2013 is 2.5.1).
   ⇒ Comply with any other additional specifications imposed by the public health jurisdiction.

Enrollment phase

4. Initiate the process by contacting the ELR point of contact or by completing an online enrollment form, if available.
5. Verify reportable disease conditions, mapping codes, messaging format with ELR point of contact for the applicable jurisdiction.
6. Prepare for data submission by determining the amount of data based on the previous year's records.
7. Set up secure electronic data transfer protocol in collaboration with the public health authority.
8. Precertification checklist
   ✓ Verify that only reportable conditions filtered.
   ✓ Validate standards: LOINC and SNOMED codes and HL7 message.
   ✓ Submit test message.
9. Certification process: This involves submission of ELR while continuing with conventional reporting until the responsible public health authority agrees that data by both systems match.

Source: Adapted from California Reportable Disease Information Exchange Electronic Lab Reporting (details available at: http://www.cdph.ca.gov/data/informatics/tech/Pages/CalREDIEELR.aspx).
Reproduced with permission of the State of California.

up-to-date version of Health Level Seven International (HL7). HL7 messaging standards allow exchange of health information to support patient care and data management [29]. Difficulties in complying with HL7 are a challenge cited by public health jurisdictions as a reason for slow progress in full implementation of ELR

[27]. California, for example, uses a certification process to ensure that all the necessary steps are met in addition to validation of submitted records (Box 19.2) [30]. Procedural challenges encountered in implementation can be reduced by practical guidelines that include links to standards (e.g., reportable condition mapping tables). Examples of guidelines that link to practical information are available on the California and Ohio health department websites [30,31].

To be useful in surveillance, case reports received through electronic reports must contain the same information that is typically included on paper reports. In addition to facilitating timely public health response, details included in cases reports (e.g., patient demographics) enable better description of distribution of cases and evaluation of surveillance systems. However, experiences in early implementation of ELR in many jurisdictions (e.g., New York, Pennsylvania) cited lack of patient address as a serious limitation [23].

Public health jurisdictions also face barriers in implementation of ELR. Costs for development and maintenance of ELR-related information technology infrastructure present an obstacle to public health authorities. Resources required for building and maintaining ELR range from $1 million to $5 million; approximately half of this money is for IT support [32]. There is a shortage of public health officials with appropriate skills to analyze data and often a lack of institutional support for implementation. Other barriers cited by public health jurisdictions include lack of robust information systems to handle ELR and surveillance systems that are incompatible with ELR [33].

Some of the costs for ELR implementation by public health jurisdictions are covered through the Affordable Care Act (ACA). In 2013, the CDC distributed over $85 million in funds appropriated as part of the ACA through the ELC funding mechanism to all 50 state health departments, six public health jurisdictions in large metropolitan areas (Los Angeles County, Philadelphia, New York City, Chicago, Houston, District of Columbia), Puerto Rico, and the Republic of Palau [34]. Although institutional support within public health departments depends largely on the leadership in specific jurisdictions, epidemiologists responsible for surveillance can help by performing analyses to demonstrate the value of ELR. For example, an evaluation of the impact of ELR on hepatitis A surveillance in New York City in 2006 documented a median decrease of 17 days in time to report, which enabled public health officials to administer post-exposure prophylaxis to 299 individuals, a fourfold increase from 2000 [35].

Experiences and lessons learned from implementation of electronic laboratory reporting in Florida

Implementation

In 2001, the Florida Department of Health (FDOH) computerized the collection and management of reportable disease case reports in Merlin, Florida's web-based reportable disease surveillance information system. Soon afterwards, implementation of electronic laboratory reporting from the state public health laboratory to Merlin began [36]. Starting in 2004, ELR data from the public health laboratory were captured through Merlin. Since then ELR for all reportable conditions has increased steadily as more laboratories have been added, reaching more than 2.5 million laboratory result records received in 2012–2013, representing 241,000 cases of reportable diseases [37]. At the end of 2013, ELR data were being received from five major regional commercial laboratories, 52 hospital laboratories, four offices of the state public health laboratory, one county health department laboratory, one transplant facility laboratory, and the New York State Public Health Laboratory. Although the ELR-reporting hospitals represent only about a quarter of the 213 licensed hospitals in Florida, the hospitals, commercial laboratories, and other reporters participating in ELR together submitted about 69% of all reportable laboratory results in Florida. (The remaining 31% that were generated in hospitals or laboratories not yet participating in ELR were submitted to local health departments via paper, fax, or phone calls, or not reported).

Initially, records were transmitted through a message format developed specifically for use with Merlin. The system's stability greatly improved in 2007 when the public health laboratories started to use a commercial off-the-shelf software solution. In 2008, Merlin was modified to receive results in these formats and vocabularies, and FDOH added an integration broker to receive all external laboratory reports, validate them, transform them according to preset rules or filters, and send them to the correct surveillance information system.

A 2006 amendment to Florida's disease reporting regulations had mandated that laboratories submit specified test results via an electronic surveillance system developed by FDHOH [38] The rule specified the type of demographic data required [24] and mandated that laboratories submit data in an up-to-date version of HL7. Initially, FDOH was not fully prepared to receive these messages, especially as laboratories had been given little information about data standards beyond the message format. However, this rule gave the health department the authority to collect required laboratory results by an electronic mechanism and assured hospital and commercial laboratories that reports submitted in this way would satisfy their legal reporting mandate.

In 2007, Florida began electronically filtering results received through the integration broker from the state laboratory and a small number of commercial laboratories. An SQL query scanned incoming results and marked those that appeared to represent cases of reportable diseases with a Data of Interest (DoI) flag. Flagged results were moved from the large database of unfiltered records to smaller databases maintained by Merlin and by its counterpart applications for sexually transmitted disease case reports (Patient Reporting Investigation Surveillance Manager [PRISM]) and for HIV/AIDS reports (Enhanced HIV/AIDS Reporting System [eHARS]).

During the first half of 2007, a software tester and a Merlin project manager were added to the team to begin testing the ELR feeds from individual laboratories and to develop an ELR Implementation Guide, which mandated the use of LOINC codes to describe test types. Later that year, Merlin began receiving results for 31 tests from the public health laboratory's new COTS LIMS; and a full-time integration broker specialist was added to the team. By July 2008, Merlin was receiving results for 82 test types from the public health laboratory through the new mechanism, and the focus shifted to commercial laboratories.

In 2008, a business analyst was added to the team with the goal of increasing electronic reporting from commercial laboratories, and an additional software tester was hired. The business analyst was responsible for obtaining a list of tests being done by each laboratory, working with the integration broker staff to establish a secure data transfer for each commercial laboratory, coordinating evaluation of test data from each lab (from both a software and content point of view), determining when to move a laboratory's ELR feed into production and periodically searching the database for new test types from laboratories in ELR production. By December 2008, FDOH was receiving results from a large national laboratory for 82 different test types and had rewritten the ELR guidance document to include placement of all required data within the HL7 format. By March of 2009, FDOH was actively soliciting and testing data from four large national laboratories and two Florida hospitals.

The 2009 pandemic of influenza caused by a novel strain of H1N1 influenza challenged FDOH to improve how it obtained, processed, and displayed results of influenza tests, both from the state public health laboratory and from commercial and hospital laboratories. Both positive and negative influenza test results were added to the ELR feeds from the three largest commercial laboratories, which were doing the bulk of H1N1 testing in the state of Florida. The number of tests performed and test positivity rates were monitored. Inclusion of negative results was gradually discontinued after the public health emergency (declared as part of the initial recognition of H1N1 influenza) was over.

During the influenza pandemic, work on other aspects of ELR slowed. Starting in January of 2010, addition of new laboratories and tests resumed. In a significant policy change, FDOH stopped requiring the use of LOINC codes and instead began to allow use of local codes for test types and results. By mid-2011, results were being received from 19 laboratories, and the number of active filters (translation tables) had grown from fewer than 600 in January of 2010 to more than 1400, with each filter representing a particular test type from one facility. FDOH was receiving and processing over 11,000 laboratory results per day. This represents about 60% of the estimated total number of reportable laboratory results for Florida. The overall strategy was to recruit and implement ELR from the largest laboratories and hospitals first. As of mid-2011, three large hospital laboratories and dozens of smaller ones were not yet participating in ELR.

Starting in 2012, hospital laboratories had an additional incentive to participate in ELR, beyond requirements of state law and administrative rule as stage 1 of the requirements to receive federal subsidies for meaningful use of electronic records went into effect [5].

Stage 1 required hospitals to implement at least two of the following three capabilities to demonstrate meaningful use: electronic laboratory reporting, syndromic surveillance, and vaccine dose administration reporting. In stage 2, ELR participation is mandatory. To date, the list of hospitals waiting to implement ELR and thus qualify for federal subsidies (as well as comply with state law) has been manageable. FDOH has not actively recruited hospitals to participate, nor has it had an excessively long waiting period before hospitals could implement reporting. FDOH works with the largest hospitals in the queue to get them ready to submit data and verify that the data submitted are useable.

Lessons learned

Experience in Florida suggests that professionals with a wide range of skills are needed to make effective use of electronic laboratory reports. Epidemiologists are the ultimate users of the data and must specify which laboratory findings should be reportable. Laboratory scientists also can assist in identifying which findings should be reportable and in choosing coding systems. Database managers are generally responsible for database design and for assuring the integrity and accessibility of the stored data. Routine and ad-hoc reports are generally designed and produced by data analysts, following direction from epidemiologists. Business analysts help the team develop system requirements and translate those requirements into programming specifications. Software programmers do the actual programming to develop working applications. There is a need for software testers who test each participating laboratory's data feed before it is put into production. Project managers can help by identifying clear tasks and timelines for their completion and by being ready to address barriers encountered. Public health informaticians, who have been trained in public health and in computer science and software development, help assure that systems are designed to meet actual public health needs.

In 2012, the Florida Department of Health began documenting, for each reported case of a reportable disease, how the local health department received its first notification (e.g., via physician report, paper lab result, ELR). The percentage of case reports received first as a laboratory report ranged widely. For meningococcal disease (for which clinicians make telephone case reports without waiting for the laboratory culture result, based on clinical findings and CSF Gram stain), only 10% were laboratory reports. For pertussis and for toxigenic *Escherichia coli* infections, 50% and 70% of reports came first from the laboratory, respectively (personal communication, Janet Hamilton, Florida Department of Health, December 10, 2013).

Keys to success of Florida's ELR efforts started with hiring the right people into the right positions. Support of the project from FDOH upper management was also essential; management set ELR as a priority for the Department of Health and supported funding requests for ELR from the CDC Public Health Preparedness and Epidemiology and Laboratory Capacity Cooperative Agreements. The project manager also fostered an environment that encouraged teamwork and innovation. There was minimal employee and contractor turnover between 2008 and 2013. This particular project was able to succeed by allowing hospitals considerable flexibility; for example, hospitals were permitted to use local codes for their results. This does require more staff time at the central office, and striking the right balance between system flexibility and health department staff time requirements is an ongoing challenge.

Challenges encountered

Practical challenges that health departments have to surmount in order to make effective use of ELR data include obtaining necessary data, especially demographics variables (e.g., patient addresses) and processing data that arrive in local codes instead of standard codes (i.e., LOINC and SNOMED codes) and in nonstandard message formats. Clinical laboratories may be able to provide missing data elements but use of standard codes and required message format is more difficult to implement. In some situations, laboratories may have a practical reason for using local codes. Thus, the public health agency receiving ELR data from such laboratories must decide whether to insist on a required data format or accept nonstandard data. Nonstandardized data can be processed with laboratory-specific translation tables or filters before being added to the health department system. If nonstandardized data are accepted, processes must be established to assure that facilities inform the receiving health department when they change codes, and automated processes should be designed to detect such submissions. The receiving agency should set up a daily monitoring process to ensure that all expected data from all reporting labora-

tories are being received and to identify any new codes being used by laboratories.

When a jurisdiction such as the state of Florida decides what to make reportable, difficult decisions relate to diseases for which laboratory results are relatively nonspecific and for illnesses that may be long-lasting such as hepatitis B or C or Lyme disease. For these conditions, a laboratory result by itself does not meet the surveillance case definition, and most laboratory results received will not represent new cases requiring public health action. If laboratories must submit all positive results, the surveillance staff must determine which results represent reportable cases, significantly increasing their workload. In 2012, Florida implemented software in Merlin allowing automated generation of case reports from certain laboratory findings for salmonellosis, hepatitis B, and hepatitis C and allowed the staff to override the automated assignment of case status. Requiring laboratories to submit other results along with the disease-specific results (e.g., liver function test results along with hepatitis C antibody results) can reduce the public health staff's workload considerably. Electronic health records have (or soon will have) the capability to make case reports in a uniform format that supports automated combination of information derived from laboratory reports with information from other parts of the medical record.

Summary

ELR can significantly improve surveillance through improved timeliness, positive predictive value, and sensitivity of deployed systems. ELR has enabled public health authorities in the United States to investigate individual cases of reportable diseases more rapidly, thus preventing further spread, and to identify outbreaks of serious infections quickly. However, the benefits of ELR to infectious disease surveillance are yet to be fully realized. In this chapter, we have addressed important considerations in the development of clinical laboratory ELR. In addition to well-known benefits of ELR, it is important to acknowledge challenges that are likely to be encountered in the implementation process as well as in operation of fully deployed systems. As demonstrated in Florida, a stepwise approach that enrolls laboratories incrementally can allow public health jurisdictions time to address practical challenges encountered in the implementation process. One of the important lessons from Florida's experience is the need for a multidisciplinary team operating as part of a stable and connected public health system.

ELR requires substantial resources including monetary investments in information systems by both clinical laboratories and public health jurisdictions. Ongoing federally led efforts to transform healthcare delivery with incentives for meaningful use of electronic health records are expected to accelerate adaption of ELR. With monetary support from the CDC, public health jurisdictions can take advantage of increased ELR to strengthen surveillance by implementing new systems or refining existing systems. To ensure that desired objectives are met, ELR systems should be designed with an eye toward the ability to generate data that can be used for system evaluation, and evaluation should be part of the strategic plan for surveillance.

STUDY QUESTIONS

1. Briefly describe why disease reporting by clinical laboratories is important in surveillance for infectious diseases.
2. Describe at least three benefits of electronic laboratory reporting in terms of attributes of surveillance systems.
3. From the perspective of a clinical laboratory, briefly discuss at least three challenges encountered in implementation of electronic laboratory reporting.
4. Lack of institutional support is often cited as a barrier to effective implementation of ELR. As an infectious disease epidemiologist in a large city health department in the United States, discuss how you would go about building institutional support.
5. Assume that you are the lead epidemiologist in a group that is responsible for advising on implementation of ELR for a medium-sized state in the United States. Provide at least five tasks that must be accomplished.
6. Electronic laboratory reports are important sources of data for Merlin, Florida's web-based reportable disease surveillance system. Discuss key factors that contributed to successful implementation of ELR in Florida.
7. Provide a perspective on why a robust disease surveillance system (e.g., Merlin) is important in effective implementation of ELR.

References

1. Chorba TL, Berkelman RL, Safford SK, et al. Mandatory reporting of infectious diseases by clinicians. *JAMA* 1989;**262**:3018–3026.
2. Roush S, Birkhead G, Koo D, Cobb A, Fleming D. Mandatory reporting of diseases and conditions by health care professionals and laboratories. *JAMA* 1999;**282**:164–70.
3. M'ikanatha NM, Lynfield R, Julian KG, Van Beneden C, de Valk H. Infectious disease surveillance: A cornerstone for prevention and control. In: M'ikanatha NM, Lynfield R, Van Beneden C, de Valk H, eds. *Infectious Disease Surveillance*. Chichester: Wiley-Blackwell Publishing; 2013: 3–20.
4. Centers for Disease Control and Prevention. Progress in increasing electronic reporting of laboratory results to public health agencies—United States, 2013. *MMWR Morb Mortal Wkly Rep* 2013;**62**:797–999.
5. Centers for Medicare & Medicaid Services. Meaningful Use Stage 2. 2012. Available at http://www.cms.gov/Regulations-and-Guidance/Legislation/EHRIncentivePrograms/downloads/Stage2_HospitalCore_14_SubLabResults.pdf (accessed November 19, 2013).
6. Centers for Disease Control and Prevention. Case definitions for infectious conditions under public health surveillance. *MMWR Recomm Rep* 1997;**46**(RR-10):1–55.
7. Centers for Disease Control and Prevention. National Notifiable Infectious Conditions. 2014. Available at http://wwwn.cdc.gov/NNDSS/script/ConditionList.aspx?Type=0&Yr=2013 (accessed April 21, 2014).
8. Council of State and Territorial Epidemiologists. Position Statement Archive. 2013. Available at http://www.cste.org/?page=PositionStatements (accessed November 19, 2013).
9. Centers for Disease Control and Prevention. Epidemiology and Laboratory Capacity for Infectious Diseases (ELC) Cooperative Agreement Epidemiology and Laboratory Capacity for Infectious Diseases: Background. 2013. Available at http://www.cdc.gov/ncezid/dpei/epidemiology-laboratory-capacity.html (accessed April 14, 2014).
10. Effler P, Ching-Lee M, Bogard A, et al. Statewide system of electronic notifiable disease reporting from clinical laboratories: Comparing automated reporting with conventional methods. *JAMA* 1999;**282**:1845–1850.
11. Wurtz R, Cameron BJ. Electronic laboratory reporting for the infectious diseases physician and clinical microbiologist. *Clin Infect Dis* 2005;**40**:1638–1643.
12. Schramm MM, Vogt RL, Mamolen M. The surveillance of communicable disease in Vermont: Who reports? *Public Health Rep* 1991;**106**:95–97.
13. Council of State and Territorial Epidemiologists. State Reportable Conditions Assessment (SRCA). Available at http://www.cste.org/search/all.asp?bst=State+Reportable

+Conditions+Assessment+%28SRCA%29 (accessed April 20, 2014).

14. Maryland Department of Health and Mental Hygiene. List of Conditions to Report and Instructions for Reporting. 2010 Available at http://phpa.dhmh.maryland.gov/SitePages/what-to-report.aspx (accessed November 21, 2013).

15. State of Oregon. Reporting Communicable diseases: Lab poster. 2012. Available at http://public.health.oregon.gov/diseasesconditions/communicabledisease/reportingcommunicabledisease/pages/reportable.aspx (accessed April 14, 2014).

16. Wyoming Department of Health Reportable Disease List. 2008. Available at http://www.health.wyo.gov/phsd/epiid/reporting.html (accessed November 22, 2013).

17. State of Connecticut. Laboratory Reporting Forms and Instructions. 2013. Available at http://www.ct.gov/dph/cwp/view.asp?a=3136&q=453838 (accessed November 22, 2013).

18. German RR, Lee LM, Horan JM, Milstein RL, Pertowski CA, Waller MN. Updated guidelines for evaluating public health surveillance systems: Recommendations from the Guidelines Working Group. *MMWR Recomm Rep* 2001; **50**(RR13):1–35.

19. Ward M, Brandsema P, van Straten E, Bosman A. Electronic reporting improves timeliness and completeness of infectious disease notification, The Netherlands, 2003. *Euro Surveill* 2005;**10**:27–30.

20. Nguyen TQ, Thorpe L, Makki HA, Mostashari F. Benefits and barriers to electronic laboratory results reporting for notifiable diseases: The New York City Department of Health and Mental Hygiene experience. *Am J Public Health* 2007;**97**(Suppl 1):S142–S145.

21. Panackal AA, M'ikanatha NM, Tsui FC, et al. Automatic electronic laboratory-based reporting of notifiable infectious diseases at a large health system. *Emerg Infect Dis* 2002;**8**:685–691.

22. Overhage JM, Grannis S, McDonald CJ. A comparison of the completeness and timeliness of automated electronic laboratory reporting and spontaneous reporting of notifiable conditions. *Am J Public Health* 2008;**98**:344–350.

23. M'ikanatha NM, Southwell B, Lautenbach E. Automated laboratory reporting of infectious diseases in a climate of bioterrorism. *Emerg Infect Dis* 2003;**9**:1053–1057.

24. Florida Department of Health. Laboratory Reporting Guidelines of Notifiable Diseases or Conditions in Florida. 2008. Available at http://hardeechd.org/forms/Laboratory%20Reporting%20Guidebook%202009-01.pdf (accessed December 12, 2013).

25. Regenstrief Institute, Inc. Logical Observation Identifiers Names and Codes (LOINC®). 2014. Available at http://loinc.org/ (accessed April 14, 2014).

26. The International Health Terminology Standards Development Organization. SNOMED Clinical Terms. 2011. Avail-

able at http://www.ihtsdo.org/about-ihtsdo/ (accessed November 24, 2013).

27. Magnuson JA. 2010 National Electronic Laboratory Reporting (ELR) Snapshot Survey. 2012. Available at http://www.coast2coastinformatics.com/2010NationalELRSurvey-Summary.pdf (accessed October 19, 2013).

28. phConnect Admin. Reportable Condition Mapping Table. 2013. Available at http://www.phconnect.org/group/rcmt (accessed November 24, 2013).

29. Health Level Seven International. About HL7. 2014. Available at http://www.hl7.org/about/index.cfm?ref=nav (accessed April 14, 2014).

30. State of California. CalREDIE Electronic Lab Reporting (ELR). 2014. Available at http://www.cdph.ca.gov/data/informatics/tech/Pages/CalREDIEELR.aspx (accessed April 14, 2014).

31. Ohio Department of Health. Electronic Laboratory Reporting. 2013. Available at http://www.odh.ohio.gov/healthstats/elr/elr1.aspx (accessed November 24, 2013).

32. Council of State and Territorial Epidemiologist. 2004–2010 National Assessment of electronic laboratory reporting in health departments. 2012. Available at http://www.cste2.org/webpdfs/ELRAssesmentBrief.pdf (accessed November 24, 2013).

33. Coast2Coast Informatics. Annual National Electronic Laboratory Reporting (ELR) survey data summary reports, 2004–2010. 2011. Available at http://www.coast2coastinformatics.com/ReferenceMaterial.html (accessed November 24, 2013).

34. Centers for Disease Control and Prevention. Epidemiology and Laboratory Cooperative Agreement—FY 2013. 2013. Available at http://www.cdc.gov/ncezid/dpei/pdf/aca-elc-fy2013-funding-8-30-2013.pdf (accessed November 24, 2013).

35. Moore KM, Reddy V, Kapell D, Balter S. Impact of electronic laboratory reporting on hepatitis A surveillance in New York City. *J Public Health Manag Pract* 2008;**14**:437–441.

36. Centers for Disease Control and Prevention. Potential effects of electronic laboratory reporting on improving timeliness of infectious disease notification—Florida, 2002–2006. *MMWR Morb Mortal Wkly Rep* 2008;**57**:1325–1328.

37. Hamilton J, Eisenstein L. Impact of Electronic Laboratory Reporting on Immediately Reportable Conditions: Is Public Health Still Receiving Phone Calls from Laboratories? Council of State and Territorial Epidemiologists Annual Conference, Pasadena, CA, June 9–13, 2013. Available at https://cste.confex.com/cste/2013/webprogram/Paper2199.html (accessed November 25, 2013).

38. State of Florida Department of State. Florida Administrative Code section 64D-3. 2006. Available at https://www.flrules.org/gateway/ruleno.asp?id=64D-3.029 (accessed April 14, 2014).

CHAPTER 20

Use of geographic information systems in infectious disease surveillance

Rebecca J. Eisen[1] and Lars Eisen[2]

[1] Centers for Disease Control and Prevention, Fort Collins, CO, USA
[2] Colorado State University, Fort Collins, CO, USA

Introduction

Maps are important tools in infectious disease surveillance. They are commonly used to depict where infectious disease cases most frequently occur and also can be used to generate hypotheses about the causes underlying the spatial distribution of disease cases. In 1854, in what has been lauded as the dawn of epidemiology, John Snow prepared maps showing the locations of cholera cases in relation to public water sources in London, England. The clustering of cases around the Broad Street water pump implicated this particular pump as the source of the agent causing the cholera cases. Snow's maps were used to support his argument that cholera was a waterborne disease, which was in striking contrast to the prevailing thinking of the time that the disease (for which the etiological agent had not yet been identified) was caused by inhaling foul air [1].

Modern epidemiology seeks answers to the same type of questions as those addressed by John Snow: Where and when are infectious disease cases occurring, how are people exposed to the causative agents, where and when are the next cases likely to occur, and how can we best prevent future cases? Geographic information system (GIS) technology has greatly increased the speed and accuracy with which spatial information on infectious disease cases can be collected and integrated with other types of geographic information to track the spread of disease cases and clarify pathogen transmission dynamics. For example, GIS technology was used to map the westward spread of West Nile virus from New York, where it was introduced in 1999, to the West Coast of the United States where the virus had become widely established by 2004 [2] (Figure 20.1). This also resulted in timely delivery of up-to-date maps to the public by the Centers for Disease Control and Prevention (CDC) and the United States Geological Survey (USGS) through GIS-based map services that provide information for West Nile virus infection in humans, domestic animals, wild birds, and vector mosquitoes [3,4]. In addition, by combining environmental variables (e.g., temperature, precipitation, elevation, land cover) with epidemiological data for West Nile virus disease within a GIS, researchers have identified environmental correlates of areas with elevated disease risk and have projected where additional cases were most likely to occur [5]. In this chapter, we provide an overview of how GIS technology is used to address fundamental questions in infectious disease surveillance: where disease cases have occurred; how the causative agents are perpetuated; and how limited surveillance, prevention, and control resources should be targeted in

Concepts and Methods in Infectious Disease Surveillance, First Edition. Edited by Nkuchia M. M'ikanatha and John K. Iskander.
Published 2014 by John Wiley & Sons, Ltd.

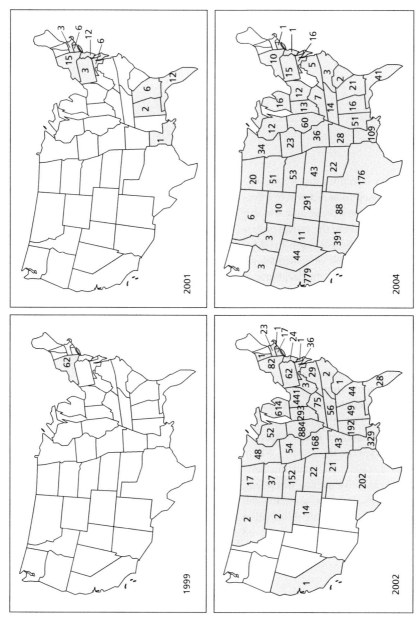

Figure 20.1 Distribution of human cases of West Nile virus disease in the continental United States, 1999–2004. Source: Adapted from http://www.cdc.gov/ncidod/dvbid/westnile/surv&control_archive.htm. Centers for Disease Control and Prevention.

space and over time to most effectively prevent future cases. We also address key challenges to the effective use of GIS in infectious disease surveillance.

An overview of geographic information system technology

A GIS is a computer-based, spatially explicit relational database with a graphical user interface that is designed to store and display spatial information and to integrate information from multiple sources for any given spatial extent [6]. A relational database is a database that is structured to join multiple pieces of information (in this case to a specific geographical location); a graphical user interface is a visual or graphical way of interacting with computer software; and spatial extent is the geographic domain encompassed by the data collection or model output. A GIS provides capacity to develop and display customized maps. Advanced GIS software typically also has extensive built-in capacity for spatial analyses. GIS technology is distinct from emerging, Internet-accessible mapping technologies, such as Google Earth, which provide access to images of the physical environment but where additional functionalities are limited to basic feature-making tools for map overlays. In a GIS, each piece of included information is captured as a data layer with associated attributes. For example, locations of disease cases, based on source location for the infection or the home address of the afflicted person, may be mapped using data obtained from global positioning system (GPS) receivers. The GPS-derived longitude and latitude of the disease case location provides a spatial reference for the case. Disease case points within such a disease case data layer can then be associated with, or overlaid upon, other spatially explicit data layers containing relevant information. Drawing upon the cholera example described above, one data layer within a GIS might contain point locations of cholera cases. Associated with this data layer, attributes such as age and sex of cases and outcome of infection may be recorded. Each cholera case point would then be displayed in relation to other data layers contained within the GIS, such as locations of water pumps, sewers, streets and houses. Each of these additional data layers might also contain relevant attribute data such as maintenance records for each pump or socioeconomic information for neighborhoods or individual households.

Spatial and temporal information (data layers and associated attributes) stored within a GIS provides a foundation for spatial and space–time analyses of infectious disease trends. Any of the data layers contained within a GIS can be displayed in map format, and spatially referenced information can be extracted from the GIS and used to perform statistical analyses (Figure 20.2). Some of the most commonly used data layers in infectious disease surveillance include (1) epidemiological data, (2) administrative boundaries (e.g., country, state, county), (3) locations of healthcare facilities, (4) socioeconomic data (e.g., census data), and (5) environmental data related to the disease of interest (e.g., locations of water sources for waterborne diseases, land-cover type and climatic variables for vectorborne diseases). Some of these data, especially those relating to the physical landscape (e.g., vegetation type, elevation, or locations of water bodies), can be obtained through the use of remote sensing technologies such as satellite imagery or aerial photography [7]. Data layers are provided through a wide variety of sources and range in cost of acquisition from free of charge to very expensive. Should critical information (e.g., different aspects of the infrastructure of developed areas, political boundaries) not already be available as a GIS data layer), it may be digitized by recording spatial coordinates from other sources, such as paper-based maps or surveys or Internet-accessible mapping technologies providing images of the physical environment.

Current uses of the geographic information system in infectious disease surveillance

After data are imported into a GIS, spatial information is used within the field of public health (1) to depict trends in disease cases in space and over time, (2) to coordinate a public health response to an outbreak, or (3) to identify spatial factors that are correlated with elevated risk for disease case occurrence and, thereafter, to extrapolate from this point-based information to develop a continuous risk map surface.

Depicting trends in space and over time
Tracking and mapping of trends of disease case occurrence or disease incidence in space and over time is a core activity in infectious disease surveillance. It allows

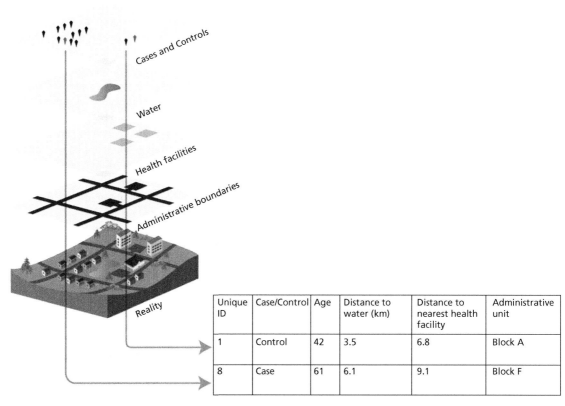

Unique ID	Case/Control	Age	Distance to water (km)	Distance to nearest health facility	Administrative unit
1	Control	42	3.5	6.8	Block A
8	Case	61	6.1	9.1	Block F

Figure 20.2 Combining different types of data in a GIS.

for targeting of surveillance and control resources to the areas and time periods where they have the greatest impact. The generated maps also can be used by individuals of the public to assess their personal risk for infection and to make informed decisions regarding the need for personal protective measures. Surveillance of vector-borne diseases also can be complemented by tracking of the arthropod vectors and the presence of the pathogen in these vectors (vectorborne pathogen surveillance). This is exemplified by the publication in 1998 of distributional maps for the primary tick vectors (*Ixodes scapularis* and *Ixodes pacificus*) of the causative agent of Lyme disease in the United States (the bacterium *Borrelia burgdorferi*) to help identify areas potentially presenting risk for infection and to assess the need for personal protection measures [8].

Rapid collection of standardized disease data is a key component of disease case tracking. To achieve this, in collaboration with state public health agencies, the United States Centers for Disease Control and Prevention has implemented a National Electronic Disease Surveillance System (NEDSS) for reportable diseases [9]. Furthermore, the recent emergence of mosquito-borne West Nile virus in North America resulted in new electronic surveillance systems for mosquito-borne arboviruses both in the United States [10] and Canada [11]. Importantly, the information for West Nile virus infections was made accessible to the public in map format (Figure 20.1) through a regularly updated website [10]. During the westward spread of the virus from 1999 to 2004 this provided critical and readily accessible information both for state and local public health entities regarding the need for setting up surveillance and control programs and for the public regarding the need for personal protection measures such as use of mosquito repellents.

The global effort to eradicate malaria also produced a major initiative to define the areas where malaria occurs and the intensity of local transmission of malaria para-sites in the Malaria Atlas Project [12]. The Malaria Atlas Project generates map-based information for a wide range of factors that can be used to inform continental or global malaria elimination or eradication strategies as well as determine the need for local malaria surveillance and control programs [13]. Key factors presented in map format include the spatial distributions of different human malaria parasites (*Plasmodium falciparum* and *Plasmodium vivax*) and their primary mosquito vectors (*Anopheles* species), the clinical burden of *Plasmodium falciparum* malaria in humans, and the *P. falciparum* basic reproductive number. (The basic reproductive number is the number of secondary infections arising from a focal infection, often referred to as R_0.)

Using spatial information to respond to outbreaks

Outbreaks, or epidemics, are defined as the occurrences of more cases of disease than expected in a given area or among a specific group of people over a particular period of time. Mapping and GIS technologies are being used increasingly to aid in emergency responses to infectious disease outbreaks. For example, access to geographic information including where disease cases have occurred in relation to the distribution of human populations and to transportation networks can greatly facilitate prevention and response activities. This was exemplified by a recent response to a poliomyelitis outbreak in the Democratic Republic of Congo (DRC) [14].

Polio, a debilitating viral disease that affects the nervous system and can lead to paralysis, is spread by direct contact between infectious and susceptible persons or through contact with infected mucus or feces [15]. By 2004, as a result of global vaccination efforts to eradicate polio, the DRC was free of polio cases. Then an outbreak occurred in 2006. In response, a massive vaccination campaign was launched to contain the spread of the poliovirus. The first phase of the vaccination campaign had little impact on containing the outbreak; and a more targeted approach (the "river strategy") was implemented after mapping of cases revealed a progression of spread along the Congo River. The river strategy sought to target vaccination efforts to populations neighboring the Congo River. In this part of the world where detailed maps of populations and transportation networks, including rivers and tributaries, are sparse and often outdated, integration of data from

satellite-derived imagery accessed through Google Earth into a GIS hastened efforts to dispatch the vaccines leading to a decline in cases in the targeted area [14].

In another example [16,17], GIS and spatial analysis played an integral role in the design of an oral rabies vaccine (ORV) distribution campaign. In the late fall of 2008, rabies, which is a viral infection that is spread primarily through bites delivered by infected animals, reappeared in foxes in the mountainous region of Italy after approximately a decade's absence. In response, authorities launched an ORV campaign designed to contain the outbreak. Given the timing of the outbreak in relation to the onset of winter and the sensitivity of the oral vaccine to freeze–thaw cycles, it was decided that the vaccine would be distributed only at elevations where temperatures would be conducive to the delivery of active vaccine (<1000 m for the winter and <1500 m for the spring). After unsuccessful attempts to manually distribute vaccine baits, a digital elevation model was used within a GIS to determine, based on elevation and topography, the optimal places for helicopters to distribute the ORV [16]. Rabies surveillance data collected subsequent to the initial vaccination effort were used to analyze spatial trends in the distribution of rabid foxes. The analysis indicated that initial efforts were effective at controlling the spread of rabies. However, case clusters were detected above 1500 m. These findings prompted officials to modify the summer vaccination campaign to include sites up to 2300 m elevation [17]. The spatial analysis had a significant impact on the efforts to control rabies because the results contradicted previous assumptions about the upper elevation thresholds for which ORV should be distributed within mountainous regions.

Identifying spatial risk factors and predicting and extrapolating spatial trends

The integration of spatial information on disease case occurrence into infectious disease surveillance systems (described above) has enabled the use of GIS and spatial analysis to identify risk factors for infectious diseases. Such spatial analyses can vary in scale from community-level to national, continental or even global spatial extents. As described below, the knowledge gained from spatial analyses is often scale dependent. Fine scale spatial analyses provide more explicit information on the underlying mechanisms of pathogen transmission compared with analyses performed at coarser scales, but development of fine-scale models is dependent on access to fine resolution epidemiological surveillance data. Recent GIS-based analyses of tuberculosis (TB) in Texas, USA [18], and cholera in Lusaka, Zambia [19], exemplify how access to fine-resolution epidemiological data and accurate fine-scale spatial data can be used to identify local risk factors for disease case occurrence. On the other hand, a fine scale model may not be accurate if attempts are made to apply it at coarser scales than the one at which it was developed [20].

TB is an airborne bacterial disease with a global distribution. Historically, increases in TB incidence have been associated with immigration, poverty, and unemployment [18]. Although mapping of TB incidence can reveal local hot spots, reporting of cases within socioeconomically or ethnically diverse city or county boundaries can obscure the ability to detect locally relevant risk factors. Within the Houston/Harris County area of Texas, TB cases were mapped to home address and census tract. Detailed information about the cases was obtained through surveys, and census-tract demographic data were obtained from the 2000 United States Census. The study identified significant clustering, with some neighborhoods showing higher case numbers than others. A geographically weighted regression analysis revealed that areas of elevated TB incidence were associated with poverty, age, race, foreign birth, and use of public transportation [18].

Similar to the Texas TB study, detailed data on the locations of households where cholera patients resided were available for Lusaka, Zambia [19]. Cases and matched controls were mapped within a GIS in relation to administrative boundaries and communal water point areas. From these data layers, detailed information was obtained regarding household demographics (e.g., size of household, monthly income), hygienic practices (e.g., hand washing, type of water storage, use of chlorination), and physical structure pertaining to waterborne transmission of the cholera-causing bacterium, *Vibrio cholera* (e.g., households with shallow wells, without latrine, without drainage). Subsequent spatial analyses revealed significant clustering of cases, which indicated that there were local environmental factors that facilitated transmission of the cholera bacterium. Specifically, cholera was more common in localities lacking latrines and drainage systems surrounding the homes. A matched case-control study revealed that chlorination of drinking water and hand washing

with soap played protective roles against infection [19]. Environmental factors associated with the locations of residences thus impacted the risk of exposure to the cholera agent, but human behavior also played an important role in determining whether or not infections occurred.

GIS-based approaches also have been used to identify specific areas within vast spatial extents, such as continental or global scales, where infectious disease cases are most likely to occur. This is especially useful for rare but severe diseases, particularly those for which pathogen transmission is associated with specific environmental, ecological or climatic conditions. Plague is a rare but potentially fatal disease caused by the bacterium *Yersinia pestis*, which is primarily spread through bites by infectious fleas or direct contact with infected animals. In the United States, 1–40 cases were reported annually in the western United States from 1971 to 1995 [21]. Mortality rates range from 50% to nearly 100% for untreated infections, but outcome of infection is improved by early diagnosis and appropriate antibiotic treatment [22,23]. The ability to predict when and where plague cases are most likely to occur can aid in targeting limited prevention and control resources.

Plague in the United States provides a best case scenario for spatial risk modeling. The epidemiological dataset is complete; and location of pathogen exposure, rather than simply location of residence, is geocoded to a fine spatial scale. Due to the severity of disease and mandatory reporting requirements, few if any cases are missing from the epidemiological surveillance records. All reported cases are laboratory confirmed, and cases are routinely investigated to determine the location of pathogen exposure. Furthermore, exposure locations are strongly associated with specific environmental and climatic conditions that are spatially referenced to an appropriate spatial scale [24]. Based on approximately 50 years of plague case data from the American Southwest, logistic regression modeling was used to identify environmental risk factors for plague; these included elevation and distance to key vegetation types. The model yielded an overall accuracy of approximately 82% and identified roughly 14% of the region to pose elevated risk for human exposure to the plague bacterium. The model also identified fine-scale heterogeneities in exposure risk that were previously obscured when data were reported as numbers of cases per county [25].

Integration of spatial information in geographic information system–based decision support systems

Decision support systems, augmented by the integration of a GIS software for map-based data visualization, are recent developments in infectious disease surveillance and control [26]. Stand-alone GIS software packages are well designed for use of existing data layers but often very cumbersome to use for entry of new data. This can be a problem for infectious disease surveillance and control programs, because they often deal with a wide range of continuously generated data, which need to be processed and analyzed in a timely manner to ensure the rapid implementation of needed control measures. A GIS-based decision support system can provide improved capacity for data entry, management, and analysis for the full range of relevant data for a specific disease or set of diseases, while still retaining the map-making benefits of the integrated GIS software.

Privacy concerns, spatial scale issues, and data quality challenges

There are ethical concerns related to the use of GIS in infectious disease surveillance. In the United States, due to privacy issues [27,28], maps showing specific locations of pathogen exposure sites or residences of humans afflicted with an infectious disease typically are not generated. One potential approach to protection of the privacy of disease case patients is to display a map with random offsets from the actual point locations, but this essentially means that an inaccurate disease case location map is presented. The most commonly used solution is to generate maps that show number of disease cases or disease incidence for spatially coarse administrative boundary units such as a state or county and, thus, ensure patient privacy. However, this may fail to account for fine-scale variability in risk patterns within these coarse administrative boundaries, as demonstrated for West Nile virus disease in Colorado where county, compared to the smaller census tract unit, was found to account for only 50% of the overall variance in West Nile virus disease incidence, and for 33% for the subset of cases classified as West Nile neuroinvasive disease [29].

Another concern with the practice of aggregating disease case counts or disease incidence to administrative boundaries is the modifiable areal unit problem, which occurs when numerical results vary when the same set of data is grouped at different levels of spatial resolution. This raises the question of which boundary unit best captures the variability of spatial infectious disease data without compromising data quality [30,31]. Spatial scale also can be a concern in GIS-based modeling if the scale of the available data layer for the dependent epidemiological variable being modeled (e.g., point locations for pathogen exposure) is dramatically different from the scale for available data layers for the independent predictor variables included to explain the distribution of disease cases (e.g., environmental factors extracted from data layers with grid sizes of several kilometers). This is especially important to consider in environmentally or climatically highly heterogeneous areas.

Perhaps the most important thing to remember when embarking on a mapping or modeling project is that the map or model outputs are only as good as the data upon which they were based. Epidemiological data have several potential weaknesses. Not all infectious diseases are notifiable, and case definitions and reporting practices for those that are notifiable may vary between different areas and also change over time. Lack of resources for laboratory confirmation of clinically diagnosed illnesses can be a major problem in areas with limited resources. Furthermore, some agents of infectious diseases, such as the mosquito-borne viruses causing dengue and West Nile virus disease, commonly result in mild or asymptomatic infections which are not captured through passive surveillance systems. Finally, the pathogen exposure location may differ from the residence of the afflicted person but not be known because no effort was made to determine where the infection occurred. These and other potential problems need to be considered when generating and displaying maps for infectious diseases, so that the maps can be accompanied with text noting the relevant caveats.

For the purpose of spatial modeling of infectious diseases, the quality of data for predictor variables also is critically important. Spatial risk models for infectious diseases have been based on associations with socioeconomic conditions or environmental factors such as elevation, soil type, vegetation type, land cover, and climatic or meteorological variables. The quality of existing data layers is generally high in the developed world; but, unfortunately, critical data layers for predictive modeling are often lacking or of poor quality in developing regions where the morbidity and mortality from infectious diseases is greatest and most disruptive to social and economic progress. Specific problems include poor quality data layers for societal infrastructure (e.g., roads, housing, health facilities), the challenge of acquiring cloud-free satellite imagery in the tropics, and the need for an enhanced meteorological observation network in developing countries to produce better GIS-based climate data. It also should be noted that data layers require updating to maintain their quality (e.g., updating of infrastructure data for rapidly growing population centers).

Case study

Plague in Uganda

Plague in Uganda was selected as a case study because the data quality challenges faced here are representative of other vector-borne diseases in developing countries. In general, the spatial distribution of vector-borne disease cases is often strongly correlated with environmental or climatic predictors, which impact the arthropod vectors or vertebrate reservoir hosts of the pathogen in question. Thus, access to data for environmental or climatic variables can aid in the prediction of spatial and temporal trends of disease case occurrence [32]. These predictions can then aid in targeting limited surveillance, prevention, and control resources. This is especially important in the developing world, because per-capita morbidity, mortality, and economic burden of infectious diseases is greatest in parts of the world where the least amount of accurate and appropriately scaled environmental and meteorological data are available, namely, tropical and subtropical regions including sub-Saharan Africa and Southeast Asia [33,34]. This case study highlights how improvements to epidemiological surveillance, access to remotely sensed environmental data, and modeling of climate data aid in the development of spatial risk models for plague in Uganda. A previous publication compared and contrasted plague modeling efforts between North America and Uganda [35].

Plague claimed the lives of millions during three historical human pandemics [36]. Improvements in sanitation have limited the scale of epidemics to focal outbreaks, and advances in diagnostics coupled with access to antibiotic therapy have reduced mortality rates [37]. However, due to the rapid progression of the disease, outcome of infection is greatly improved by early detection and treatment [23]. Plague has a worldwide distribution; but in recent decades, the majority of cases and the greatest plague-attributable mortality have been reported from East Africa and Madagascar [37]. Within these geographic regions, plague is restricted to foci where ecological and climatic conditions are conducive for persistence of *Y. pestis*. However, in many instances, adequate surveillance for the disease is lacking, resulting in a coarse delineation of the spatial distribution and temporal occurrence of disease cases.

Within the West Nile region of Uganda, which is located in the northwestern corner of the country bordering the DRC (Figure 20.3), an average of 199 suspected plague cases per year were reported by the Ugandan Ministry of Health from 1999 to 2007. An epidemiological database that identified case patients to their village of residence was developed based on a review of health records from a total of 31 health facilities in the West Nile region [38]. Prior to 2008, diagnosis was based on clinical presentation. Beginning in 2008, clinical samples were collected from suspected case patients and confirmed using standard laboratory diagnostics. The locations of households of confirmed cases were then mapped using GPS receivers [39].

Statistical modeling within a GIS framework was used to identify when and where humans were at greatest risk of exposure to *Y. pestis* [38,39]. The first attempt to model the spatial distribution of plague cases and to identify landscape level risk factors for case occurrence focused on suspected plague cases reported to the parish spatial scale. A parish represents the smallest administrative boundary that was geocoded for the area and encompasses numerous households and villages and often is ecologically highly diverse. Although clinics reported the village of residence of plague cases, geographic extents of villages had not been mapped. Due to a paucity of georeferenced data for this area, input variables for the initial spatial analysis were limited to a digital elevation model and single-scene satellite images from which indices of soil, vegetation, and wetness were derived. Nonetheless, the model accurately classified parishes by incidence (overall accuracy of 74%) and identified parishes where cases may be underreported and where enhanced surveillance and

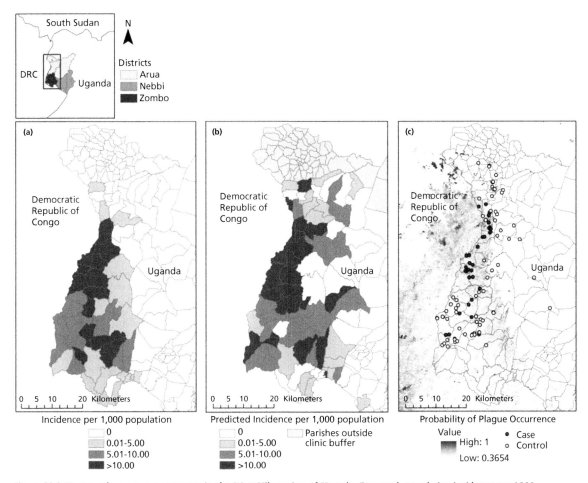

Figure 20.3 Human plague case occurrence in the West Nile region of Uganda. Reported cumulative incidence per 1000 population (1997–2007) by parish [38]. (A) Model prediction of parishes characterized as elevated risk [38]. (B) Subparish-level model of areas predicted to pose an elevated risk of exposure to *Y. pestis* [39]. (C) Location of the area of interest is shown as an inset. Source: Reproduced with permission of The American Journal of Tropical Medicine and Hygiene [38].

prevention measures could be implemented (Figure 20.3). Furthermore, it identified several landscape level risk factors for plague, including elevation, and remotely sensed indices of soil and vegetation that were likely indicative of growth of annual crops.

The greatest drawbacks of the parish-level model were: (1) It did not reveal spatial heterogeneities within parishes, making it difficult to allocate resources to villages at greatest risk; and (2) because population data per administrative boundary was needed to extrapolate the incidence-based model and such information was lacking from neighboring regions of the DRC, spatial extrapolation was not possible. A second model was

developed subsequently using laboratory-confirmed cases that were geocoded to the location of residence, rather than only the parish of residence [39]. Controls were selected based on similar access to health care. Although similar predictive variables were included in this second model, overall accuracy of the model was improved (overall accuracy of 81%), spatial heterogeneities in risk were revealed within parish boundaries, and the model was extrapolated to an area of the neighboring DRC with similar environmental and climatic conditions (Figure 20.3). The spatial extrapolation showed the West Nile region to represent the eastern edge of the plague focus with areas of elevated risk also within the DRC to the west, where civil unrest has prevented consistent surveillance activities.

Although it is well documented that the spatial distribution of plague cases is often correlated with climatic conditions [32], lack of accurate and appropriately scaled climatic data prevented their use as predictive variables. Recently, a dynamically downscaled climate model was created for the West Nile region and was made available as a GIS layer [40]. When the point-based model that had been developed using laboratory-confirmed cases was reconstructed with the inclusion of climate data, the overall accuracy of the model was improved (overall accuracy of 94%); and the climate variables provided a better fit to the data than the satellite-derived variables which, although they included estimates of moisture, represented a temporal snapshot of the environmental wetness [41]. Improving the quality of both the epidemiological data and also of the environmental data associated with the underlying pathogen transmission dynamics thus were needed to improve the quality of the risk assessment model.

Summary points

- Advances in mapping and GIS technologies provide new opportunities for surveillance and control of infectious diseases.
- GIS-based risk modeling has proven an effective tool to develop risk surfaces (maps) to inform policy makers, control programs, and the public.
- Spatial modeling results are often scale-dependent.
- Perhaps the most important thing to remember when embarking on a mapping or modeling project is that map or model outputs are only as good as the data upon which they are based.

STUDY QUESTIONS

1. How can GIS enhance infectious disease surveillance?
2. What are the main obstacles to use of GIS in infectious disease surveillance?
3. What do spatial models add to simply mapping disease case locations?
4. Why is it important to determine pathogen exposure locations?

References

1. Koch T, Denike K. Essential, illustrative, or…just propaganda? Rethinking John Snow's Broad Stree map. *Cartographica* 2010;**45**:19–31.
2. Kramer LD, Styer LM, Ebel GD. A global perspective on the epidemiology of West Nile virus. *Annu Rev Entomol* 2008;**53**: 61–81.
3. Centers for Disease Control and Prevention. West Nile Virus data and maps. Available at http://www.cdc.gov/ncidod/dvbid/westnile/index.htm (accessed March 19, 2012).
4. United States Geological Survey. West Nile Virus historical. Available at http://diseasemaps.usgs.gov/wnv_historical .html (accessed March 19, 2012).
5. Winters AM, Bolling BG, Beaty BJ, et al. Combining mosquito vector and human disease data for improved assessment of spatial west nile virus disease risk. *Am J Trop Med Hyg* 2008;**78**(4):654–665.
6. Cromley EK, McLafferty SL. *GIS and Public Health*. New York: The Guilford Press; 2002.
7. Jensen JR. *Remote Sensing of the Environment: An Earth Resource Perspective*, 2nd ed. Upper Saddle River, NJ: Pearson Prentice Hall; 2007.
8. Dennis DT, Nekomoto TS, Victor JC, et al. 1998. Reported distribution of *Ixodes scapularis* and *Ixodes pacificus* (Acari: Ixodidae) in the United States. *J Med Entomol* 1998;**35**: 629–638.
9. Centers for Disease Control and Prevention. National Electronic Disease Surveillance System. Available at http://www.cdc.gov/phin/tools/NEDSS/ (accessed March 19, 2012).
10. Centers for Disease Control and Prevention. Arbonet maps. Available at http://www.cdc.gov/ncidod/dvbid/westnile/USGS_frame.html (accessed March 19, 2012).
11. Gosselin P, Lebel G, Rivest S, Douville-Fradet M. The Integrated System for Public Health Monitoring of West Nile Virus (ISPHM-WNV): A real-time GIS for surveillance and decision-making. *Int J Health Geogr* 2005;**4**:21.
12. Hay SI, Snow RW. The malaria Atlas Project: Developing global maps of malaria risk. *PLoS Med* 2006;**3**(12):e473.
13. Malaria Atlas Project. MAP. Available at http://www.map.ox.ac.uk/ (accessed March 19, 2012).
14. Kamadjeu R. Tracking the polio virus down the Congo River: a case study on the use of Google Earth in public health planning and mapping. *Int J Health Geogr* 2009;**8**:4.
15. Modlin JF. Poliovirus. In: Mandell GL, Bennett JE, Dolin R, eds. *Principles and Practice of Infectious Diseases*. Philadelphia: Elsevier Churchill Livingstone; 2009:2345–2352.
16. Mulatti P, Ferre N, Patregnani T, Bonfanti L, Marangon S. Geographical information systems in the management of the 2009–2010 emergency oral anti-rabies vaccination of foxes in north-eastern Italy. *Geospat Health* 2011;**5**(2): 217–226.

17. Mulatti P, Muller T, Bonfanti L, Marangon S. Emergency oral rabies vaccination of foxes in Italy in 2009–2010: Identification of residual rabies foci at higher altitudes in the Alps. *Epidemiol Infect* 2011 Jul 11;**140**:1–8.

18. Feske ML, Teeter LD, Musser JM, Graviss EA. Including the third dimension: A spatial analysis of TB cases in Houston Harris County. *Tuberculosis (Edinb)* 2011;**91**(Suppl 1): S24–S33.

19. Sasaki S, Suzuki H, Igarashi K, Tambatamba B, Mulenga P. Spatial analysis of risk factor of cholera outbreak for 2003–2004 in a peri-urban area of Lusaka, Zambia. *Am J Trop Med Hyg* 2008;**79**(3):414–421.

20. Winters AM, Eisen RJ, Lozano-Fuentes S, Moore CG, Pape WJ, Eisen L. Predictive spatial models for risk of West Nile virus exposure in eastern and western Colorado. *Am J Trop Med Hyg* 2008;**79**(4):581–590.

21. Centers for Disease Control and Prevention. Plague fact sheet. Available at http://www.cdc.gov/ncidod/dvbid/plague/facts.htm (accessed March 19, 2012).

22. MMWR. Human plague-four states, 2006. *MMWR Morb Mortal Wkly Rep* 2006;**55**:1–3.

23. Poland JD, Barnes AM. Plague. In: Steele JH, ed. *CRC Handbook Series in Zoonoses Section A: Bacterial, Rickettsial and Mycotic Diseases*, Vol. I. Boca Raton, FL: CRC Press Inc.; 1979:515–559.

24. Eisen RJ, Enscore RE, Biggerstaff BJ, et al. Human plague in the southwestern United States, 1957–2004: Spatial models of elevated risk of human exposure to *Yersinia pestis*. *J Med Entomol* 2007;**44**(3):530–537.

25. Eisen L, Eisen RJ. Using geographic information systems and decision support systems for the prediction, prevention, and control of vector-borne diseases. *Annu Rev Entomol* 2011;**56**:41–61.

26. Lozano-Fuentes S, Barker CM, Coleman M, et al. Emerging information technologies to provide improved decision support for surveillance, prevention, and control of vector-borne diseases. In: Jao C, ed. *Efficient Decision Support Systems—Practice and Challenges in Biomedical Related Domain.* Rijeka, Croatia: InTech—Open Access Publisher; 2011: 89–114.

27. VanWey LK, Rindfuss RR, Gutmann MP, Entwisle B, Balk DL. Confidentiality and spatially explicit data: Concerns and challenges. *Proc Natl Acad Sci U S A* 2005;**102**(43):15337–15342.

28. 104th Congress. Health insurance portability and accountability act of 1996. Available at http://www.cms.hhs.gov/HIPAAGenInfo/Downloads/HIPAALaw.pdf (accessed March 19, 2012).

29. Winters AM, Eisen RJ, Delorey MJ, et al. Spatial risk assessments based on vector-borne disease epidemiologic data: Importance of scale for West Nile virus disease in Colorado. *Am J Trop Med Hyg* 2010;**82**(5):945–953.

30. Openshaw S. *The Modifiable Areal Unit Problem*. Norwich, UK: Geo Books; 1984.

31. Rytkonen MJP. Not all maps are equal: GIS and spatial analysis in epidemiology. *Int J Circumpolar Health* 2004;**63**: 9–24.

32. Gage KL, Burkot TR, Eisen RJ, Hayes EB. Climate and vectorborne diseases. *Am J Prev Med* 2008;**35**(5):436–450.

33. Gubler DJ. Resurgent vector-borne diseases as a global health problem. *Emerg Infect Dis* 1998;**4**(3):442–450.

34. Murray CJL, Lopez AD. Mortality by cause for eight regions of the world: Global Burden of Disease Study. *Lancet* 1997;**349**(9061):1269–1276.

35. Mak S, Eisen RJ. Use of GIS and spatial analysis in infectious disease surveillance in North America and East Africa: A case study. In: Mikanatha NM, Lynfield R, Van Beneden CA, de Valk H, eds. *Infectious Disease Surveillance*. Oxford: Wiley-Blackwell; 2014:558–564.

36. Gage KL, Kosoy MY. Natural history of plague: Perspectives from more than a century of research. *Annu Rev Entomol* 2005;**50**:505–528.

37. Tikhomirov E. Epidemiology and distribution of plague. In: Dennis DT, Gage KL, Gratz N, Poland JD, Tikhomirov E, eds. *Plague Manual: Epidemiology, Distribution, Surveillance and Control*. Geneva: World Health Organization; 1999: 11–37.

38. Winters AM, Staples JE, Ogen-Odoi A, et al. Spatial risk models for human plague in the West Nile Region of Uganda. *Am J Trop Med Hyg* 2009;**80**(6):1014–1022.

39. Eisen RJ, Griffith KS, Borchert JN, et al. Assessing human risk of exposure to plague bacteria in northwestern Uganda based on remotely sensed predictors. *Am J Trop Med Hyg* 2010;**82**(5):904–911.

40. Monaghan AJ, MacMillan K, Moore SM, Mead PS, Hayden MH, Eisen RJ. A regional climatography to support human plague modeling in West Nile, Uganda. *J Appl Meteorol Climatol* 2012;**51**:1201–1221.

41. MacMillan K, Monaghan AJ, Apangu T, et al. Climate predictors of the spatial distribution of human plague cases in the West Nile region of Uganda. *Am J Trop Med Hyg* 2012; **86**(3):514–523.

SECTION IV

Cross-cutting issues in
infectious disease surveillance

CHAPTER 21

Communication of surveillance findings

Brian G. Southwell[1] and Bridget J. Kelly[2]

[1] RTI International, Research Triangle Park, NC, USA
[2] RTI International, Washington, DC, USA

Introduction

In a survey of U.S. residents at the start of the 2009 H1N1 flu pandemic, 55% of respondents had never heard the term "H1N1 virus" and only 20% thought the term meant the same thing as swine flu. Despite a large volume of media coverage related to how the disease was transmitted, 29% mistakenly reported that they could get the virus from someone standing 30 feet away and 13% incorrectly answered that they could contract the virus by eating pork [1]. While infectious disease professionals undoubtedly were inundated with daily news about the emergent disease, there was a substantial amount of misinformation circulating among the public.

Such an example highlights the importance of clear and effective communication about infectious disease during times of outbreak, in order to correct misinformation and disseminate accurate facts about how to slow transmission. In 2005, the World Health Organization (WHO) declared, "It is now time to acknowledge that communication expertise has become as essential to outbreak control as epidemiological training and laboratory analysis" [2]. The utility of communication expertise extends beyond just outbreak control to infectious disease surveillance more broadly, as communication planning should begin during periods when there is no crisis.

While communication of information appears to be crucial in coping with communicable disease, many public health officials are insufficiently trained to plan, conduct, and evaluate communication efforts. The primary objective of this chapter is to describe ways that current and future public health professionals can successfully engage media organizations as partners, use media technologies as tools, and involve laypeople as an audience and as collaborators. Rather than focusing exclusively on the work of public health professionals, however, we will take a broader approach, also emphasizing the larger information environment and the ways in which public health officials fit into that environment. We will illustrate concepts in this chapter with three distinct groups: public health professionals, mass media professionals, and lay audiences. Once we begin to understand the interactions of these three groups, it will become evident that infectious disease communication can succeed or fail on many different planes. To promote future success and minimize failure, we will highlight lessons learned from past efforts and provide some practical guidelines for effective communication.

Three essential partners: public health professionals, the mass media, and lay audiences

Public health professionals

Whether operating at the local, state or federal level, public health professionals are faced with a number of constraints and challenges that can hinder communication efforts. Some of these might be obvious in an era of government budget cuts: Decreased budgets or lack

Concepts and Methods in Infectious Disease Surveillance, First Edition. Edited by Nkuchia M. M'ikanatha and John K. Iskander.
© 2015 John Wiley & Sons, Ltd. Published 2015 by John Wiley & Sons, Ltd.

Table 21.1 World Health Organization Outbreak Communication Guidelines.

In 2005, the World Health Organization introduced guidelines for outbreak communication. They emphasized five areas for consideration, as follows:	
Trust	The overriding goal for outbreak communication is to communicate with the public in ways that build, maintain, or restore trust. This is true across cultures, political systems, and level of country development.
Early announcement	The parameters of trust are established in the outbreak's first official announcement. This message's timing, candor, and comprehensiveness may make it the most important of all outbreak communication efforts.
Transparency	Maintaining the public's trust throughout an outbreak requires transparency (i.e., communication that is candid, easily understood, complete, and factually accurate).
The public	Understanding the public is critical to effective communication. It is usually difficult to change pre-existing beliefs unless those beliefs are explicitly addressed, and it is nearly impossible to design successful messages that bridge the gap between the expert and the public without knowing what the public thinks.
Planning	There is risk communication impact in everything outbreak control managers do, not just in what is said. Risk communication should be incorporated into preparedness planning for major events and in all aspects of an outbreak response.

Source: Adapted from the World Health Organization Outbreak Communication Guidelines.

of staffing resources limit the ability of many programs to employ staff whose main purpose is to oversee communication efforts. Other challenges are more subtle. One obstacle faced by disease surveillance staff involves the elusive nature of trust among populations served by public health workers. Trust and credibility are essential factors in communication about risk; without trust between audiences and officials, no amount of encouragement to heed official announcements likely will be very successful [3]. Trust, in fact, is one of five key areas for consideration that are highlighted in the WHO's guidelines for outbreak communication (see Table 21.1). However, several trends in public perceptions currently pose major hurdles, as confidence in government, traditional social institutions, and industry has eroded in the United States and elsewhere in recent decades, because of factors like conflicting information and political infighting [4,5].

So how might trust be restored? We know that perceptions of empathy and caring, competence, commitment, and accountability on the part of message sources contribute to trust [6,7]. Note that sheer expertise is only part of this list of factors. Having access to credible information does not guarantee optimal trust among lay laypeople. Because many people have viewed public health institutions negatively at various points in recent history [8], it is especially important for such organizations to defy negative stereotypes by providing transpar-

ency and balanced information in a consistent and timely way.

Solidifying and building trust can be especially important *before* an outbreak unfolds, or as it is unfolding. Quinn et al. [9] have argued that pre-existing trust (or mistrust) in institutions may be especially important during unprecedented or unfamiliar events. For example, inconsistent messages from government officials and faulty information in the past contributed to widespread mistrust during the 2001 anthrax attack. As Reynolds and Seeger succinctly note, "Organizations that fail to develop credible, trusting relationships prior to a crisis will have an exceptionally difficult time doing so after a [disease outbreak] occurs" [3].

A related challenge, inherent to the field of infectious disease surveillance, is the difficulty posed by uncertainty. In any disease epidemic, there is some degree of uncertainty. At the beginning of an outbreak, we may not know exactly which populations are most at risk, the potential severity of the epidemic, or the odds of mutation to a more virulent strain, for example. It is important to be explicit about the sources and dimensions of such uncertainty rather than to hide such information. Consider the example in which a reporter poses the question of how many people are infected with an emerging illness. One might be tempted to answer, "We cannot answer that question." But think about the implications of that response compared to this one : "We are not certain at this point because we are awaiting test results to confirm some probable cases. We expect to have better estimates of the number of people who have been infected in a few days." When you don't have the answer, try to describe the process (e.g., the laboratory tests take up to 2 days because ...). Being explicit about the reasons for any uncertainty and when such uncertainty may be resolved can help to bolster confidence in an agency or spokesperson's expertise and authority.

Another aspect of the life of public health workers relevant to our discussion is the dynamic (rather than static) nature of the information available during an outbreak. Recommendations have a tendency to evolve. Failure of public health professionals to prepare reporters or laypeople for such changes can result in loss of credibility as advice or estimates change midstream. In contrast, transparency about why a recommendation is changing (e.g., new information has come to light that suggests case numbers are higher than expected because some states submitted revised reports) can help prevent the perception that public health officials made a mistake or are simply indecisive.

In the last few years, the proliferation of digital and social media has made the timeliness of communication more important than ever before. Consider the case of a meningococcal outbreak in a school in the United Kingdom in 2010 [10]. On a Friday evening, two cases of the disease were identified. The following Monday, letters were issued to all students and parents. In the meantime, over the weekend, most parents had already found out about the outbreak through phone conversations, online instant messaging, or text messaging. Those who attempted to contact the school said they did not receive much information. Many students did not want to attend school on Monday for fear of catching the disease [10]. Results of qualitative research suggest that rumors circulating over the weekend caused confusion and anxiety that may have been alleviated through earlier communication by health officials or school administrators. For example, a message could have been sent to all parents via email or automated telephone message. As outlined in Box 21.1, early communication is crucial to alleviating unwarranted fears about disease outbreaks. Much as we have seen in other arenas, rumors thrive when a trickle of sensational news is followed by a vacuum of official response [11,12]. Chapter 3 provides details on surveil-

---

Box 21.1 Practical recommendations for public health officials on infectious disease outbreaks.

- Communicate early and often to prevent rumors from running rampant before the facts are explained.
- Acknowledge uncertainty, and be explicit about the reasons for it. When possible, provide a timeframe for when answers or updates may be available.
- Express empathy for fears or concerns. A simple statement such as, "We recognize that this situation is frightening," can go a long way to earning trust.

---

lance systems at national, state, and local levels, and Chapter 15 describes approaches used to conduct infectious surveillance globally.

Mass media organizations and professionals

Public health officials are routinely engaged with media professionals, but there has been no shortage in recent years of critique, commentary, and complaint about media coverage of health [13–15]. Media coverage of the controversy regarding the measles, mumps, rubella (MMR) vaccine, sparked by a study that has now been retracted and deemed fraudulent [13,16], discouraged parents from obtaining the vaccine for their children and contributed to a documented decline in vaccine uptake [13].

Some public health organizations nonetheless have actively embraced the opportunity to work with media outlets. The National Public Health Information Coalition, for example, serves as a support network for public information specialists in health agencies and annually recognizes excellence in interactions between public health professionals and media organizations. In 2011, the North Dakota Department of Health was awarded for its breaking news release regarding the first measles case in that state since 1987. The Virgin Islands Department of Health received recognition for its Dengue Fever outbreak campaign [17].

Defining "mass media" increasingly offers a challenge, however; we are no longer in an era when media channels are limited to television, radio, film, and printed material. The emergence of digital technology has changed that, offering an array of content platforms and devices. We now have information delivered to our mobile phones and streamed to our Internet-capable televisions. Moreover, the typical content contributor also has evolved; instead of reading well-researched investigative work by a health reporter at a large metropolitan newspaper, many people now encounter the work of freelance bloggers and other members of the public who post their thoughts. For our purposes, then, we can consider mass media to be those information technologies and forums that draw large and heterogeneous groups of people. Despite these changes, news media organizations and journalism professionals still need to be central to our discussion. Theoretically, such media outlets offer an efficient way of contacting mass audiences with crucial warnings and recommendations. People still frequently name mass media as a prevalent source of information about health and science [18,19].

However, there are challenges to accurate reporting of infectious disease information. Schwitzer [14] has assessed television news coverage of health and noted a number of tendencies that he found troubling, including a disturbing lack of data to back up sensational claims, use of hyperbole, reliance on single sources for stories, and brevity in stories that deserve a longer format. He notes a scarcity of full-time health journalists working at television news departments and points out the lack of primary investigation by local journalists (as opposed to simply repackaging information from wire services or press releases). While television news is often cited as a particularly striking example, critics have raised similar complaints about news organizations across the array of mass media. For example, data from the Pew Research Center suggests that because of a shortage of resources in the last several years, fewer newspapers are tailoring national stories to their local communities [20].

Health and science news professionals are constrained by at least four primary factors: source availability, the need to portray a story's newsworthiness, the difficulty of communicating science to the public, and the need to demonstrate a balance in perspectives with particular incentive to present conflicting or opposing views [21]. All of these factors are useful to consider in preparing to work with journalists. Designating official media contacts in public health agencies and making them as accessible as possible, for example, can address the issue of source availability, making the lives of journalists easier and also helping to ensure reporting of key mes-

Box 21.2 Practical guidelines for working with media professionals.

- Respect journalists' deadlines. If you want to see your story in tomorrow's paper, you have to give them enough time to write it. If you know when those deadlines are and can release statements accordingly, working with the media will be a much more rewarding experience.
- Understand the importance of newsworthiness. Journalists will not cover this year's seasonal flu just because you want them to. The story has to have a new impact or relevance to their readership/audience (e.g., is it affecting a new or different age group more seriously? Is the flu vaccine recommended for a new group of people this year?).
- Consider formal media training. This service, which may be available through internal or external training sources, can help you, as a spokesperson, deliver your message in a way that is more likely to resonate with your audience.
- Try to frame new studies in the context of broader information. If this is the first study to find a link between an exposure and a disease where many others have found no association, be sure to point out the large body of previous literature.

sages that are consistent with health-agency goals. Sometimes this contact will not be an infectious disease subject matter expert, but a designated public information officer. (See Box 21.2 for a summary of practical guidance for working with media professionals.)

The need for newsworthiness is perhaps the force affecting news coverage of health that is least appreciated by public health officials. Routine disease surveillance is not necessarily newsworthy. However, outbreaks—particularly those that are more severe—are. News organizations see their main job as production of a regularly updated window onto current events. That window reflects recent events, not necessarily long-term trends, and tends to highlight people, events, and ideas that are already well-known. A single celebrity being diagnosed with a disease is often more likely to generate front page coverage than 100 people contracting the disease every year. Consider the classic example of Magic Johnson's infection with HIV.

Research suggests his announcement of his HIV status in 1991 increased awareness, as well as increasing the number of persons getting tested for HIV and the desire to obtain more information about HIV and AIDS [22]. Much of the explanation for the coverage that ensued lies in Johnson's celebrity status, as much as the importance of the public health story.

One factor that affects a topic's longevity (or ability to maintain its newsworthiness) is the ephemeral nature of news, stemming from the emergence of a 24-hour news cycle in which the sheer abundance of new stories limits the ability of any particular story to get sustained attention. In 2003, severe acute respiratory syndrome (SARS) emerged in south China and other parts of the world. Intense and sustained mass media coverage followed for several months. Stories focused on various aspects of the phenomenon beyond epidemiology, including the potential economic impact and the controversial interventions by some governments around the world such as China's decision to slaughter civet cats or that country's initial suppression of information about the disease, which slowed WHO's investigation [23]. For a short period, any new information about SARS was newsworthy, in part because there had been so much recent coverage of the disease. Following the drop in new cases that year, however, much discussion of the disease—and, importantly, discussion of what to do about it—also disappeared. Scientists hoping to focus public debate on infectious disease had to wait until a new syndrome emerged on the nightly news.

A third constraint is the difficulty of translating scientific information—and specifically, information related to infectious disease, which is often inherently complex—to the public. Most health and medical reporters have little or no formal education in medical terminology or related topic areas and have learned what they know about health on the job. As a result, it is not surprising that they sometimes get the facts wrong.

Reporters' emphasis on providing more than one viewpoint, while ostensibly a useful ideal, is often problematic in the realm of public health, where sometimes there are either many more than two sides to a story or where there are two sides that are not equally deserving of coverage. The aforementioned controversy regarding the MMR vaccine is a good example. While some might argue that coverage of original research that linked

vaccine use with the development of autism was justified, the subsequent accumulation of evidence against that claim suggests that perhaps the more appropriate approach would have been to report a broader view of the topic, rather than to focus on a single study. Some would argue that by simply reporting the controversy, without framing it in a broader context, the perceptual damage was done; and the unintended consequence of suppressing vaccine uptake, even in the face of other evidence of its safety, was set in motion.

Journalists are not the only media professionals with an opportunity to present information on disease. In addition to formal news outlets, entertainment programming also routinely portrays information relevant to infectious disease. Television programs such as *ER*, *Grey's Anatomy*, and *Private Practice* in the United States have emphasized the importance of relevant behaviors such as safe sex practice, hand washing and immunization. Public health officials cannot necessarily rely on such a strategy as a means of promoting particular messages, though, as there are serious limitations with this approach. Entertainment producers often look for even more dramatic and arousing fare than do reporters, writers for such programs may have a limited understanding of scientific research, and the programming available may be intended for an audience that differs from the target group. Perhaps most importantly, the lead time necessary to incorporate relevant information into a movie, television show, or popular song probably rules out this approach for emerging disease situations in which information must be presented quickly. What is probably more useful is for public health professionals instead to monitor entertainment programming and to assess how infectious disease is framed and presented. Many laypeople understand the difference between entertainment programming and news and will likely recognize that a story regarding a specific infectious disease may be overdramatized and not entirely realistic or representative. Nonetheless, general awareness of what is currently circulating in the information environment can be helpful.

In addition to news media and entertainment programming, the proliferation of digital and social media has revolutionized surveillance and public health communication in the last several years. Text messaging (i.e., using a short message service [SMS] or texting) is a promising tool for infectious disease surveillance in international settings [24], allowing public health offi-cials to collect data from remote areas very quickly. It is also possible to mine data from user-generated sites or even search engines to identify clusters of disease. Google.org Flu Trends has had promising results, detect-ing regional outbreaks 7–10 days earlier than traditional surveillance systems [25]. There is evidence that rapid dissemination of prevention information via text mes-saging has also helped to mitigate the effects of some disease outbreaks [26]. Despite the promise of these new tools, there are some features specific to social media that must be considered, lest they create chal-lenges for effective communication.

Unlike their print and broadcast media counterparts, digital and social media offer opportunities for two-way communication. While the ability to communicate directly with the target audience can be appealing, it is important to consider whether the option is realistic, as it requires having the resources to handle real-time responses to potentially very large numbers of people. In addition, the user-generated nature of sources like YouTube and Facebook means that messages can be altered or edited before they are forwarded to others; and, thus, public health officials must be willing to relinquish control of the content to some degree. While the same could be said of professional news media, the role of fact-checkers, editors, and producers as gate-keepers provides some insurance about accuracy.

Lay audiences

People do not uniformly engage, retain, or act upon all the information they encounter. In other words, people are imperfect communication partners who do not always receive the exact messages that are presented to them [27]. Sometimes, people simply do not under-stand what we are trying to tell them. Sometimes, the information people need in order to act does not match the information that is provided, which means that simply repeating the message will not achieve any addi-tional behavioral compliance. Factors including scien-tific and health literacy, as well as emotions, can be barriers to effective message processing.

Consider the public health communication challenges presented by the 2005 earthquake in Kashmir. Health workers needed to promote basic sanitation messages; and yet, because of the state of the infrastructure, finding an appropriate way to frame that message was difficult. Many residents of these areas were trauma-tized and in such physically demanding situations that what they needed most was practical information as to how exactly they *could* comply. How could they keep their hands clean if clean water was not available? Rather than focusing on dramatic persuasion efforts, investing in getting instructional guides into everyone's hands might have been a useful approach.

A variety of factors influence audience engagement with information and intention to act on that informa-tion. Any successful attempt to persuade audiences to comply with future health behavior recommendations, for example, is likely to require careful consideration of existing beliefs. Consider the impact of pre-existing cul-tural ideas about sexual relations that might infringe on a person's decision to wear a condom. People also harbor information-processing constraints; we know that fast-paced messages, cluttered with lots of graphics, can infringe on learning and memory, even though we see those practices regularly in cable television news programs on CNN and Fox News [28].

Health literacy also can be an important barrier to audience engagement. Scientific jargon abounds in disease-related media coverage and likely will not be well understood by a lay audience. While considering education or literacy levels is a good first step in devel-oping clear, appropriate messages, it is also important to consider whether the audience is likely to understand specific health concepts that are crucial to the message (such as how a virus is transmitted or why it is impor-tant to cover your cough). When considering which channels to use, it may also be important to think about the audience's computer literacy or limitations in their use of digital media.

In addition, risk communication experts agree it is very important in times of outbreak—particularly severe outbreaks—to consider the role that emotion plays in receptivity to recommendations. We know from the health communication literature that fear can interfere with message processing or even result in rejection of the message [29,30]. Epidemiologists have particular reason to be cautious, given how frightening the pros-pect of disease transmission can be. This problem can be mitigated by including behavioral recommendations the audience generally considers efficacious as part of the message (Box 21.3). In other words, if a message increases the perceived level of risk, it should also contain some recommendation for how to prevent or reduce it [29].

Box 21.3 Practical guidelines for reaching public
audiences directly.

- Set aside resources to monitor social media
  conversations. Just as one might hire a clipping service
  to monitor traditional media coverage of an outbreak,
  similar organizations can be contracted to monitor
  online and social media conversations. Where
  resources are limited, monitoring may consist of staff
  members occasionally scanning Facebook messages or
  blog posts.
- Avoid using jargon. Phrases like "case fatality rate,"
  "transmissibility," and "herd immunity" will not be
  well understood by a lay audience. The general public
  does not always need to know the technical term. If
  you can explain something in simpler language, do so.
- Put numbers in context. For example, explaining that
  the seasonal flu results in as many as 36,000 deaths
  every year can help to provide perspective on the
  importance of getting an annual flu vaccine.

Lessons learned and recommendations

Partnerships with journalists

When public health officials fail to plan ahead for communication activities, the result can be chaos and difficulty in providing the media and the public timely, accurate information. In one example, at the start of a large rural outbreak of Legionnaires' disease in the United Kingdom, health officials initially had no communication plan. Media coverage was intense and inquiries came 24 hours a day. Officials had to respond to ad-hoc media inquiries, which took them away from leading the investigation and management of the outbreak. Eventually, staff members began to develop press releases to coincide with copy deadlines, to set up a press hotline, to post press material on the Internet, and to schedule staff members to be on call so that at least one person was available to do live interviews at various points across 12 hours each day [31].

Public health officials can attempt to plan in advance for communication activities, both with regard to routine surveillance and in response to specific outbreaks. Observations about the nature of health news suggest a series of recommendations for such planning. Media organizations are not likely to change in struc-

ture or tendency anytime soon. What is perhaps more useful at this stage is for public health officials to take the lead to work constructively within the media constraints described previously. When public health officials and journalists collaborate, exceptional coverage is possible. In the early 1990s, efforts of the U.S. Centers for Disease Control and Prevention (CDC) to work with reporters at the *Atlanta Journal Constitution* to highlight the emergence of antibiotic resistant organisms led to a Pulitzer Prize [32]. Such cooperation does require active planning and foresight, but the result can be message communication of a sort unmatched by other techniques.

Establishing goals for message presentation

In addition to encouraging greater coordination with journalists, epidemiologists can strive for specific goals in their communication planning and message presentation. Heeding cultural differences can help create messages that resonate with audience members' perspectives on disease and interpersonal relations. Instead of simply translating a child immunization message from English into Somali to reach recent immigrant mothers, for example, staff may want to ensure that materials address the whole family and are respectful of possible sensitivity regarding traditional Somali gender roles.

Providing action steps should be another goal. A message about preventing a foodborne illness, such as *Escherichia coli*, should be accompanied by specific recommendations. A message that simply states the illness is thought to be spread by contaminated spinach will not be as useful as one that explains how washing the produce can reduce risk of infection. The numbing effect of repeated exposure to warning messages that include no steps for practical action can diminish the impact of the message over time.

Selecting mass media channels or outlets

Which channels should public health professionals use in trying to reach audiences? Evidence suggests that the most effective communication efforts are those that engage multiple channels of information [33]. Choices about which channels to emphasize in communication planning should focus on which combination of channels to use rather than on which single channel to employ. Best practices for ensuring the audience is exposed to your content involve conducting formative research to determine from the target audience which channels they are most likely to use.

New media technology and surveillance

Social media tools offer exciting options for rapid dissemination of information. However, the user-generated nature can provide challenges if health officials lose control of the content. In some cases, public health professionals may need to have a plan for correcting misinformation. In others, it may be best to allow that misinformation to be corrected by other users so as not to seem heavy-handed or too authoritarian.

Case study

CDC's use of Facebook during H1N1 pandemic

Reynolds [8] provides an example of the self-correcting nature of Facebook from messages posted on CDC's page during the H1N1 pandemic:

> Facebook is a self-correcting environment and CDC understood that individuals should be free to post their beliefs and concerns, some of which were counter to CDC's science and recommendations. As is the custom, individuals on Facebook offered corrective information, not the agency.
>
> Here are excerpts from CDC's Facebook H1N1 discussions regarding the value and safety of flu vaccination:
>
>> Female 1:…Oh and my uncle just got his h1n1 shot and got sick with the flu within 1 weeks' time.
>> Female 2: what flu did he get sick with? Was it confirmed h1n1? If he got sick within a week his inoculation was too late, it takes two weeks before the antibodies make you immune to the virus.
>
> Within a short time, an individual in the community helped dispel a recurring misperception—that the flu shot can cause the flu.

Summary

The success of communication efforts regarding surveillance and outbreaks is a function of the simultaneous behavior of several groups, including health professionals, mass media professionals, and the public. The experience of each group offers both opportunities and constraints for improving communication. The key to effective communication during epidemics is that we must continue to build local and national information networks *before* acute episodes occur. Journalists and media professionals do not always discuss infectious disease optimally, but they are constrained by time and budget considerations and can benefit from proactive effort on the part of health agencies to help them cover emerging issues. Members of the general public are vulnerable to the perception-warping effects of dramatic examples, their own limitations in understanding complex scientific and health information, and emotionally provocative messages. At the same time, they often seek accurate and straightforward information in times of crisis. By being cognizant of these communication issues, public health professionals can begin to tap the impressive but perplexing power of contemporary mass media and digital and social media to mitigate harm from infectious diseases.

Acknowledgment

Parts of this chapter have been adapted with permission from: Southwell, BG, Reynolds, BJ, and Fowlie, K. [34]. Communication, media relations, and infectious disease surveillance. In M'ikanatha N, de Valk H, Lynfield R, and Van Benden C, eds, *Infectious Disease Surveillance* (2nd ed.). Oxford: Wiley-Blackwell Publishing.

STUDY QUESTIONS

1. Imagine you have just been hired by a state department of health to lead the state's infectious disease surveillance efforts. You would like to do some communication planning to prepare for potential disease outbreaks in your state. What are some organizational training or planning initiatives you might propose?

2. Name some constraints that might affect a journalist's ability to cover a public health story. What are some ways that you might work with the media to help them overcome those constraints in order to more accurately report on infectious disease stories?

3. At the start of an emerging disease outbreak, a member of your communication team recommends using social media to disseminate information more quickly. What are some factors you should consider in deciding whether this is the appropriate strategy?

4. What are the most essential factors to consider in determining which media channels to use to disseminate a message about infectious disease?

5. Assume you are a public health professional for a local health department that has come under fire in recent months for withholding important information from the public about a potential outbreak of an emerging infectious disease. What are some ideas you might consider implementing to help bolster trust when the next outbreak occurs?

6. Assume that you have been invited to a surveillance and epidemiology seminar to offer some perspective on challenges encountered by public health officials in communication. In your response, discuss why trust and credibility and uncertainty about the evolving nature of outbreaks are important considerations.

7. A newly appointed commissioner of a large city public health department in the U.S. Midwest has consulted you about an effective public health communication strategy. Provide justification why consideration for each of the following groups is important: public health professionals, mass media professionals, and the lay public

References

1. Harvard School of Public Health. Survey finds nearly half of Americans concerned they or their family may get sick from swine flu. 2009. Available at http://www .hsph.harvard.edu/news/press-releases/survey-americans -concerned-swine-flu/ (accessed April 14, 2014)

2. World Health Organization. WHO Outbreak Communication Guidelines. 2005. Available at http://www.who.int/ csr/resources/publications/WHO_CDS_2005_28/en/ (accessed April 21, 2012).

3. Reynolds B, Seeger M. Crisis and emergency risk communication as an integrative model. *J Health Commun* 2005; **10**:43–55.

4. Peters RG, Covello VT, McCallum DB. The determinants of trust and credibility in environmental risk communication: An empirical study. *Risk Anal* 1997;**17**:43–54.

5. Reynolds B, Crouse Quinn S. Effective communication during an influenza pandemic: The value of using a crisis and emergency risk communication framework. *Health Promot Pract* 2008;**9**:S13–S17.

6. Izard CE. Translating emotion theory and research into preventive interventions. *Psychol Bull* 2002;**128**:796–824.

7. Reynolds B, Galdo J, Sokler L. *Crisis and Emergency Risk Communication*. Atlanta, GA: Centers for Disease Control and Prevention; 2002.

8. Reynolds B. Building Trust through social media: CDC's experience during the 2009 H1N1 influenza response. *Mark Health Serv* 2010;**30**:18–21.

9. Quinn SC, Thomas T, McAllister C. Postal workers' perspectives on communication during the Anthrax attack. *Biosecur Bioterror* 2005;**3**:207–215.

10. Taylor-Robinson D, Elders K, Milton B, et al. Students attitudes to the communications employed during an outbreak of meningococcal disease in a UK school: A qualitative study. *J Public Health (Oxf)* 2010;**32**:32–37.

11. Weeks B, Southwell B. The symbiosis of news coverage and aggregate online search behavior: Obama, rumors, and presidential politics. *Mass Commun Soc* 2010;**13**: 341–360.

12. Weeks BE, Friedenberg LM, Southwell BG, et al. Behavioral consequences of conflict-oriented health news coverage: The 2009 mammography guideline controversy and online information seeking. *Health Commun* 2012;**27**: 158–166.

13. McGreevy D. Risks and benefits of the single versus the triple MMR vaccine: How can health professionals reassure parents? *J R Soc Promot Health* 2005;**125**:84–86.

14. Schwitzer G. Ten troublesome trends in TV health news. *BMJ* 2004;**329**:1352.

15. Wilkins L. Plagues, pestilence, and pathogens: The ethical implications of news reporting of a world health crisis. *Asian J Commun* 2005;**15**:247–254.

16. Eggertson L. Lancet retracts 12-year-old article linking autism to MMR vaccines. *CMAJ* 2010;**182**:E199–E200.

17. National Public Health Information Coalition. 2011 Awards of excellence in public health communications. 2011. Available at http://www.nphic.org./conferences/2011/ awards-all-entries (accessed May 14, 2012).

18. National Science Board. Science and Engineering Indicators 2010. NSB 10-01. Arlington, VA: National Science Foundation; 2010.

19. Wallack L. Mass media and health promotion: Promise, problem, and challenge. In: Atkin C, Wallack L, eds. *Mass Communication and Public Health: Complexities and Conflicts.* Newbury Park, CA: Sage; 1990:41–51.

20. Pew Research Center's Project for Excellence in Journalism. The State of the News Media 2012: An annual report on American Journalism. 2012. Available at http:// stateofthemedia.org/2012/ (accessed May 14, 2012).

21. Turner RH. Media in crisis: blowing hot and cold. *Bull Seismol Soc Am* 1982;**72**:s19–s28.

22. Casey MK, Allen M, Emmers-Sommer T, et al. When a celebrity contracts a disease: The example of Earvin "Magic" Johnson's announcement that he was HIV positive. *J Health Commun* 2003;**8**:249–265.

23. Lev T. UN groups says China's errors hurt SARS fight. *The Chicago Tribune.* 2003, April 29. Available at http://articles.chicagotribune.com/2003-04-29/news/ 0304290266_1_henk-bekedam-world-health-organization -investigators-sars (accessed May 14, 2012).

24. Freifeld CC, Chunara R, Mekaru SR, et al. Participatory epidemiology: Use of mobile phones for community-based health reporting. *PLoS Med* 2010;**7**:1–5.

25. Carneiro HA, Mylonakis E. Google trends: A web-based tool for real-time surveillance of disease outbreaks. *Clin Infect Dis* 2009;**49**:1557–1564.

26. Yen M-Y, Wu T-SJ, Chiu AW-H. Taipei's use of a multichannel mass risk communication program to rapidly reverse an epidemic of highly communicable disease. *PLoS One* 2009;**4**:1–10.

27. Southwell B. Risk communication: Coping with imperfection. *Minn Med* 2003;**86**:14–16.

28. Southwell BG. Between messages and people: A multilevel model of memory for television content. *Commun Res* 2005;**32**:112–140.

29. Witte K. Putting the fear back into fear appeals: The extended parallel process model. *Commun Monogr* 1992;**59**: 329–349.

30. Yzer MC, Cappella JN, Fishbein M, Hornik R, Ahern RK. The effectiveness of gateway communications in antimarijuana campaigns. *J Health Commun* 2003;**8**:129–143.

31. Kirrage D, Hunt D, Ibbotson S, et al. The Hereford Legionnaires' Outbreak Control Team. Lessons learned from handling a large rural outbreak of Legionnaires' disease: Hereford, UK 2003. *Respir Med* 2007;**101**:1645–1651.

32. Freimuth V, Linnan HW, Potter P. Communicating the threat of emerging infections to the public. *Emerg Infect Dis* 2000;**6**:337–347.

33. Hornik R. Public health education and communication as policy instruments for bringing about changes in behavior. In: Goldberg ME, Fishbein M, Middlestadt SE, eds. *Social Marketing: Theoretical and Practical Perspectives*. Mahwah, NJ: Lawrence Elrbaum Associates; 1997:45–58.

34. Southwell BG, Reynolds BJ, Fowlie K. 2013. Communication, media relations and infectious disease surveillance. In N. M'ikanatha, H. de Valk, R. Lynfield, and C. Van Benden (Eds.), *Infectious Disease Surveillance* (2nd ed.). Oxford (UK): John Wiley & Sons. 607–617.

CHAPTER 22

Lessons learned in epidemiology and surveillance training in New York City

Elizabeth Chuang[1] and Carolyn Greene[2]

[1] *Montefiore Medical Center, Bronx, NY, USA*
[2] *New York City Department of Health and Mental Hygiene, Queens, NY, USA*

Introduction

Infectious disease surveillance is a complex and continuously evolving practice, requiring coordinated efforts of highly trained public health professionals. Early in the 1900s, as the first schools of public health were established in the United States, early leaders in public health education recognized the value of field experience as a counterpoint to coursework. In 1915, the Rockefeller Foundation published the seminal Welsh-Rose report, which called for the close collaboration of these schools with local, state, and federal agencies to ensure adequate training of future health professionals [1]. The New York City (NYC) Department of Health and Mental Hygiene (DOHMH) was an ideal setting for such collaboration because of its history of innovation, including controlling cholera and typhus by using the first municipal laboratory to test and quarantine passengers arriving by ship into New York Harbor in the 1890s. Other innovations included controlling diphtheria by providing free antitoxin to the poor in 1906 and initiation of the largest-ever rapid vaccination campaign to thwart a smallpox epidemic in 1947 [2].

DOHMH currently runs four formal training programs. The Public Health/ Preventive Medicine Residency Program is a 2-year postgraduate training program for physicians. The Health Research Training Program (HRTP) provides year-round field opportunities in public health for undergraduate and graduate students from a variety of disciplines. The Epi Scholars Program is a summer internship in applied public health research for graduate students in epidemiology, and the Surveillance Scholars program offers summer internships in applied surveillance to graduate students at the Columbia Mailman School of Public Health (MSPH). In addition to running local training programs, DOHMH hosts trainees from national public health training programs including the Centers for Disease Control and Prevention's (CDC) Epidemic Intelligence Service (EIS) and the Council of State and Territorial Epidemiologists' (CSTE) Applied Epidemiology Fellowship (Table 22.1).

The shifting of public health priorities over time continues to offer compelling training experiences: fighting the HIV/AIDS epidemic since the 1980s, controlling a resurgence of tuberculosis in the 1990s, identifying risk factors for chronic diseases, and preparing for bioterrorism threats in the twenty-first century. Even as the increasing burden of noncommunicable diseases has led to seismic changes in public health priorities [3], the DOHMH has recognized the imperative to maintain the capacity to conduct rigorous infectious disease surveillance. Field experience at DOHMH allows all trainees to begin to appreciate the rewards and challenges of conducting public health surveillance at the local level and inspires many to pursue careers in applied public health.

Concepts and Methods in Infectious Disease Surveillance, First Edition. Edited by Nkuchia M. M'ikanatha and John K. Iskander.
© 2015 John Wiley & Sons, Ltd. Published 2015 by John Wiley & Sons, Ltd.

Table 22.1 Formal training programs available at the New York City Department of Health and Mental Hygiene.

Program	Organizing institution	Eligible participants	Size
Public Health/Preventive Medicine Residency	NYC DOHMH	Physicians who have completed a medical degree and at least 1 year of postgraduate clinical training	6–8 first- and second-year residents
HRTP	NYC DOHMH	Undergraduate and graduate students with an interest in public health	Approximately 150 students per year
Epi Scholars	NYC DOHMH	Graduate students pursuing masters and doctorate degrees in epidemiology	Approximately 10 students per year
Surveillance Scholars	NYC DOHMH	Students from Columbia's Mailman School of Public Health pursuing master's and doctorate degrees in epidemiology	2–3 students per year
EIS Program	CDC	Physicians with at least 1 year of clinical training, doctoral-level scientists, medical professionals, and veterinarians with an MPH or equivalent public health experience	2 officers at any given time
CSTE Applied Epidemiology Fellowship	CSTE	Recent master or doctoral level graduates in epidemiology or related fields	2–5 fellows at any given time

Note: CDC: Centers for Disease Control and Prevention; CSTE: Council of State and Territorial Epidemiologists; DOHMH: Department of Health and Mental Hygiene; EIS: Epidemic Intelligence Service; HRTP: Health Research Training Program; MPH: Masters in Public Health; NYC: New York City.

The Public Health/Preventive Medicine Residency Program: training physicians in public health theory and methods

The Public Health/Preventive Medicine Residency Program, originally accredited in 1959, is one of the oldest such programs in the country [4]. The residency works in partnership with the MSPH at Columbia University, which enables residents to obtain a Masters in Public Health (MPH) degree during their 2 years of residency training. The aims of the program are to train physicians in health promotion and disease prevention on a population level and to develop leaders in epidemiological and clinical research, public health practice, and clinical preventive medicine. Applicants to the program must have completed a medical degree and at least 1 year of postgraduate training in a clinical residency program.

Residents are expected to gain competency in conducting surveillance; analyzing data; planning, implementing, and evaluating disease prevention and control initiatives; communicating with the public, policymakers, and health-care providers; promoting health and preventing disease in healthcare institutions and the community; and formulating policy [5]. Residents gain these competencies through a combination of hands-on experience, observation and didactic sessions. While they are enrolled in the MSPH master's program during both years of residency, they conduct several short-term projects in various work units of the DOHMH during the first year and complete a year-long practicum during the second year.

Examples of surveillance activities

The DOHMH provides unique opportunities for residents to participate in infectious disease surveillance projects. For example, the DOHMH initiated the Primary Care Information Project (PCIP) in 2005, which allows the department to receive de-identified aggregate data from primary care practices that have adopted electronic health record systems with the department's assistance. One resident piloted a project to link laboratory-confirmed influenza cases with outpatient visits for influenza-like illnesses. She coordinated with four PCIP primary care sites to collect data and specimens from patients with influenza-like illness. Specimens were analyzed in the DOHMH public health laboratory by reverse transcription polymerase chain reaction (RT-PCR) for the presence of influenza virus. The resident ensured accurate data collection, reported aggregate data to the CDC weekly, and distributed weekly epidemic curves for use by the DOHMH.

Residents also have the opportunity to work with many of the rich data sets available at the DOHMH, including NYC's Citywide Immunization Registry (CIR). One resident used the CIR to determine the geographic distribution of underimmunized children. Initiated in 1997, the CIR combines birth information from vital records with mandatory vaccine administration reports from pediatric providers. The resident used the data in the CIR to map immunization coverage by zip code using geographic information systems (GIS). She identified the 10 zip codes with the lowest immunization coverage for targeted outreach by the DOHMH.

Residents also have the opportunity to lead at least one outbreak investigation and to participate in tuberculosis contact investigations. One resident completed a practicum project on a tuberculosis cluster investigation. Since 2001, the DOHMH has used genotyping to enhance cluster investigations and to distinguish between reactivation and exogenous reinfection. Using genotyping, the resident was able to show probable transmission of tuberculosis within NYC in 2009, which informed the activities of the Bureau of Tuberculosis Control.

Many other resident projects have involved aspects of infectious disease surveillance and epidemiology. Two residents assisted on a quality improvement project for cause-of-death reporting on death certificates. As a result of this project, overreporting of heart disease deaths and underreporting of other causes of death including pneumonia and influenza were corrected [6]. This helped residents understand the importance of monitoring the quality of data sources for surveillance. Another resident created a report on the epidemiology of meningococcal disease in NYC, and one resident used hospital discharge data to document the rising incidence of community-onset, methicillin-resistant *Staphylococcus aureus*.

The on-call experience

Residents spend time on call for the DOHMH on some weekends and evening hours, allowing them to experience first-hand how to respond to a wide variety of questions and reports that the health department receives from the provider community. On-call experiences frequently allow residents to participate in the initial response to an outbreak. In 2001, a resident was on call when the first case of cutaneous anthrax was reported to the DOHMH and was able to participate in the earliest stages of the investigation. During the H1N1 pandemic of 2009, when providers began to report multiple cases of influenza, an on-call resident assisted in collecting and recording information for analysis by the swine flu investigation team. These activities gave residents experience in communicating during public health emergencies, and they demonstrated the role of the local health department in high-profile infectious disease control.

In addition to learning from hands-on experience, there are numerous formal and informal didactic opportunities for residents. Residents are required to take introductory epidemiology and biostatistics courses for their MPH degree and some elect to take advanced infectious disease epidemiology coursework. Coursework often directly informs the residents' ongoing work at the DOHMH, and residents choose elective courses that build the necessary skill sets to complete their practical experience. In addition, the residency holds weekly formal didactic sessions that include journal club, presentations of public health topics by outside speakers and preparation for certification tests. Residents are encouraged to attend the DOHMH Division of Epidemiology grand rounds and methods seminars in the Bureaus of HIV/AIDS and Tuberculosis Control where they learn how data are interpreted and used and see first-hand how surveillance data influence activities of the department.

Lessons learned

The success of the residency program is dependent on the development of projects that meet residents' interests and skill sets and that complement their coursework while fostering professional competency. Projects must be feasible with respect to time and resources available. Public Health/Preventive Medicine Residents must balance a full-time MPH course load with their work at the DOHMH and are not always available to work daily on time-sensitive projects such as outbreak investigations. Residency directors have learned to carefully screen projects for feasibility and ensure that preceptors document the expected time commitments for projects carefully prior to accepting the project.

The residency director collaborates closely with the MSPH to ensure that residents take appropriate courses that build the skill sets necessary for successful completion of their projects. This requires regular communication as curricula and course content are frequently updated. Funding for resident stipends must be pursued. For example, since 2004, one resident per year has been funded through a grant from the American Cancer Society.

Program impact

Several graduates of the public health/preventive medicine residency program currently serve in leadership positions within DOHMH. Others have gone on to work for other local health departments, international non-governmental organizations, academic medical centers, public hospitals and schools of public health [5]. Some graduates return to clinical medicine where they may be more likely to participate in public health initiatives and to apply population health principles in their practices.

The Health Research Training Program: fostering interest in public health across disciplines:

Building on the success of the Public Health Preventive Medicine Residency, HRTP was created in 1960 in order to include undergraduate and graduate students from a variety of disciplines. The current aims of the program are "to orient students to the principles and practices of public health planning, policy, research, administration and evaluation; to broaden students' concept of public health by increasing their awareness of needs, challenges and career opportunities in the field; and to assist the DOHMH in recruiting skilled, professional candidates with proven potential" [7]. HRTP accepts about 30 part-time interns for each of the fall and spring sessions, and 70–100 full-time interns for the summer session. Applicants are undergraduates in any field and graduate students from varying disciplines including public health, nursing, and occasionally even law school.

HRTP interns participate in applied public health projects and didactic sessions. Eligible projects are those

that will develop core public health skills such as data collection, data analysis, survey design, health promotion, community health outreach, program planning, and evaluation. The summer weekly didactic sessions provide a robust curriculum and are taught by DOHMH staff members who volunteer their time. Lectures cover the agency's priority public health initiatives. Workshops include SAS statistical software training, program evaluation and GIS. Additionally, interns are invited to attend a career panel comprised of a diverse group of public health professionals. Some students attend staff, agency, and citywide task force meetings that give them a better understanding of the scope of local public health work. HRTP also promotes networking among interns through an interactive orientation, a midsummer feedback session and other events.

Examples of surveillance activities

In recent years, the number of projects involving non-communicable diseases has increased, yet the DOHMH continues to offer numerous infectious disease–related training opportunities. One HRTP intern has been involved in maintaining the DOHMH's hepatitis A database. Other HRTP interns have contributed to the DOHMH's enhanced surveillance for salmonellosis. The DOHMH uses the Minnesota protocol under which a centralized team conducts rapid assessment of effected individuals using hypothesis-generating telephone interviews as soon as possible after cases are reported through NYC laboratories to the DOHMH. In order to reach cases quickly during foodborne outbreaks, interns conduct patient interviews both during and after regular business hours. Interns also develop databases for data entry, clean and analyze the data, and write outbreak reports. These experiences allow interns to understand how surveillance systems operate from case identification through analysis to data dissemination.

Lessons learned

Formalizing and centralizing the internship experience through HRTP has significant benefits for both interns and the DOHMH. HRTP staff members identify and recruit exceptionally skilled and dedicated preceptors. HRTP monitors the quality of intern projects by requiring potential preceptors to submit a project summary that is explicit about the skills the trainee will bring to the project and the skills the trainee will develop. In addition, providing a formal didactic curriculum allows interns to make connections between their course work and practical experience.

Having a centralized program also makes it easier for programs to bring in high-quality interns, because the formal, rigorous application and selection process for all trainees is standardized and handled by HRTP staff. HRTP encourages paid internships, because this allows the DOHMH to recruit talented interns who might not otherwise be able to participate due to financial constraints.

Program impact

HRTP is a highly successful program. In 2011, the department contacted 343 HRTP alumni for whom contact information was available. Of the 238 (69%) who confirmed participation in HRTP and responded to questions about their experience, the vast majority indicated that HRTP had assisted them in their educational goals (94%) and their career goals (90%); 95% stated that HRTP had positively influenced their career. Of the 178 (52%) who answered questions related to employment, 74% were employed in a public health agency, 59% were employed in the local public health setting, and 37% had been employed at DOHMH at some point in their career after completing HRTP [8].

Because of the program's longevity, professionals at the DOHMH are familiar with HRTP and are experienced in initiation of discrete projects that benefit both the intern and the program. Since many HRTP interns have subsequently been hired by DOHMH, these graduates of the program serve as ideal mentors for new students. Many DOHMH projects are only completed because of the availability of highly motivated HRTP interns. HRTP is a model for successfully integrating field training into public health education.

The Epi Scholars Program: providing hands-on training for future epidemiologists

The World Trade Center and anthrax attacks of 2001 led to a renewed national interest in investing in public health infrastructure, setting the stage for expanding

training [9]. In 2007, DOHMH secured funding from the Josiah Macy, Jr. Foundation to launch the Epi Scholars Program. This program accepts graduate students in epidemiology to work closely with a mentor at the DOHMH on an analytic project during a 12-week paid summer internship. The program aims to cultivate leadership in applied epidemiology, to advance public health research at DOHMH and other participating health departments, to provide applied public health research experience to epidemiology graduate students, and to attract graduate epidemiology students to public health as a career choice [10].

Over the first 5 years of the program, 43 trainees have participated in the Epi Scholars Program. The program has continued to grow under new grants from the de Beaumont Foundation. The number of participating schools of public health has increased from 8 to 15; and two locations outside of DOHMH have been added—the Los Angeles County Department of Public Health and the Seattle & King County Public Health. Demand for the program remains high, indicating that further expansion is possible.

In addition to working on their analytic project, scholars attend didactic sessions, which include workshops on questionnaire design, program evaluation, searching the public health literature, scientific communication, focus groups, outbreak investigation, new media, grant writing, and using statistical packages such as SAS, SPSS, SUDAAN, and GIS [11]. Scholars must present their work in a formal presentation at the end of the internship and are encouraged to publish their work in peer-reviewed publications.

Examples of surveillance activities

Epi Scholars work on various aspects of infectious disease surveillance and epidemiology. An outbreak investigation of tuberculosis in NYC public housing residents prompted the Bureau of Tuberculosis Control to apply for an Epi Scholar to investigate the incidence of tuberculosis in public housing residents. The Epi Scholar, who reviewed all cases of tuberculosis among NYC residents from 2001 to 2009, found that among U.S.-born New Yorkers, those living in public housing were at higher risk for tuberculosis than nonpublic housing residents. This is because they were more likely to have underlying risk factors such as recent substance abuse and older age, a finding that has programmatic implications for DOHMH and the New York City Housing Authority.

Several scholars have worked with the Bureau of HIV/AIDS. One participated in launching new online and in-person surveys of sexual risk factors for HIV infection among young men who have sex with men. These surveys will be repeated several times a year to track the impact of DOHMH HIV prevention campaigns. The scholar's analysis described significant differences in reported sexual behaviors between online and in-person respondents, highlighting the ways in which the survey mode influences response.

Scholars also have the opportunity to help characterize emerging infectious diseases. One student used influenza surveillance data to conduct a case-control study to explore the risk factors for severe pandemic influenza A (H1N1) disease. The student conducted interviews of hospitalized cases and ambulatory controls with influenza to obtain demographic and clinical data. Analysis of these data revealed that socioeconomic status, as measured by education level and neighborhood poverty, was associated with hospitalization for influenza, even after controlling for access to care and underlying medical conditions.

Lessons learned

Didactic sessions provide an important complement to analytic projects. However, adult learners who are relatively advanced in their studies work best in settings that are interactive and incorporate self-directed learning [12]. Whenever possible, these didactic sessions are presented as interactive workshops. For example, in the scientific communication workshop, scholars are expected to work on a manuscript based on their own analyses.

Funding for trainee stipends must be aggressively pursued. One important component of the Epi Scholars Program has been the implementation of an alumni-tracking system from the very beginning of the program. Tracking scholars' careers and successes allows the DOHMH to demonstrate program impact to potential funders.

Program impact

The most recent survey was conducted in 2011, and 27 of the 43 graduates (63%) responded. Of the respondents, 78% indicated that the program enhanced their interest in pursuing a career at a local health department [11,13] A recent review of the surveys conducted during 2007–2010 among graduates of the Epi Scholars Program and their mentors found that five Epi scholars have continued to work in public health for the DOHMH, CDC, National Institutes of Health, and the Environmental Protection Agency, and three have chosen to pursue a doctorate after completing a master's degree in epidemiology [14]. Among the 32 Epi Scholar mentors who completed program evaluation surveys from 2007 to 2010, 81% indicated that mentoring a scholar enabled them to complete work that could not have been completed without the scholar [14].

This young program has been well received by students, mentors, and faculty alike. All 11 of the 2011 NYC scholars that responded to a follow-up survey indicated that participating in the program improved their analytical and epidemiological skills and their ability to conduct research in an applied setting. Respondents indicated that the summer curriculum complemented their academic work. All would recommend the program to a peer. Similarly, all 2011 mentors responding to the follow-up survey stated they would mentor another Epi Scholar in the future if given the opportunity [11]. The popularity and success of the Epi Scholars Program highlight the value of collaboration between local public health agencies and schools of public health.

Surveillance Scholars: partnership with the MSPH at Columbia University

In 2008, the DOHMH was approached by faculty at MSPH who had received feedback from employers indicating that their graduates lacked hands-on experience in surveillance. DOHMH agreed to reserve 2–3 HRTP surveillance-related projects annually for MSPH students participating in a new Surveillance Scholars track. It was quickly noted that Surveillance Scholars would benefit from the didactic curriculum and the formal project presentations designed for the Epi Scholars Program. In the summer of 2012, the Surveillance Scholars program merged with the Epi Scholars Program.

This program serves as an example of an efficient continuous feedback loop whereby employers such as the DOHMH identify critical gaps in the skills of public health school graduates, and then the school and the employer collaborate to create experiences that will build these skills and ultimately produce employees that are more effective. Nearly 100 years after the Welch-Rose report, collaboration between graduate schools and public health agencies on public health professional training through field experience is still vital and relevant.

EIS officers and CSTE applied epidemiology fellows: DOHMH involvement in national training programs

Epidemic Intelligence Service

The CDC began field training for postgraduate health professionals in 1951 with the Epidemic Intelligence Service (EIS) fellowship, and DOHMH has participated since 1959. This is a 2-year program designed to give health professionals—such as physicians, veterinarians, and dentists—hands-on training in epidemiologic methods and applied public health practice. Fellows are recruited and accepted through CDC and matched to CDC programs or state or local health departments.

Typically, the DOHMH has two EIS officers at any given time—one working in the Bureau of Communicable Disease on infectious disease surveillance and epidemiology and another working in the Division of Epidemiology. These positions are among the few EIS positions at a local, urban health department. Since the DOHMH is one of the oldest and largest public health agencies in the country, EIS officers have the potential to be exposed to numerous subject matter experts and diverse projects in communicable and noncommunicable disease, environmental health, mental health, and public health policy, among others. The DOHMH employs many EIS alumni who can serve as supportive and experienced mentors. Since the DOHMH has an institutional familiarity with the EIS program, EIS officers are often given significant autonomy, especially during their second year. Finally, NYC provides a challenging and exciting place to practice public health given the diverse population and the city's support for innovative public health initiatives.

Officers complete 3 weeks of training at CDC prior to deployment. They then complete several specific activities during their 2 years at their training site, including participating in a field investigation; designing, conducting, and interpreting an epidemiologic analysis using public health data; designing, implementing, or evaluating a public health surveillance system; and writing and submitting a scientific manuscript to a peer-reviewed journal [15]. CDC provides one supervisor for the fellow, and the Department provides primary and secondary local field supervisors. The primary field supervisor must have completed the EIS Program or have prior EIS supervisory experience. With CDC approval, equivalent supervisory experience, training experience, or recent EIS-conference attendance can be substituted for this requirement (WR Daley, personal communication, March 15, 2013). Meeting this requirement might be challenging for some local health departments that, unlike the DOHMH, may not employ numerous EIS alumni. EIS officers have contributed substantially to DOHMH's efforts to implement new infectious disease surveillance systems. EIS officers made a significant contribution to the 1999 investigation of West Nile meningoencephalitis in the NYC metropolitan area, which first documented this virus in the Western Hemisphere (Figure 22.1) [16]. Additionally, in 2005,

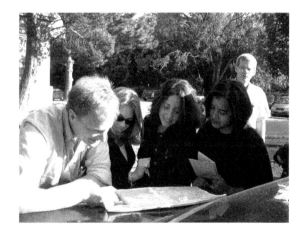

Figure 22.1 Dr. Michael Phillips, EIS 2000 (far left), consults a map of Staten Island with epidemiologists Beth Maldin, Anne Labowitz, and Debjani Das (from left to right). Dr. Phillips, as a member of the Bureau of Communicable Disease of the NYC Department of Health, led the West Nile virus serosurvey in the fall of 2000, a year after the virus was first recognized in the Western Hemisphere. Source: Reproduced with permission of Don Weiss, Director of Surveillance, Bureau of Communicable Disease, New York City Department of Health and Mental Hygiene.

DOHMH implemented the CDC's Serologic Testing Algorithm for Recent HIV Seroconversion to estimate the incidence of new HIV infection in NYC. The evaluation by the EIS officer revealed that although the system was relatively simple, timely, and acceptable to stakeholders, data quality did not reach CDC standards [17]. This work provided important insight into areas HIV surveillance that needed improvement and exposed the fellow to the challenges of implementing new surveillance protocols in a real-world setting and provided experience in applying the CDC's surveillance evaluation guidelines.

The CDC has championed electronic laboratory reporting, or ELR, as a means for improving the timeliness and completeness of reporting and for broadening surveillance capacity. An EIS officer evaluated the NYC experience with this transition. She found that completeness of data was high and even improved for some diseases like giardiasis and salmonellosis and that ELR decreased data entry burden for some diseases. However, ELR required a commitment of time and resources for data cleaning and quality assurance. In addition, complex diseases, such as tuberculosis and syphilis, which require interpretation of laboratory results and clinical data to identify new cases, do not lend themselves to automation. This study helped the EIS officer gain a deeper understanding of the practical implementation of surveillance at the local level [18].

Given previous public health successes, there are fewer large outbreaks of infectious diseases in the NYC than in the past, making it more difficult for trainees to gain field experience in outbreak investigation. Still, EIS officers will have the opportunity to participate in the outbreak investigations that arise during their hands-on training. Recently, an EIS officer participated in the initial outbreak investigation and follow-up after pandemic influenza A (H1N1) spread rapidly through a high school in Queens. She designed and implemented a survey of household members of cases and coordinated collection of nasopharyngeal swabs in order to determined rates of household transmission and transmission risk factors [19,20]. This officer also conducted an outbreak investigation of healthcare-associated viral hepatitis, which led to development of a systematic approach to investigation of cases of possible healthcare-associated viral hepatitis infections using scarce public health resources [21].

EIS officers' practical experience managing infectious disease surveillance at the local level prepares them for leadership positions in public health. The EIS training is often a career-changing experience, transforming clinicians into public health practitioners. At the DOHMH, many EIS officers have stayed on to spend their careers at the department. About 40 former EIS officers currently are employed at DOHMH, providing leadership and direction for the department. The majority of officers who recently completed training at DOHMH are working in public health for the CDC, the U.S. Army, DOHMH, other local health departments, international organizations, and schools of public health. EIS officers at the DOHMH benefit from many years of collaboration between the CDC and the DOHMH on this program and high-level support from former EIS officers in leadership positions.

Council of State and Territorial Epidemiologists Applied Epidemiology Fellowship

In 2002, the CSTE, CDC, Health Resources and Services Administration, and Association of Schools of Public Health collaborated to form an Applied Epidemiology Fellowship, a 2-year training modeled after the EIS program. The goals of the program are to provide experience in applied epidemiology to recent master or doctoral level graduates in epidemiology or related fields, and the program seeks to strengthen the local and state epidemiology capacity by placing more epidemiologists in state and local health departments for long-term careers. This nationally centralized program recruits fellows and places them in positions in local health departments through a matching process. The DOHMH began participating in 2005 and typically has several fellows at a time, with two working in the Bureau of Communicable Diseases. CSTE fellows reap the benefits of working in a large, urban health department with an outstanding staff as outlined above. The CSTE provides 1 week of training at the beginning of the fellowship. Fellows are then expected to gain competency in epidemiologic methods through their work at DOHMH, including designing and evaluating surveillance systems and interpreting surveillance data.

One CSTE fellow evaluated the effect of increasing electronic reporting from 2000 to 2006 on hepatitis A surveillance and on the provision of post-exposure prophylaxis (PEP) with immune globulin within the 14-day window when PEP is effective. In 2000, when reports were made by phone, fax or mail, the median reporting time from case diagnosis to receipt of the report by DOHMH was 27 days, making it difficult for DOHMH to provide timely PEP. In fact, in 2000, only one person received PEP for about every 10 cases of acute hepatitis A in NYC. In 2006, use of ELR decreased the median reporting time to 6 days, allowing DOHMH to provide PEP to an average of 2.4 people per case of acute hepatitis A [22]. Documenting this kind of success helps build the case for continued modernization of surveillance practices.

Fellows also implement new surveillance systems. NYC was known to have higher rates of antibiotic resistance in *Shigella* isolates than the rest of the United States. In order to further characterize resistance patterns, a CSTE fellow implemented enhanced surveillance of *Shigella* by collaborating with the public health laboratory to test all isolates from 2006 to 2009 for antimicrobial resistance and by following up with all cases to assess treatment. She found that NYC isolates had a greater probability of resistance to several common antibiotics than observed nationally. Additionally, 11% of NYC patients were treated with an antibiotic to which their isolate was resistant. These findings led to recommendations against routine empiric treatment of *Shigella* infection and for susceptibility testing prior to antimicrobial therapy [23]. Another fellow applied for and obtained grant funding from OutbreakNet to develop enhanced surveillance for *Salmonella* in NYC [24].

The CSTE fellowship experience gives fellows hands-on training in surveillance methods that is difficult to obtain elsewhere. Although the program began recently, DOHMH has already hired several former CSTE fellows. The major challenge for this program is finding sustainable funding for fellows interested in infectious disease surveillance. More outside funding is available for healthcare-associated infection and noncommunicable disease surveillance, and local health departments may be hard-pressed to find funding for a fellow without grant support.

Lessons learned

EIS officers and CSTE fellows are required to present and publish the work they are engaged in during their fellowship. This helps to disseminate the work of the department to a broader audience and to attract grant funding.

Other programs

In addition to the 2-year residency program, medical students and residents of other programs in the United States and abroad are invited to participate in 1-month elective rotations at the DOHMH. Preventive medicine residents are required to complete a rotation at a public health department and most residents from local programs fulfill this requirement at the DOHMH. These trainees often work on outbreak investigations or HIV surveillance projects, and they are invited to the weekly residency didactic sessions.

The DOHMH also hosts trainees from other programs such as the CDC's Public Health Associate Program and Public Health Prevention Service (PHPS). One recent PHPS trainee worked on a study of pandemic influenza A (H1N1) vaccine effectiveness in children. Other recent trainees from these programs have been assigned to the Bureau of Immunizations and the Bureau of Tuberculosis Control.

DOHMH is committed to improving the public health competency of the clinical provider community and the public at large. To this end, the Division of Epidemiology makes surveillance data available to the public online through EpiQuery (https://a816-healthpsi.nyc.gov/epiquery/). This site allows researchers, clinicians and the public to access aggregate surveillance data from large databases created by the annual Community Health Survey, the annual NYC Youth Risk Behavior Survey, the NYC Health and Nutrition Examination Survey conducted in 2004, the World Trade Center Health Registry, the Communicable Diseases Surveillance System, and Vital Records. DOHMH also regularly publishes *City Health Information*, a publication for clinicians that uses local surveillance data to inform and encourage best practices on clinical topics of public health significance (http://www.nyc.gov/html/doh/html/chi/chi.shtml).

Summary of lessons learned

Based on DOHMH experience, there are three fundamental attributes that make field training at a local health department successful. First, the DOHMH has a strong leadership commitment to training. Dr. Leona Baumgartener, a public health education champion and NYC Health Commissioner in the late 1950s and early 1960s, initiated a long tradition of commitment to excellence in public health training at the DOHMH. Second, DOHMH maintains a robust and compelling research agenda that provides quality projects and attracts top trainees. Finally, DOHMH has created the Bureau of Public Health Training (BPHT), which is dedicated solely to public health training.

BPHT is charged with the responsibility of assessing public health training needs and collaborating with internal and external groups to develop curricula, training content, and training opportunities. BPHT runs the HRTP, Epi Scholar, and Surveillance Scholars programs. BPHT also offers online modules and classroom-based courses to DOHMH staff that address competence in fundamental public health skills. These courses are often made available to trainees both within and outside of DOHMH.

Having a unit dedicated to the development of the public health workforce brings benefit to DOHMH for several reasons. BPHT offers expertise in creating competency-based training that addresses nationally established public health competencies. It works with agency subject matter experts to develop trainings that are instructionally sound, interactive, and appropriate for adult learners. BPHT maintains a current awareness of public health training opportunities and resources that are available locally and nationally. Further, it cultivates relationships with academic institutions and other health departments. Finally, the bureau has expertise in the evaluation of training programs that allows it to improve course content and structure based on feedback received.

BPHT ensures that DOHMH can face the challenges associated with providing outstanding field experiences. The Bureau has developed strategies to recruit high-quality trainees, develop curricula and identify feasible projects that meet the educational needs of trainees and maintain quality in the face of periodic budget cuts. Some of these strategies include developing recruitment materials; assigning dedicated staff to attend professional meetings and travel to professional schools to advertise the programs; and developing a formal, rigorous application and selection process for all trainees. Additional strategies are identifying and maintaining relationships with talented mentors and providing mentor training; implementing a formal review process to identify compelling, appropriate projects; creating a formal curriculum in addition to promoting informal educational opportunities; and conducting regular evaluations that are used to improve the programs.

While trainees often provide a valuable service at low costs, projects become scarce as programs trim their activities. If DOHMH professionals must perform more duties due to staffing cutbacks, less time is available for mentoring and project development. During times of financial strain, it is especially important for training program staff members to meet regularly with department leaders to promote training programs and to encourage potential preceptors to think about working with trainees. DOHMH has learned that projects that are carefully planned and have clear objectives allow trainees to contribute as a resource instead of being a burden. Even during times of reduced public funding, the DOHMH has found that there are benefits to providing staff the time to mentor and teach didactic sessions. Such opportunities offer professional satisfaction, boost morale, and allow staff to stay abreast of current public health methods and theory.

Despite many challenges, DOHMH has developed and maintained high-quality public health training through decades of changes that included ebbs and flows of public and private investment in public health education and extensive shifts in public health priorities.

Conclusion

Although chronic diseases demand increasing resources, public health still depends upon health departments' abilities to detect and respond to infectious disease outbreaks; to prevent new cases of infections that lead to chronic diseases such as HIV, as well as hepatitis B and C; to monitor and prevent new cases of tuberculosis and sexually transmitted diseases; and to detect emerging infectious diseases and agents of bioterrorism. DOHMH's commitment to public health training through field experience ensures that the future public health workforce is well equipped to face the infectious disease challenges to come.

STUDY QUESTIONS

1. How does field experience inform and enhance professional training in public health?
2. Why is it important to provide field training experiences at the local level?
3. Does educating the community of practicing physicians on public health practices benefit local health departments?
4. Why might it benefit public health agencies to offer training opportunities to students with a wide variety of educational backgrounds including undergraduates and graduate students in fields outside of health and medicine?
5. What are the benefits and drawbacks for students of completing fieldwork through formal programs such as Health Research Training Program?
6. Whose responsibility is it to ensure that public health professionals such as epidemiologists receive appropriate field training?
7. Should local, state, and federal agencies or other public health employers influence what is taught in schools of public health? In what ways do schools of public health influence the practices of local, state, and federal agencies or other public health employers?
8. What are the benefits for state and local health departments of participating in national training programs compared to developing training programs internally?
9. Why is it important for public health organizations to maintain a commitment to public health training during times of financial difficulties?

References

1. Delta Omega Honorary Public Health Society, Fee E. The Welch-Rose Report: Blueprint for public health education in America. 1992. Available at http://www.deltaomega.org/documents/WelchRose.pdf (accessed April 30, 2012).
2. New York City Department of Health and Mental Hygiene. Protecting Public Health in New York City: 200 Years of Leadership. 2005. Available at http://www.nyc.gov/html/doh/html/bicentennial/bicentennial-booklet.shtml (accessed August 18, 2012).
3. World Health Organization. Action Plan for the Global Strategy for the Prevention and Control of Noncommunicable Diseases. 2008 Contract No.: A61/8.
4. Accreditation Council for Graduate Medical Education. List of ACGME Accredited Programs and Sponsoring Institutions. 2012. Available at http://www.acgme.org/adspublic/ (accessed May 24, 2012).
5. New York City Department of Health and Mental Hygiene. Public Health Residency Program. 2014. Available at http://www.nyc.gov/html/doh/html/career/phmrp.shtml (accessed April 17, 2014).
6. Bureau of Vital Statistics. Summary of vital statistics 2010: The City of New York. New York New York City Department of Health and Mental Hygiene; 2011.
7. The Health Research Training Program (flier). New York: New York City Department of Health and Mental Hygiene; 2012.
8. Department of Health and Mental Hygiene. Health Research Training Program Alumni Survey: Data Snapshot. New York: New York City Department of Health and Mental Hygiene; 2011.
9. Committee on Assuring the Health of the Public in the 21st Century. *The Future of the Public's Health in the 21st Century.* Washington, D.C.: The National Academies Press; 2002.
10. New York City Department of Health and Mental Hygiene. Epi Scholars Program. 2014. Available at http://www.nyc.gov/html/doh/html/career/epi-scholar.shtml. (accessed May 17, 2014).
11. Rose J, Blake J. 2011 Epi Scholars Annual Report—deBeaumont Foundation. New York: New York City Department of Health and Mental Hygiene; 2011.
12. Conlan J, Gabowski S, Smith K. Adult learning. In: Orey M, ed. *Emerging Perspectives on Learning, Teaching, and Technology.* Bloomington, IN: Association for Educational Communications and Technology; 2003. Available at http://projects.coe.uga.edu/epltt/ (accessed August 18, 2012).
13. Department of Health and Mental Hygiene. NYC Epi Scholars Alumni Snapshot, 2007–2011. New York: New York City Department of Health and Mental Hygiene; 2011.
14. Blake J, Choden T, Hemans-Henry C, Koppaka R, Greene C. NYC Epi Scholars Program: Promoting applied health disparities research in an urban public health department—A program model. *J Public Health Manag Pract* 2011;**17**(4): 313–315.
15. Centers for Disease Control and Prevention. Epidemic Intelligence Service. Atlanta, GA: 2010. Available at http://www.cdc.gov/EIS/More.html (accessed April 19, 2012).
16. Nash D, Mostashari F, Fine A, et al. The outbreak of West Nile virus infection in the New York City area in 1999. *N Engl J Med* 2001;**344**:1807–1814.
17. Nair H, Torian L, Forgione L, Begier E. Evaluation of HIV incidence surveillance in New York City. *Public Health Rep* 2011;**126**:28–38.
18. Nguyen T, Thorpe L, Makki H, Mostashari F. Benefits and barriers to electronic laboratory results reporting for

notifiable diseases: The New York City Department of Health and Mental Hygiene experience. *Am J Public Health* 2007;**97**(S1):S142–S145.

19. France AM, Jackson M, Schrag S, et al. Household transmission of 2009 influenza A (H1N1) virus after a school-based outbreak in New York City, April–May 2009. *J Infect Dis* 2010;**201**:984–992.

20. Jackson ML, France AM, Hancock K, et al. Serologically confirmed household transmission of 2009 pandemic influenza A (H1N1) virus during the first pandemic wave— New York City, April–May 2009. *Clin Infect Dis* 2011;**53**: 455–462.

21. Bornshlegel K, Dentinger C, Layton M, Balter S, France AM. Investigation of viral hepatitis infections possibly associated with health-care delivery—New York City, 2008–2011. *MMWR Morb Mortal Wkly Rep* 2012;**61**(19): 333–337.

22. Moore K, Reddy V, Kapell D, Balter S. Impact of electronic laboratory reporting on Hepatitis A surveillance in New York City. *J Public Health Manag Pract* 2008;**14**: 431–441.

23. Wong M, Reddy V, Hanson H, et al. Antimicrobial resistance trends of Shigella serotypes in New York City. *Microb Drug Resist* 2010;**16**:155–161.

24. New York City Department of Health and Mental Hygiene, Farley T. Team Salmonella. New York: 2012. Available at https://a816-healthsslvpn.nyc.gov/sites/HUB/Blog/Lists/Categories/,DanaInfo=healthshare+Category.aspx?Name=Food%20Safety (accessed May 24, 2012).

Additional resources

Council of State and Territorial Epidemiologists Fellowship.
   Website: http://www.cste.org/?page=Fellowship
Epidemic Intelligence Service.
   Email: EIS@cdc.gov
   Website: http://www.cdc.gov/eis/index.html
Epi Scholars Program
   Website: http://www.nyc.gov/html/doh/html/career/epi-scholar.shtml
   NYC Epi Scholars Program
   Email: Epischolars@health.nyc.gov
   LA Epi Scholars
   E-mail: EpiScholars@ph.lacounty.gov
   Seattle Epi Scholars
   E-mail: Epischolars@kingcounty.gov
Health Research Training Program
   Email: hrtp@health.nyc.gov
   Website: http://www.nyc.gov/html/doh/html/career/hrtp.shtml
   Application: https://www.formstack.com/forms/?1216914-RFJNeG9Xrq
Public Health Associate Program: http://www.cdc.gov/phap/
Public Health Prevention Service: http://www.cdc.gov/PHPS/
Public Health/Preventive Medicine Residency
   Email: healthrp@health.nyc.gov
   Website: http://www.nyc.gov/html/doh/html/career/phmrp.shtml

Index

Note: Page entries in *italics* indicate figures; tables are noted with *t*; boxes are noted with b.

Concepts and Methods in Infectious Disease Surveillance, First Edition. Edited by Nkuchia M. M'ikanatha and John K. Iskander.
© 2015 John Wiley & Sons, Ltd. Published 2015 by John Wiley & Sons, Ltd.

Printed and bound by CPI Group (UK) Ltd, Croydon, CR0 4YY

27/10/2024

14580288-0003